Epidemic Urbanism

Epidemic Urbanism

Contagious Diseases in Global Cities

EDITED BY

Mohammad Gharipour and Caitlin DeClercq

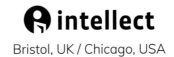

Bristol, UK / Chicago, USA

First published in the UK in 2021 by
Intellect, The Mill, Parnall Road, Fishponds, Bristol, BS16 3JG, UK

First published in the USA in 2021 by
Intellect, The University of Chicago Press, 1427 E. 60th Street,
Chicago, IL 60637, USA

Cover designer: Alex Szumlas
Cover image: Swan Hill Hospital, diphtheria tent, photograph by George
Hamilton, 1910 (Courtesy of the Swan Hill Regional Library) and Social
distancing circles at Domino Park, New York City (Photograph by
Jaclyn Skidmore, March 2021)
Copy editors: Angela Andersen and Newgen
Production manager: Mareike Wehner
Typesetting: Newgen

Hardback ISBN 978-1-78938-467-3
Paperback ISBN 978-1-78938-470-3
ePDF ISBN 978-1-78938-468-0
ePub ISBN 978-1-78938-469-7

Printed and bound by Gomer, UK

To find out about all our publications, please visit our website.
There you can subscribe to our e-newsletter, browse or download our current catalogue,
and buy any titles that are in print.

www.intellectbooks.com

This is a peer-reviewed publication

Dedication

We dedicate this book to the global community of scholars, practitioners, policymakers, and members of the public who are part of the Epidemic Urbanism Initiative (EUI). As COVID-19 traversed cities across the world and put into stark and urgent focus the need for new solutions to effectively and equitably respond to current and future pandemics, in March 2020, Mohammad Gharipour and Caitlin DeClercq established the EUI to create an interdisciplinary community of scholars whose work explores the history of cities and epidemics, innovate new methods and approaches for teaching history and public health, and educate the public and policymakers on the relevance of history to contemporary issues and challenges regarding COVID-19 and its social and spatial impacts. Through the convening of four international symposia and ongoing online conversations with experts and practitioners from diverse fields including architecture, medicine, public health, art, history, and architectural history—all of which are publicly accessible online—the EUI has grown to be a dynamic community of more than 1,600 participants from more than 90 countries as of March 2021. This volume is in honor of this community.

Contents

PART 4: URBAN DESIGN AND PLANNING: 240
INTERVENTIONS AND IMPLICATIONS

CONTENTS

Preface

Mohammad Gharipour and Caitlin DeClercq

The outbreak of the coronavirus disease (COVID-19) in late 2019 and its rapid spread in early 2020 gave impetus to this project. In May 2020, while sheltering in place due to COVID-19, we convened eighteen scholars from across the world to participate in an online symposium, "Epidemic Urbanism: Reflections on History," and share case studies that showcased how past epidemics have affected urban life and space across diverse time periods and geographies. The work of this symposium and the subsequent worsening of the COVID-19 pandemic put into stark, urgent perspective the need to study epidemics and pandemics as a means to understanding and responding to the many crises provoked by the societal, institutional, infrastructural, and professional impacts of contagious diseases within urban settings, and to engage public, practitioner, and academic audiences in this discourse.[1]

Indeed, outbreaks of COVID-19 had a disproportionate impact on the populations of global cities and profoundly changed the way people were permitted to inhabit, use, and move through urban spaces. Responses to this pandemic called into question precisely which urban interventions might be necessary to mitigate severe viral illnesses and prevent future outbreaks. The need to consider cities as both vectors of illness and sites of prevention and intervention is not new—both the biological and sociocultural phenomena that drive and respond to contagion are embedded in human settlements and cities themselves, from private latrines and municipal sewers to hospitals and quarantine stations. COVID-19 is just one of a series of historical and recent pandemics, including the bubonic plague, Severe Acute Respiratory Syndrome (SARS), and Ebola, which have forced an examination of the impact of epidemic illness on urban life and exposed the vulnerabilities of the societies they ravage alongside the bodies they infect.[2]

Many scholars have written about the social trajectory of past epidemics and pandemics from medical, sociological, and even religious studies perspectives, exploring how patterns of illnesses are first observed and defined, the anxiety that accompanies outbreaks of contagious illnesses, and the identification of certain practices, communities, and places as pathological and disease-causing; the analysis in the literature reveals the ways in which these factors illuminate or obscure the vectors of illness and the ways in which underlying issues like racism, segregation, and political strife and distrust exacerbate the impact and spread of epidemic illnesses. The case studies in this volume extend and amplify these observations by focusing on the built environment across a range of global contexts from the 14th to the 21st centuries.

This emphasis on the physical environment is a primary contribution of the chapters in this volume, which collectively demonstrate that connection, commerce, inequity, and neglect emerge as determinants of illness and foci of intervention. Indeed, biological pathogens and vectors of illness like fleas and mosquitoes gain a significant advantage when they are carried along trade routes and across transnational transportation networks, allowed to take root in overcrowded housing and neighborhoods, and nurtured by neglected infrastructure. A long and broad continuation of these same patterns across time and geography has sustained our collective susceptibility to infectious illness. Further, increased global connections and pronounced social inequities have made urban humanity even more vulnerable to epidemic illness.

The coexistence and commingling of people and pathogens in cities is one part of a story that also includes the rationale for design intervention and the experience and efficacy of a built environment that is similarly shaped by factors that include and expand upon scientific expertise. Parts of this volume read as tales of scientific and medical innovation during times of pestilence, and one interpretation of these case studies might be that medical "progress"—the cycles of observation, discovery, and intervention, and, in some cases, eradication (or at least management) of infectious disease—is possible. Yet there are cautionary accounts here, too, about the limits of this progress-oriented thinking. The persistence of infectious illnesses in urban environments is due, at least in part, to the relative neglect of the distal social and built environment factors that render marginalized communities vulnerable to illness. Interventions are at times misguided, reactionary, or rendered incomplete due to discrimination, economic greed, colonial hubris, impulsive design approaches, social pressure, government mismanagement, or a combination of all these factors. By centering physical urban environments in our study of epidemics, we offer insight into these issues that build upon social and political analysis. The long-lasting local and global implications of place and space help us pose new questions, confront assumptions, and configure interpretations about illness and the contexts of disease interventions, responses and outcomes.

The scope of this volume

It is our contention that history matters as an academic practice as well as a social and public health practice. Our goal for this volume is to present scholarship gathered from a range of disciplines and contributed by authors who present urban case studies from across the globe. Each chapter shares the story of a city or region, an outbreak of illness, and the urban response to an epidemic outbreak. In this way, we see each chapter as offering a rich case study in its own right, yet one that is further enriched when read in dialogue with other chapters and seen within the context of the book's main themes. This convergence of urban and architectural history perspectives on epidemics demonstrates how cities are the primary sites of exposure and quarantine as well as locations and instruments of intervention. In this way, the built environment is a medium through which to provide an understanding of the current COVID-19 crisis and to better anticipate and respond to inevitable future epidemics. The contributors to this volume are historians, public health experts, art and architectural historians, sociologists, anthropologists, doctors, and nurses. All have deliberately spoken to an audience that includes the public, practitioners, and academic readers, and the case studies they share reveal a diverse range of urban interventions that are connected to the impact of epidemics on society and urban life, and the conceptualization of and response to disease.

Understanding epidemics of the past, we believe, will enable us to make better, more just, and more effective decisions now and in the future. With that in mind, we have called upon the authors to address some specific questions: Where have notable interventions or actions have been implemented and with what effect? What impact have epidemics had on urbanism, urban design, and urban planning? How do epidemics shape architecture in the short and long term? And, finally, what impact have built environments had on epidemics and the experience of illness? Each chapter begins with a brief introduction to the geographical, social, and historical context for the outbreak of an infectious illness, which highlights the local and transregional factors that amplified the spread of disease. From there, authors embrace a case study through which they explore urban interventions and their justifications. A critical eye is turned toward the social, cultural, political, and built environment factors that thwarted epidemic responses and the post-outbreak experience and to the inefficacy of policies, infrastructure, and social and cultural shifts toward racialized segregation, hygiene, class, and community. The chapters conclude by synthesizing the broader implications from each case study.

There is clear benefit to be derived from looking at regionalized histories of public health, local sources of knowledge, and accounts of experience and impact that include traditional ways of dispersing information and caring, gendered experiences of disease, tensions between state and local governmental bodies, and economic by-ways as well as modern, clinical theories of disease within the global narrative. Contributors engage oral interviews, archival records, correspondence, press accounts, political cartoons, building plans, landscape designs, postcards, works of art, diaries, standing architecture, and more, all of which have given rich insights into the social and physical context of urban epidemics.

This broad view demonstrates how epidemic illnesses, along with city residents' responses to them, exploit and amplify social inequality in urban communities—this is a particularly important contribution made by this book, given the systemic racism and entrenched social inequities that continue to subjugate so many. It is not a coincidence that protesters came out in force against racial and social injustice around the world at the same time that COVID-19 was killing infected people from racial minorities, migrant communities, Indigenous, and other historically marginalized groups at a disproportionate rate. When viewed across more than five hundred years of history, it is apparent that, with every new epidemic outbreak comes novel interventions, new vaccines or treatments, and new insights about public health; yet in nearly every case, the same, persistent, and pernicious social inequities are little changed and even potentially exacerbated by so-called colonial improvements, or ostensibly modern city planning schemes. Epidemics expose the vulnerabilities of the societies they befall; however, despite centuries of outbreaks and interventions we have yet to truly implement changes based on this lesson.[3]

This book foregrounds important distal, contextual factors of epidemics by centering the role of urban environments in the study of past epidemics. There is a need for and value in built and infrastructural interventions that help to prevent illness and promote health and resilience. Above all, the built environment should not do harm to inhabitants. By focusing on the built environment, this book creates a space to confront persistent assumptions about epidemic illness. Physician and public health expert Richard J. Jackson has observed that it is all too easy to attribute disasters, including epidemics, to random acts of God.[4] Yet, the case studies in this volume iterate that there is very little that is random in the environments and social structures within which epidemics are the most common, and the most virulent and deadly.

Frank Snowden's seminal work on the social contexts of epidemics, *Epidemics and Society*, called into question the popular refrain that infectious pathogens are the great equalizer—that they, unlike the people who host them, do not discriminate, and that everyone is equally susceptible.[5] This volume shows further evidence that susceptibility to disease is determined by factors such as zoning practices, housing quality, infrastructure access, and health-support availability. Importantly, all of these are *designed* aspects of the urban environment, meaning that they are not natural, not random, and far from equally accessible. In this way, a built environment-centered perspective confronts any solely biological definition of epidemic illness, for it is clear that epidemics are also social, political, and urban phenomena—to overlook this is to miss important elements of the origin and eradication of epidemic disease. The discussions in this book dispel any notion that urban epidemics might be brought to a conclusive end and show instead that little has actually been done to redesign cities to prevent or mitigate the impacts of disease.

Increased globalization, climate change, and social inequities have impacted the profound and complex ways that urban experiences, urbanism, and the built environment have responded to epidemics around the world.[6] Epidemics have necessitated the design or redesign of urban spaces with health concerns in mind, and many of these interventions have had lasting salutogenic impacts. This project makes clear that investing in infrastructure, ensuring access to health care, and prioritizing affordable and adequate housing for all will be significant steps toward a world in which health-centered, health-promoting design is the norm. It is possible to design cities to prevent and mitigate epidemic illness, and this book offers some clues for how to undertake this process. By the time this volume is published, many around the world will have had access to a vaccine for COVID-19 that will prevent the deaths of millions and slow the economic ruin caused by pandemic shutdowns. Yet, as this book reminds us, the cities we inhabit and the vulnerabilities and resources our societies offer will continue to resonate with lessons and important implications for the next inevitable outbreak.

Contents of this volume

This volume includes 36 chapters that deploy interdisciplinary approaches to the analysis of the mutual relationship between epidemics and the built environment. The chapters share the story of an epidemic in a particular city or region from five continents and are organized in four sections to convey the mechanisms of change that affect vulnerabilities and responses to epidemic illnesses: Urban Governance, Urban Life, Urban Infrastructure, and Urban Design and Planning.

The first section, "Urban Governance: Politics and Management," consists of case studies from present-day Romania, India, Mexico, England, Italy, China, the United States of America, and Kenya. These chapters foreground official policies and practices that shaped the very definitions of diseases and responses to observed illnesses. Policy also informed, justified, and mobilized a range of epidemic interventions, many of which centered on the built environment. By beginning with the topic of urban governance, we introduce a broad understanding of the built environment, which necessarily includes the mechanisms that foster, justify, and legitimize built interventions into urban settings. Together, these case studies probe and interrogate assumptions about how urban interventions such as quarantine and vaccination programs were justified in the name of medical expertise, societal progress, or the public good. Authors explore how, where, and for whom interventions were carried out across uneven social structures. Such responses to epidemics had both intended and unintended effects. In exploring these themes, the chapters in this section foreground the factors that necessitate and shape official responses to urban epidemics and the elements that make official responses to plague at the local, state, and international levels effective or not: power and powerlessness, trust and mistrust, action and reaction, compliance and resistance.

The second section, "Urban Life: Culture and Society," emphasizes social practices and structures and foreground the social context and implications of space and spatial intervention in the volume's conception of the built environment. The chapters examine how different communities experienced and navigated epidemics amid interventions that exploited and amplified social divisions. Case studies from England, the present-day Czech Republic, the United States of America, Iraq, Italy, Iran, Ghana, and Brazil demonstrate how daily life is profoundly disrupted by epidemics and associated interventions like quarantine, mask-wearing, and vaccinations. Authors foreground the importance of social spaces and cultural and religious practices as sources of resilience and support during times of pestilence and in the face of such disruptions. The case studies also reveal the pernicious and persistent themes of displacement, discrimination, and othering, and of deeply entrenched inequalities that exacerbate the effects of illness, especially among vulnerable populations. So, while the first section of this volume is about official responses to epidemics, this section engages the power of the public and the unofficial and everyday responses to infectious diseases.

The third section, "Urban Infrastructure: Permanence and Change," examines built urban forms, socio-economic systems, governing bodies, and other types of infrastructures and how they were created, mobilized, and/or modified in response to epidemics. The chapters in this section include study cases from Portugal, Spain, Mexico, Bangladesh, Brazil, India, Vietnam, the Philippines, and Australia. The main contribution of this section is the exploration of the role of infrastructural public health interventions that aim to quell and manage epidemics but at times actually exacerbate illness. In many societies, governments have initiated large, urban projects with public hygiene and disease prevention in mind, not only in response to pestilence but also as a measure of authority and a symbol of good governance. Other communities have relied upon features in the natural landscape or long-standing traditions around sites and spatial practices to provide infrastructural responses to disease transmission. Both physical and social urban infrastructures that are seemingly durable or permanent can be porous, transgressed, and used in unpredictable ways. The very presence or absence of physical and ephemeral infrastructure is a commentary on the societal prioritization of epidemic response.

The fourth and final section of the volume, "Urban Design and Planning: Interventions and Implications," examines the role of urban design practices and concepts implemented during epidemics and the factors that shaped and codified each. These factors range from the application of biomedical expertise and bureaucratic standards and codes, which may on the surface appear neutral or benign in their aims, to the motivations and practices of profiteers, which reveal themselves more overtly as prejudicial and nefarious. The chapters in this section explore Italy, England, Japan, China, the Philippines, Senegal, Nigeria, and Mauritius and provoke questions about who makes key decisions about and benefits from large-scale epidemic interventions. The long-term implications of changes to urban forms including housing, sewer systems, hospitals, and public parks as well as changes to urban practices like zoning and building standards persist long after a single epidemic subsides. These urban interventions often shape and reflect social interactions for select groups of people, some of whom benefit, but many of whom suffer as a consequence. Built interventions demonstrate the long-term implications of foregrounding health in urban design and planning practices, but they also disclose the potential for place to become a factor in the colonial occupation, economic control, and segregation of populations in the name of public health.

Physician and epidemiologist Sandro Galea opens the book with a prologue on urban health to frame these provocations and explore the mechanisms that contribute to the inherent susceptibilities of cities to illness—and of the structures for resilience that are present in urban settings. In response to these ideas, and the additional provocations explored in the ensuing case studies, Richard J. Jackson's epilogue closes the book with a call to action with a health and equity-centered vision for the future of urbanism in the post-COVID-19 age. Both prologue and epilogue highlight essential elements of built and social environments that promote resilience, prevention, and equity and remind us of the benefits of integrating urban and built environment issues and medical intervention in the successful response to and prevention of epidemics.

In sum, the chapters presented in this volume highlight distinct, historical studies on selected epidemic illnesses in an encyclopedic format. Rich ideas from diverse geographies, epidemics, and time periods are covered in these interdisciplinary chapters, but it is important to note that this is not a universal nor a comprehensive total accounting of the many ways and contexts in which epidemics have shaped global cities. The earliest case included in this volume is from the 15th century, and most of the studies are largely focused on the past few centuries, but there is much to be learned from the epidemics faced during earlier periods.

Likewise, there is further opportunity to explore the relationship of some of the most recent epidemics and pandemics, including AIDS, SARS, and Ebola, with the built environment. Despite our best intentions and efforts to reach scholars working in these regions, we were unable to represent select geographical areas such as South Africa and Scandinavia in this volume. To work across these broad disciplines, geographies, and time scales is necessarily a practice of translation. We have balanced the richness of these perspectives with the need to present an accessible and coherent volume with simplified translations, transliterations, and contemporary place names. We have also implemented a uniform format in appreciation of the nuances of an interdisciplinary volume with 45 authors from various fields. Historic images, including maps, paintings, postcards, and photographs contribute to providing proper coverage of epidemics in both textual and visual media.

Implications

Historian Mark Honingsbaum argues that recent epidemics have offered sobering lessons about the increasing vulnerability of our global society to infectious illnesses, the perniciousness of fear invoked by the onset of infectious disease, the fallibility of public health practice, and the need to continually anticipate the next outbreak.[7] We hope the questions the case studies in this volume provoke can inspire and guide readers to make sense of other case studies they encounter and experience.

Indeed, historical examples of disease find echoes in the COVID-19 pandemic that dominated the lives of all who contributed to this book during the writing and editing process. Although some things were learned about the transmission of COVID-19 and the efficacy of mask-wearing and social distancing in 2020, biomedical knowledge of the virus did little to change the spread of the pandemic until the successful development of a vaccine. In large urban centers like New York City, the same neighborhoods that suffered the impact of the arrival of the virus in March 2020 were still the most vulnerable to COVID-19's continued spread later that year. As a result of sociocultural and governance factors in the United States, including the politicization of the pandemic response itself, large portions of the public remained skeptical about basic science, and policies were instituted unevenly across cities and states. Ultimately, while a leader in the medical sciences, the United States nevertheless remained a primary contributor to the global pandemic. Like the historical epidemics that preceded it, COVID-19 has shown the vulnerability of even technologically advanced societies with well-established governmental and built infrastructure to epidemic illness. There is more to learn from COVID-19, let alone from the past five hundred years of urban epidemic history represented in this volume.

Our intentional engagement of public, practitioner, and interdisciplinary academic audiences in dialogue about past epidemics will help us to respond to this and future epidemics more effectively and equitably with responsible, thoughtful approaches. Ideally, there must be investment in adequate and affordable housing for all citizens to help reduce the crowded, unsafe, and unsanitary conditions that can lead to or exacerbate the effects of infectious disease. Communication must happen across state, regional, and national borders to coordinate interventions in the public interest. Political aims detrimental to public health must be addressed and eliminated. Financial aid must be made available to counter the significant economic impacts of epidemics for those who have lost income or who have been saddled with medical care costs. Continual preparation and planning for pandemics must be prioritized on a global scale as well as in local practice. Health-promoting practices and spaces, including vaccines and curative remedies and efforts beyond these medical interventions, must be part of the vision for a healthy society. The best preventative and remedy for urban epidemics, in other words, is to work toward more equitable social and built environments.

This is perhaps the most profound and urgent hope of this volume: that it inspires and informs action for a variety of audiences. For some, this action might look like seeing news coverage of the epidemics through a broader lens, to be attuned to the very real promise of spatial, medical, and social interventions like quarantine, vaccination, and social distancing, and of the equally salient threats of racism, distrust, and exploitation that too often accompany disease outbreaks. For others, this action might take the form of individual actions toward self-care, toward community organizing, or toward advocating interventions that benefit all citizens—and especially the most vulnerable. For others, this action might be the adoption of a public health lens in teaching about the built environment, or of a built environment lens when teaching about public health, to illuminate new and necessary opportunities to think about implications and interventions. And still for others, this action might mean seeing personal or professional responsibility to intervene, in other words, to recognize the urgent role that citizens, educators, historians, and designers can—and should—play in helping to anticipate and respond to future epidemics.

Acknowledgments

We would like to thank the authors for their hard work during the preparation of this manuscript. We are also grateful to the Society of Architectural Historians and the Global Architectural History Teaching Collaborative, specifically to Pauline Saliga, Victoria Young, and Eliana Abu-Hamdi for their support in organizing our online conferences that provided the foundation for this publication, and to Ellie Goodman for being an early supporter and advocate of this volume. We would also like to express our gratitude to Angela Andersen for her amazing work in editing this volume, Meridith Murray for making an excellent index, Andrew Bui and Caroline Makary for their research and design assistance, Jaclyn Skidmore for her wonderful aerial photography, anonymous readers for generously sacrificing their holidays to read this volume and providing very helpful comments, Tim Mitchell for expertly managing this publication from the beginning, and Mareike Wehner for so beautifully bringing this publication to print. This volume would not have been possible without the generous funding provided by the Global Architectural History Teaching Collaborative and we are grateful to them for their trust and continuous support.

NOTES

1. The spread of COVID-19, as well as outbreaks of many of the infectious diseases presented in this volume, can be defined as *pandemics*, given their broad reach across multiple global geographies. The term *epidemic* describes an infectious disease outbreak within a specific geographic setting, more limited than a pandemic. However, it is important to note that epidemic disease outbreaks can eventually grow to be pandemics. See the Glossary for more on these and other key terms from this volume.

2. See, e.g.: John Duffy, "The Social Impact of Disease in the Late 19th Century," in *Sickness and Health in America*, 3rd ed., ed. Judith Walzer Leavitt and Ronald N. Numbers (Madison: University of Wisconsin Press, 1997), 418–25; Mark Honingsbaum, *The Pandemic Century: One Hundred Years of Panic, Hysteria, and Hubris* (New York: W. W. Norton, 2019); and Frank M. Snowden, *Epidemics and Society: From the Black Death to the Present*, revised ed. (New Haven, CT: Yale University Press, 2020).

3. Snowden, *Epidemics and Society*, ix.

4. Richard J. Jackson, "Foreword," in *Extreme Weather, Health, and Communities*, ed. Sheila Lakshmi Steinberg and William A. Sprigg (Switzerland: Springer International, 2016), v–ix.

5. Snowden, *Epidemics and Society*.

6. Honingsbaum, *The Pandemic Century*, 361–68.

7. Ibid.

Prologue:
Pandemics and Urban Health

Sandro Galea

Cities are where people congregate and, as a direct result, where infectious diseases take hold and become epidemics. Fifty-five percent of the world's population lives in cities today, and 68 percent is projected to live in cities by 2050. Yet, in the year 1800, just 3 percent of the world's population was urban. Cities have often been at the forefront of the world's cultural and political movements, inspiring the emerging ideas of the Renaissance, laying the foundations for modern-day pluralistic democracies through the revolutions that took hold in the 18th century, and generating many of the scientific advances that today shape all aspects of our health. Urban epidemics transform how we live both during an outbreak and long after that outbreak has passed. It is hard to think of the impact that epidemics have on society without thinking of them through the lens of cities, and conversely, it is hard to think of cities without understanding how epidemics have shaped their growth over the centuries. This book offers an absorbing series of case studies that discuss each of these points, ranging from the construction of urban hospitals in Lisbon, Portugal, to public-health policies in post-influenza Lagos, Nigeria. Such examples point to the variety of experiences from countries and cities that are substantially different from one another but also to the commonalities shared by disparate contexts, leading to the root of why it is that cities are inseparable from our understanding of epidemics and pandemics.

Ways of thinking about pandemics and urban living can be grounded in the study of urban health. The field of urban health seeks to understand how characteristics of cities shape the health of populations and to help us organize our thinking about what precisely it is about cities that ultimately shapes our health. This points the way, of course, to the design of healthier cities. By way of highlighting this thinking in regard to pandemics and urban life, I comment here on a few sentinel features of cities that shape health, doing so most dramatically in times of pandemics. Thus, I lean on the COVID-19 pandemic to offer some illustrations that emerge from the moment at which I am writing.

Put simply, cities are urban environments where a lot of people, by living together, create density in the population. These worldwide definitions of the city often rest not on the absolute number of people living in an area but on the relative density of the urban population compared to the surrounding region. For example, there is little disputing that the center of Yellowknife in northern Canada is a city. Even if its total population is under twenty thousand people, Yellowknife is a city by virtue of its density relative to the surrounding Northwest Territories, which are sparsely populated. Cities simply have more people, living closer to one another, which makes them the perfect place for epidemic spread. While we can make the fundamental observation that the viruses or bacteria that drive epidemics easily move from person to person in close proximity, this is a vast simplification of the role that the social environment plays in shaping health generally—and responses to epidemics specifically—in cities. While dense populations are definitional, these same populations have different characteristics that shape the extent to which they facilitate or mitigate pandemic spread.

Social norms are one central emergent property of urban social environments. Norms are a product of both formal rules and regulations, and of the public conversations that determine how groups interact with one another. Social norms can encourage or discourage group cohesion; the extent to which they do so are determinative for the spread of an epidemic. For example, social norms that encourage group cohesion can prepare urban populations for the swift responses required to mitigate spread during pandemics, while norms that encourage mistrust and division can present nearly insurmountable barriers to collective action in the face of a rapidly moving threat. The fractured social norms sowed by decades of racial divisions in the United States have created substantial mistrust of the health care system on the part of minority groups who, at best, do not believe that the collective has their best interests in mind, or, at worst, that this collective is out to harm them. These anxieties create suspicion surrounding efforts to introduce a novel vaccine, or to impose behavioral modifications that can potentially benefit all, including social distancing measures that may last for years. A cohesive social environment can create the conditions conducive to the sacrifices that may be necessary to slow the spread of a pandemic. An ancillary but related factor within urban social environments is equality or, conversely, inequality and the distribution of assets that may make sacrifices appear possible or reasonable.

Urban environments are characterized by the heterogeneous spread of assets, through which the rich are typically given access to more health-producing resources than the poor. Cities with extreme inequality tend to present little opportunity for social mobility to those who have less, or to provide supportive resources to help create a social safety net for the poorer segments of the population. This has a direct impact on cohesive social norms and the ability of cities to respond effectively to a pandemic. It also creates the practical problem of isolating the groups with limited access to resources into reservoirs that provide ready opportunities for pathogens to spread. The infection then disseminates throughout the city. This was the case during the early phases of the COVID-19 pandemic in cities like Singapore, where outbreaks among migrants, often living apart from the rest of society with fewer resources, influenced the spread of the pandemic.

Cities are densely populated social environments, but they are also human-made, physical places with a population of people who require housing and places to work, play, worship, and carry out the functions of daily life. Multiple aspects of a city's physical design can facilitate, mitigate, or influence the spread of pandemics. The urban built environment may be organized and heavily regulated by laws and government policies as it is in Manhattan, or it may develop informally as a settlement, like the urban slums of Dhaka. In all cases, the nature of buildings contributes to disease spread and its prevention. Efforts to provide clean water and thereby increase public hygiene for growing cities led the Romans to build aqueducts across the empire, and the British Public Health Act of 1848 brought order to chaotic and unhygienic urban physical environments in industrial-age London to substantially reduce morbidity and mortality.

The COVID-19 pandemic still weighs heavily on the world at the time of this writing. Urban spaces can create opportunities for preventative physical distancing or remove opportunities for maintaining space between people to limit viral transmission. Marginalized groups all over the world have been more likely to develop COVID-19 in no small part because they have not had access to physical environments that have enabled distancing from others. Dense housing with multiple occupants sharing a single room is conducive to epidemic spread once just one member of the household is infected. It is obviously far easier to distance oneself in spacious surroundings that make staying isolated in the "personal" space of the home little hardship at all.

Urban public spaces typically bring residents together but take on particular significance in the context of a pandemic when such spaces may also be used to keep people apart. The physical characteristics of cities have an aesthetic component, but they also play a clear role in health and disease determination. In non-epidemic times, the design of public physical environments determines whether urban residents can exercise and have access to nutritious food, both of which are directly linked to the risk of chronic diseases. In epidemic times, the evidence of the relation between the shared urban environment and health is even more acute. Well-designed public spaces present opportunities for congregation, but urban dwellers may need to be both outside and distant from one another during an epidemic. The squares of many European towns, designed with different needs in mind, permit this use today. By contrast, poorly designed and overcrowded public spaces present opportunities for random, inevitable, and dangerous contact in the context of a pandemic. It is not at all surprising that several recent epidemics—including SARS and COVID-19—are believed to have originated in public urban markets, where humans mixed chaotically and close proximity with other species enabled zoonotic transmission of infections.

The service environment encompasses the way the delivery of health and social services unfold within cities and the extent to which urban dwellers have access to these services. This has always been a central part of urban function and the relation of cities to health, and is perhaps particularly so during pandemic times. Of sentinel interest (indicating the presence of disease) are the access to and availability and delivery of health services. In European and North American urban centers, responses to the COVID-19 pandemic were shaped almost entirely by concerns about health services and the potential inability of health services to be adequate to the task of caring for sick patients. Global efforts to limit mobility in cities through a range of stay-at-home or lockdown orders ultimately intended to reduce transmission in order to limit the number of ill persons who might require and subsequently overwhelm health services. Driving all other urban functions, the service environment and its limitations have come to exemplify their own centrality in this rather extreme context. The complexity of the service environment and its interaction with urban life is also evident in the emerging evidence about excess mortality from non-COVID-19-related causes during the pandemic. This may have been driven in part by the reduced number of people turning to the health care system for assistance with their other illnesses, thereby increasing their risk of death from those conditions. Social services and other services that support the urban infrastructure determine the intersection of cities and public health during pandemics. The extent to which social services can continue to function under stress is enormously determinative of public trust in leadership and whether the general population will heed directives to mitigate viral spread.

Confusion about what is safe and what is unsafe during the COVID-19 pandemic has colored public discourse, casting doubt on a full range of decisions that inform public thinking and action. One example is presented in the challenges faced by many countries regarding whether to open, or not open, schools in the public education system. Fundamentally, urban environments function on the strength of their network of shared services, from health care, to education, to sanitation, to parks and recreational venues, and all of these have to respond in some way to the pandemic, and in so doing shape the lives of urban residents. This emphasizes, in no small part, the extreme dependence that urban dwellers have on organized services for their daily routines. In contrast with rural dwellers who have substantially more autonomy over what they do and how they engage with a much more sparsely populated world, urban dwellers' experiences are inextricably bound with their service environment—as they are with their social and physical environments—making the effectiveness of these services a *sine qua non* of urban function and in turn of health in urban areas.

The service environment experienced by urban dwellers has not provided homogenous access to the services that shape health, both generally and during pandemics. Extreme urban social stratification most affects persons who have limited assets or are from racial minority groups. This has been illustrated by the consequences of COVID-19 when elements of the social environment come into play. Workers required to be present in their physical workplace environment, such as food service and factory employees, are at increased risk of acquiring COVID-19. Those living in lower socio-economic groups frequently have limited personal physical infrastructure, resulting in more time spent in shared physical spaces. The service environment is again determinative, as different levels of social service availability shape urban dwellers' likelihood of having protection from the risk of COVID-19 transmission. The quality of health care itself has also likely contributed to pandemic mortality. Therefore, the service environment adds a third dimension to the elements of the urban environment that shape overall health, and heterogeneity of health, during pandemics.

Three formal elements of urban form and function—the social, physical, and service environments—are helpful organizing constructs for considering the production of health in cities. The same forces that shape health in non-pandemic times are more apparent during a pandemic, creating the contexts within which urban dwellers live and within which they may be vulnerable to disease. It is important to note that while these environments shape health in the pandemic context, the pandemic context also inevitably shapes these environments long after the pandemic has passed.

Pandemics centuries ago shaped social environments, introducing quarantines and ways of curing food to limit the spread of disease. It remains to be seen how the current COVID-19 pandemic will shape our social, physical, and service environments. In the United States, early signs point to seismic shifts in workplace patterns and changes in the extent that urban dwellers might use worksites like offices versus working remotely. That shift itself could result in altered urban social environments, as substantial numbers of people who historically lived in cities near their work can potentially choose to live in less populated, more affordable areas as they carry out the same job functions. It is also likely that we shall see a restructuring of physical environments to allow for physical distancing in public spaces and renewed investment in service systems that promote resilience to future pandemics. All in all, these changes signal reciprocity in the relation between cities and pandemics, whereby urban social, physical, and service environments shape, and are shaped by, disease. The chapters in this book reinforce these observations through the particular lenses of the authors and speak to how cities have evolved with pandemics.

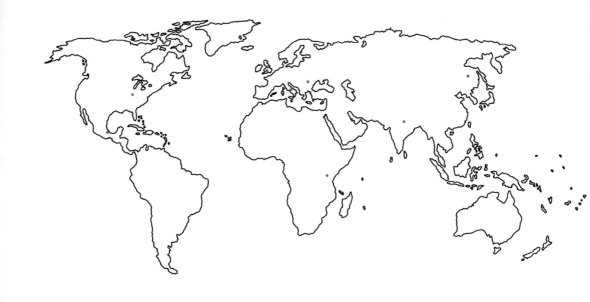

PART 1
Urban Governance:
Politics and Management

Case Studies for Urban Governance

Present-day cities and countries

1. Sibiu, Romania (Plague, 1510)
2. Agra, India (Plague, 1618–1619)
3. Bristol, England (Plague, 1665–66)
4. Veracruz, México (Smallpox, 1826)
5. York, England (Cholera, 1832)
6. Naples, Italy (Cholera, 1860–1914)
7. Harbin, China (Plague, 1910–1911)
8. Terre Haute, USA (Smallpox, 1902–03)
9. Nairobi, Kenya (Plague, 1895–1910)

This page: Map indicating the locations of case studies in this section of the book. (Map in the public domain, with annotations drawn by Andrew Bui.)

Right page: A man sitting at a table examining passports, during a plague epidemic in Mandalay. Photograph, 1906. (Courtesy of the Wellcome Collection.)

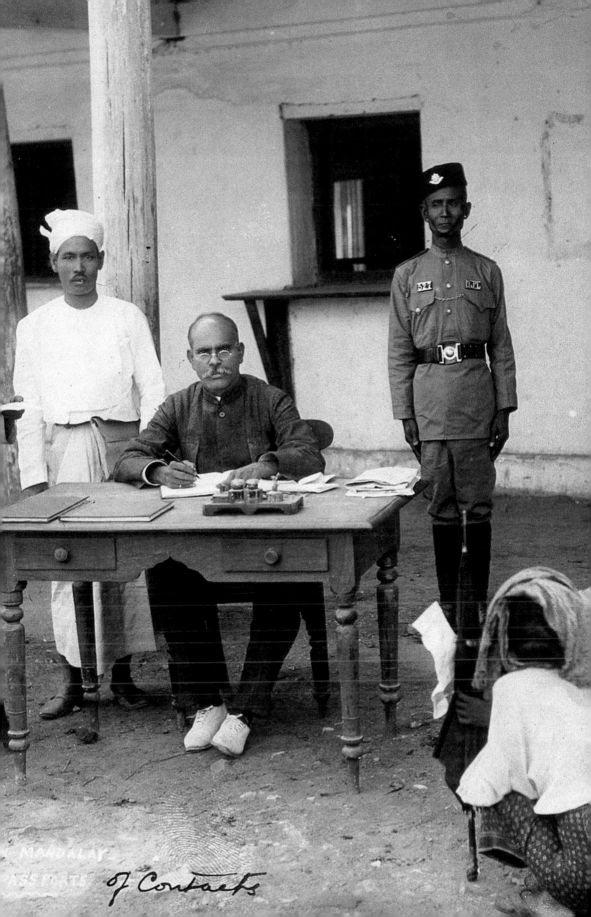

MANDALAY

ASSMATE   of Contacts

1

Plague in Sibiu and the First Quarantine Plan in Central Europe, 1510

Katalin Szende and Ottó Gecser

The eastern fringes of ancient and medieval Central Europe served as a trade crossroads for land routes that linked Europe and Asia. Beginning in the 14th century, the region facilitated the transport of precious Levantine wares and commodities such as silk and spices, a role that earned privileges for the urban communities en route. Traders from the Balkans to the Baltic moved from Istanbul via Edirne and Nikopol to Kraków, Toruń, and Gdańsk.[1] An important stretch of this route led through the eastern half of the Kingdom of Hungary, crossing the range of the Carpathian Mountains coming both from Transylvania (presently part of Romania) in the south, and the modern-day Slovak-Polish border in the north. The names of the most important stopovers on this stretch, Sibiu (Szeben, Hermannstadt), Brașov (Brassó, Kronstadt), Cluj (Kolozsvár, Klausenburg), Oradea (Várad), and Košice (Kassa, Kaschau) took many forms, indicating the multiethnic populations of towns.

Trade routes across Hungary facilitated the movement of goods, but they also enabled the spread of infections. This was well known to the Bishop of Transylvania in 1497, who complained that "Oradea was again infected by those coming from Brașov."[2] In addition to disease, public health ideals and models of charity also spread along these trade routes and were increasingly reflected in the distribution of small, municipally funded leper houses (*leprosaries*) placed on the outskirts of cities and towns. Typically, patients were separated and provided with material and spiritual care, not with medical cures, as leper houses recorded priests on their payroll, not doctors. These sites were the first urban institutions of communal care suitable for isolation practices. After the decrease of leprosy in the late 15th century, they were converted for use during epidemics identified by contemporaries with plague or with other contagious diseases.[3]

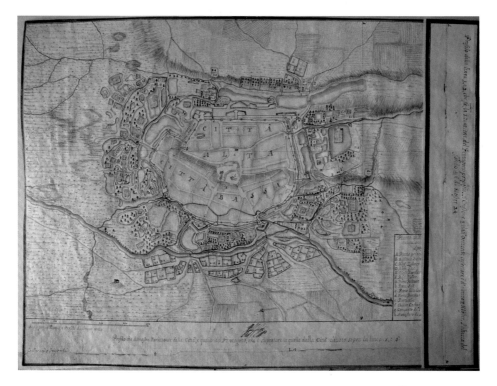

FIGURE 1.1: Ground plan of Sibiu, 1699, Giovanni Morandi Visconti. (Österreichisches Staatsarchiv Wien, Kriegsarchiv, Kartensammlung. Inland C VI. Hermannstadt Nr. 2.)

Early 16th-century Sibiu was a wealthy merchant city in the Kingdom of Hungary with approximately six thousand inhabitants, most of them Germans, the so-called Transylvanian Saxons (Figure 1.1).[4] The city was the key entry point for the land route of the Levantine trade across the Carpathian Mountains via the Turnu Rosu Pass (Figure 1.2). The city authorities invested a significant portion of their trade wealth in communal welfare. The municipal almshouse was built in 1292, an early date for such an institution in Hungary. Other specialized institutions dedicated to public welfare included a leper house from 1475, a town pharmacy called the Black Eagle built in 1494, and a hospital for syphilitic patients, constructed in 1501. Sibiu was also among the first urban centers in East Central Europe to employ municipal physicians. Little is known of most of these professionals, but they were formally trained at universities in the practice of medicine and often came from distant or even foreign places of origin such as Austria and Italy. By employing these municipal physicians and offering handsome salaries, the city imported up-to-date medical knowledge and expertise.[5]

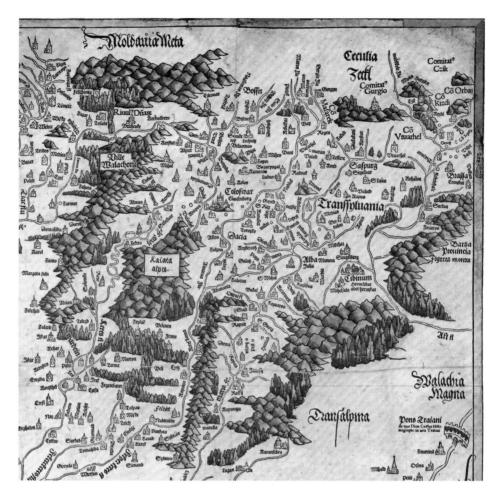

FIGURE 1.2: Map of Transylvania on the *Tabula Hungariae* of Lazarus secretarius, one-leaf engraving, Ingolstadt, 1528, detail. The map is oriented to the northwest, Sibiu is marked as Cibinium. (Public domain, Wikimedia Commons.)

Case study: Plague in Sibiu, 1510

In 1510, a severe outbreak of the plague spread across Hungary. King Wladislas II (*r.* 1490–1516) and his children fled Buda, the capital, and the diet had to be interrupted. Plague and subsequent famines were reported closer to Sibiu in the region of the Timiş (Temes) River.[6] Hans Saltzman of Styria (*d.* 1530), Sibiu's town physician at the time, was an Austrian who had previously studied in Vienna and Ferrara and practiced medicine in Moravia.[7] The appearance of the plague in the Transylvanian city was the impetus for Saltzman's text "A little work on the prevention of the plague and its cure, just as useful as necessary, explained accurately for the use of the common man" (Figure 1.3).[8] Saltzman completed the Latin booklet in August 1510 and had it printed in Vienna in November of that year, dedicating it to the royal judge Johannes Lulay (*d.* 1521) and Sibiu's city council.[9]

Saltzman prepared a German edition of his work for use in Styria eleven years after the initial Latin printing.[10] By that time, the author was a member of the medical faculty of the University of Vienna and the court physician of Ferdinand, Archduke of Austria (*r.* 1521–1564; from 1556 also Holy Roman Emperor as Ferdinand I), who sponsored the publication of the translated and revised booklet in the wake of a new plague outbreak in 1521 (Figure 1.4). The trade-route setting of Styria paralleled that of Sibiu in many ways. Situated in the northern foreground of the Alps and crossed by an important commercial artery between the Adriatic and the Danube valley, Styria was exposed to the dangers of infections carried by

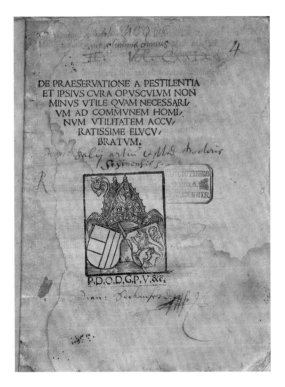

FIGURE 1.3: Title page, Johannes Saltzman, *De praeservatione a pestilentia et ipsius cura opusculum non minus utile quam necessarium ad commune hominum utilitatem accuratissime elucubratum [A little work on the prevention of the plague and its cure, just as useful as necessary, explained accurately for the use of the common man]*, Vienna: Hieronymus Vietor, 1510. (Bayerische Staatsbibliothek München, 4 Path. 321, urn:nbn:de:bvb:12-bsb00011759-9.)

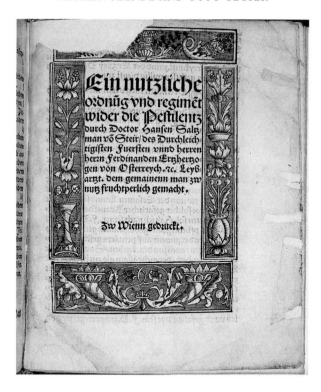

FIGURE 1.4: Title page, Hans (Johannes) Saltzman, *Ein nutzliche ordnung vnd regiment wider die Pestilentz durch Doctor Hansen Saltzman von Steir ... dem gemainenn man zw nutz fruchtperlich gemacht* [*A useful regulation against the plague by Doctor Hans Saltzman from Styria ... explained for the use of the common man*], Vienna: Singriener, 1521. (Moravian Library Brno, ST2-0695.728, přív.2.)

long-distance merchants moving from Venice through Villach and Graz to Vienna and beyond (Figure 1.5).

Saltzman's booklets fit into a long tradition of more than three hundred such plague tracts that have survived from the years between the Black Death of 1347–50 and 1500.[11] Given the characteristics of Hippocratic-Galenic medicine, medieval plague tracts were typically written with the needs of individual patients in mind. However, with the diffusion of the office of municipal physicians and the emergence of urban health boards, these publications began to address an audience of magistrates and other territorial authorities as well. The genre reached Hungary after some delay: the earliest plague tract known from medieval Hungary was copied in 1473 by János Gellértfi of Aranyas, a cleric in the Spiš (Szepesség, Zips)

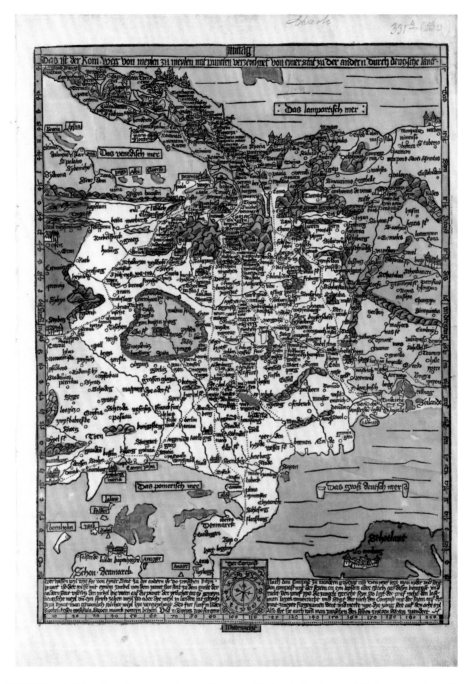

FIGURE 1.5: Map for pilgrims going to Rome, with Styria in the top left (map is oriented to the South); Erhard Etzlaub, single-leaf colored woodcut, Nuremberg, *c*.1500. (Public domain, Wikimedia Commons.)

region in modern-day Slovakia (then northeastern Hungary).[12] The original was composed by Johannes Jacobi, a professor of medicine at Montpellier (*d.* 1384).

Most plague outbreaks in premodern Europe have left behind few local sources, and this is also the case for the course and consequences of the 1510 plague in Sibiu. However, Saltzman's two booklets, when taken together, offer a well-educated physician's insights into the medical scenario. There are notable differences between the two texts. The Latin version of 1510 concentrates on the general causes of the infection and gives advice to individuals on how to prevent, diagnose, and eventually cure the disease. Apart from its dedicatory preface to the magistrates of Sibiu, it follows the usual pattern of earlier plague tracts. The German version printed in 1521 was written in the vernacular (and therefore potentially more accessible to the general public) and was complemented by a set of recommended public health measures for implementation by the civic authorities. According to Saltzman, such measures had led to the successful protection of the Transylvanian city eleven years earlier. The additional elements in the second version likely reflected Saltzman's growing practical experience and accumulated knowledge.

The preventive measures that Saltzman proposed were pragmatic in nature. For individuals, he repeated the age-old advice "*cito, longe, tarde*" (fly quickly, go far, return slowly). Needless to say, very few could afford to do so. The measures proposed for the community, however, fit more realistically into an urban context. Since the contamination of air was identified as the main cause of the disease, sanitary measures intended to protect the air quality from corruptive fumes and smells appear most prominently. Saltzman suggested that "prudent leaders of cities must make sure that all the streets and houses are kept clean, the dung removed, slaughterhouses and shambles supplied with running water and cleaned daily; pigs kept far away from the city, altogether do away with foul air as much as possible." Rules for self-isolation were introduced so that one might "avoid the gathering of crowds such as at annual fairs, weddings, baths, meeting in small churches, in the boys' schools, and in general in congested and closed spaces." He also gave strict orders to deny entrance to anyone coming from infected places or who had been in touch with infected clothes or food. Saltzman advocated for the conscious use of quarantine with a call to "assign one or more houses at a safe distance from the city or town where those coming from infected places can stay, and use fumigation to cleanse them and their clothes. They can be let into the city after having stayed in good air for twenty days."[13]

The measures described in the 1521 booklet, and reported to have been successfully applied at Sibiu, can be grouped in four major categories: first, movement restrictions (closing borders to persons coming or returning from infected regions, as well as to strangers in general); second, social distancing (enforced both on an individual level and through bans on any sort of gathering); third, isolation at home or in plague hospitals (*lazarettos*), to protect the healthy and take care of the sick; and fourth, quarantine (temporary retention of persons with unknown health conditions during the longest-known incubation period).[14]

The proposal of not merely the first three types of measures but also the fourth one, the quarantine—applied, remarkably, both to those coming from outside regions and to the households of the contaminated—was perhaps the most important novelty of Saltzman's plague tract.[15] To be sure, detention in quarantine had already been applied in Dubrovnik in 1377 and later in Venice and other harbor cities. However, in landlocked Central Europe, large-scale quarantining was previously unknown and posed great logistical challenges. It has yet to be determined where such a quarantine establishment might have been located on the outskirts of Sibiu.[16] The city walls, reinforced in 1500 to fend off assaults by the Ottoman army, were certainly sufficient to prevent uncontrolled entrance into Sibiu (see Figure 1.1).[17]

Conclusion

In his German pamphlet, Saltzman proudly announced that "in 1510, having followed my advice, the largest city of Transylvania called Hermannstadt [Sibiu] was completely saved so that nobody got sick during this period"; he added that "all other surrounding cities and market towns that did not stick to this regime were hard hit by the plague."[18] In the preface of the Latin version, dedicating the work to the city council, he also emphasized that Sibiu had to be saved so that it could continue to function as the "Shield of Europe" and the "Bulwark of Christianity"—a reference to the ideological topos of Hungary defending (western) Christendom, meant here to serve flattery and justification at the same time.[19]

More broadly speaking, the case of Hans Saltzman and Sibiu exemplifies how health was becoming a public value and how public health was emerging on the agenda of local as well as state authorities. This process of transformation unfolded with significant variation in different parts of late medieval Europe, but always on the municipal level first and on that of the state only later. Merchant cities along trade arteries reaped the profits of long-distance commerce, but they were subsequently forced to invest these earnings back into the handling of adverse consequences. The municipal authorities in some of these cities hired the best medical expertise available and subsequently stood at the forefront of developments in urban health. The innovation of printing as a method of disseminating knowledge was also utilized. Sibiu both fostered and benefitted from these circumstances.

While the dedication of the 1521 German-language booklet remarked on the need for sovereigns to take responsibility (as they did in Styria but not yet in

Transylvania), measures had to be adopted and implemented by the municipalities. This led to stronger municipal authorities and, under ideal circumstances, to the increased sanitation of the urban townscape. As cities grew, infections continued to be a challenge. Coordination between communities was often lacking and those with less resources were easily passed by, as Saltzman notes. Saltzman's justification for protecting Sibiu because it was "the shield of Europe" is a reminder that saving a city from an epidemic was not simply a humanitarian concern but also part of the utilitarian considerations of strategic and commercial goals.

NOTES

1. Zsigmond Pál Pach, "Hungary and the Levantine Trade in the Fourteenth-Seventeenth Centuries," *Acta Orientalia Academiae Scientiarum Hungaricae* 60, no. 1 (2007): 9–31; Katalin Szende, "Kraków and Buda in the Road Network of Medieval Europe," in *On Common Path: Budapest and Kraków in the Middle Ages*, ed. Judit Benda, Virág Kiss, Grażyna Lihończak-Nurek, and Károly Magyar (Budapest: Budapesti Történeti Múzeum, 2016), 31–37.

2. Gyula Magyary-Kossa, *Magyar orvosi emlékek: Értekezések a magyar orvostörténet köréből. III. kötet: Adattár 1000–1700-ig* [Hungarian Medical Records: Treatises on Hungarian Medical History, vol. 3: Repertory 1000–1700] (Budapest: Magyar Orvosi Könyvkiadó Társulat, 1931), 116 (no. 461).

3. Judit Majorossy and Katalin Szende, "Hospitals in Medieval and Early Modern Hungary," in *Europäisches Spitalwesen: Institutionelle Fürsorge in Mittelalter und Früher Neuzeit*, ed. Martin Scheutz, Andrea Sommerlechner, Herwig Weigl, and Alfred S. Weiß (Vienna: Oldenbourg, 2008), 409–54.

4. Mária Pakucs-Willcocks, *Sibiu-Hermannstadt: Oriental Trade in Sixteenth-century Transylvania* (Cologne: Böhlau, 2007).

5. Magyary-Kossa, *Magyar orvosi emlékek* 102 (no. 406), 133 (no. 520), 136 (no. 533), 147 (no. 589), 152 (no. 615).

6. Ibid., 135–36.

7. Robert Offner, "Johannes Saltzmann, der Stadtarzt von Hermannstadt, ließ 1510 in Wien seine Pest-Ordnung drucken," *Kaleidoscope* 2, no. 2 (2011): 127–32.

8. Johannes Saltzman, *De praeservatione a pestilentia et ipsius cura opusculum non minus utile quam necessarium ad commune hominum utilitatem accuratissime elucubratum* (Vienna: Hieronymus Vietor, 1510). Saltzman's Latin booklet, together with its later German version (see below), are the only known sources of the epidemic of 1510. We present them in some detail in order to put them in context and assess their reliability.

9. Ágnes Flóra, *The Matter of Honour: The Leading Urban Elite in Sixteenth-century Transylvania* (Turnhout: Brepols, 2019), 158.

10. Hans Saltzman, *Ein nutzliche ordnung vnd regiment wider die Pestilentz durch Doctor Hansen Saltzman von Steir ... dem gemainenn man zw nutz fruchtperlich gemacht* (Vienna: Singriener, 1521).

11. Samuel K. Cohn, *The Black Death Transformed: Disease and Culture in the Early Renaissance* (London: Edward Arnold, 2002).

12. Ottó Gecser, "Understanding Pestilence in the Times of King Matthias: The Plague Tract in the Manuscript of János Gellértfi of Aranyasi," in *Matthias Rex 1458–1490: Hungary at the Dawn of the Renaissance*, ed. István Draskóczy et al. (Budapest: Eötvös Loránd University Faculty of Humanities, Centre des hautes études de la Renaissance, 2013), http:// renaissance.elte.hu/wp-content/uploads/2013/10/Otto-Gecser-Understanding-Pestilence-in-the-Times-of-King-Matthias-The-Plague-Tract-in-the-Manuscript-of-Janos-Gellertfi-of-Aranyas.pdf (accessed September 14, 2020). The Spiš region was another stopover on the Istanbul-Kraków-Gdańsk axis.

13. Saltzman, *Ein nutzliche ordnung*, fol. b Ir–b IIv.

14. Ibid., fol. b IIr–b IIIr.

15. Ibid., fol. b IIv. See Jane Stevens Crawshaw, "The Renaissance Invention of Quarantine," in *Society in an Age of Plague*, ed. Linda Clark and Carole Rawcliffe (Woodbridge: Boydell, 2013), 161–73.

16. If the *leprosorium* was used for this purpose, then it must have been located east of the city, just outside the St. Elizabeth Gate. Special thanks to Dr. Júlia Derzsi, Institute of Social Sciences and Humanities of the Romanian Academy in Sibiu, for sharing these latest results.

17. Radu Lupescu, "The Medieval Fortifications of Sibiu," in *"Vmbringt mit starken turnen, murn:" Ortsbefestigungen im Mittelalter*, ed. Olaf Wagener (Frankfurt am Main: Peter Lang, 2010), 351–62.

18. Saltzman, *Ein nutzliche ordnung*, fol. b IIr.

19. Saltzman, *De praeservatione a pestilentia*, fol. A1. Cf. Pál Fodor, *The Unbearable Weight of Empire: The Ottomans in Central Europe – a Failed Attempt at Universal Monarchy (1390–1566)* (Budapest: Research Centre for the Humanities, Hungarian Academy of Sciences, 2016), 54.

2

Mughal Governance, Mobility, and Responses to the Plague in Agra, India, 1618–19

Mehreen Chida-Razvi

Various outbreaks of illness occurred during the Mughal Empire's (1526–1857) rule over much of South Asia (Figure 2.1). In 1616, during the reign of Emperor Jahangir (r. 1605–27), plague broke out in the empire and reoccurred each winter over the next eight years. Jahangir referenced the three epidemics that took place in the winters of 1616, 1617–18, and 1618–19 in his memoirs, the *Jahangirnama*. The symptoms he described reveal that these were outbreaks of bubonic plague and of septicemic plague, its more serious, progressive form.[1] The plague epidemic of 1618–19 is of particular interest as it directly affected Jahangir's movement through the empire and the site from which he chose to govern.

In early 1618, Jahangir and his court left Malwa to return to the imperial capital city of Agra after almost five years away.[2] After receiving word en route that the plague was endemic in the capital, Jahangir chose to establish himself and his court in the city of Ahmadabad in Gujarat until it was safe to return to Agra.[3] Jahangir departed again for the capital in the beginning of September. In December, having reached the environs of the city of Fatehpur Sikri, approximately 24 miles west of Agra, Jahangir and his retinue were informed that the plague was again resurgent there. The emperor therefore decided to stay at Fatehpur Sikri, in the palace built there by his father, until it was safe to travel on to Agra.

The Mughal Empire encompassed a vast geographical area and had established imperial capital cities, Agra being the most important at this time. However, the Mughal court was peripatetic and the seat of government moved with the person of the emperor. As Jahangir was the apex of the administrative structure, even while the plague was rampant in Agra in 1618–19, the government continued to operate at full capacity, portraying strength and exuding reassurance in Jahangir's ability to rule, regardless of where he happened to be. Being able to continuously

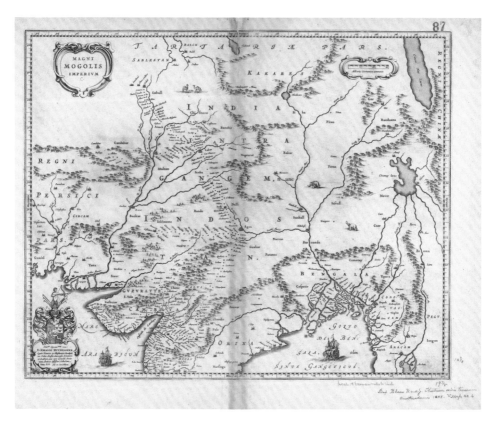

FIGURE 2.1: Map of the Mughal Empire, *Magni Mogolis Imperium*, 1640. Joan Blaeu (1596–1673) and Cornelis Blaeu (1610–1648). Norman B. Leventhal Map Center Collection G1015. C65 1630. (Courtesy of the Norman B. Leventhal Map & Education Center at the Boston Public Library.)

project imperial authority was a vital part of Mughal ruling ideology, and wherever he was, Jahangir made administrative and governing decisions, or was aware of those that were made by his local and provincial governors and officials. These administrators also kept him constantly appraised of the plague in Agra and its severity during the months he traveled to reach the capital.

Case study: Plague in Agra, 1618–19

During Jahangir's reign, the city of Agra was on its way to becoming the largest urban center in the empire; Agra's population reached approximately 500,000 people in 1609, and between 1629 and 1643 roughly 660,000 people were

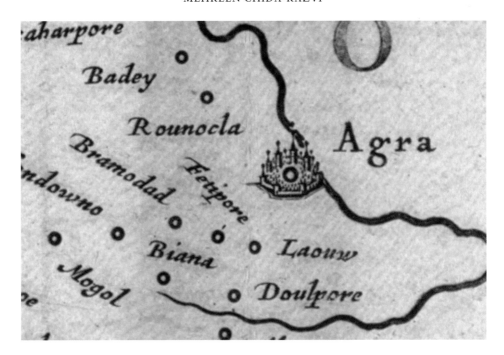

FIGURE 2.2: Detail showing Agra and proximity to Fatehpur Sikri, marked as "Fetipore." Map of Mughal Empire, *Magni Mogolis Imperium*, 1640. Joan Blaeu (1596–1673) and Cornelis Blaeu (1610–1648). Norman B. Leventhal Map Center Collection G1015.C65 1630. (Courtesy of the Norman B. Leventhal Map & Education Center at the Boston Public Library.)

estimated to have lived there.[4] The urban density very likely contributed to the rampant spread of the plague when it reached the city.[5] Jahangir described an extremely virulent strain that passed from person to person and between species with the slightest touch.[6] The plague made a resurgence in the city and the surrounding region for the third consecutive winter in 1618–19, yet it does not appear to have spread further west than the village of Amanabad, 5 miles east of Fatehpur Sikri (Figure 2.2).[7] This geographical halt in disease transmission was likely because Amanabad and its immediate surroundings were completely deserted after the two previous bouts of plague.[8] It is known, however, that even during the earlier outbreak in 1616, Fatehpur Sikri was spared while Agra was badly affected, as a member of the East India Company left Agra for Fatehpur Sikri to escape the "vehement rage of the plague."[9] Either Fatehpur Sikri's population was sparse enough at that time to limit transmission, or, more likely, the distance between the city and Amanabad was enough to prevent the epidemic from spreading to the immediate environs of Fatehpur Sikri.

One of the most effective methods for containing and dealing with the plague in Mughal South Asia was to abandon houses, villages, and towns and to relocate to safer regions. Removing any possible human vector was a recognized means of fighting epidemics. Mughal imperial historian and biographer Mu'tamad Khan (*d.* 1639) recorded responses to plague in the Doab in 1616 in his *Iqbal-nama Jahangiri* (a history of Jahangir's reign). He wrote that a family could avoid succumbing to disease by immediately leaving their home to go "away to the jungle" upon seeing signs of the illness.[10] Although no reason is explicitly stated in the sources for why the abandonment of such urban and rural centers led to disease control, several reasonable assumptions can be made. First, abandoning living quarters resulted in limiting—and ultimately halting—the possibility of transmission between human populations. Second, abandonment of population centers also prevented the disease from entering a community from an outside source, be it human or animal. As a last point, reduced human populations, or a lack of them entirely, within a defined spatial area meant minimal or no food sources for creatures through which the plague could be transmitted, denying the possibility of interspecies spread.

The evacuation of affected rural and urban areas as a means of controlling the spread of the plague was likely effective due to the provincial geographical planning established during the reign of Jahangir's father, Emperor Akbar (*r.* 1556–1605). Prior to Mughal rule, villages had been constructed approximately three kilometers apart. During Akbar's reign, Mughal towns were constructed 25–30 kilometers apart within this framework of villages to serve as intermediate centers for trade and the movement of agricultural produce. Provincial capitals were placed at the very center of these planned geographical systems.[11] The upper half of a painting of a royal procession, described in an accompanying text as traveling between Lahore and Agra, portrays this geographical arrangement of settlements and the distances between them (Figure 2.3).[12] The painting also presents a visualization of the difference in the urban density of the walled-in cities as opposed to that of smaller towns and villages in the countryside. The plague was transmitted along routes used by people of all classes and the disease thus moved between urban and rural areas.[13] Abandoning villages was therefore an essential means of controlling the spread of the plague outside of Agra.

The effectiveness of this approach is made clear by the fact that Jahangir and his retinue, and sometimes even members of the Harem, undertook frequent hunting expeditions during their stay at Fatehpur Sikri, sometimes to the limits of the village of Amanabad, with no ill effects.[14] While it may appear these were solely for pleasurable pursuits, hunting was not merely a sporting activity for Mughal rulers. The hunt was a presentation of political and military strength to subjects of all classes; it was a way of surveying one's kingdom and of reassuring the public that

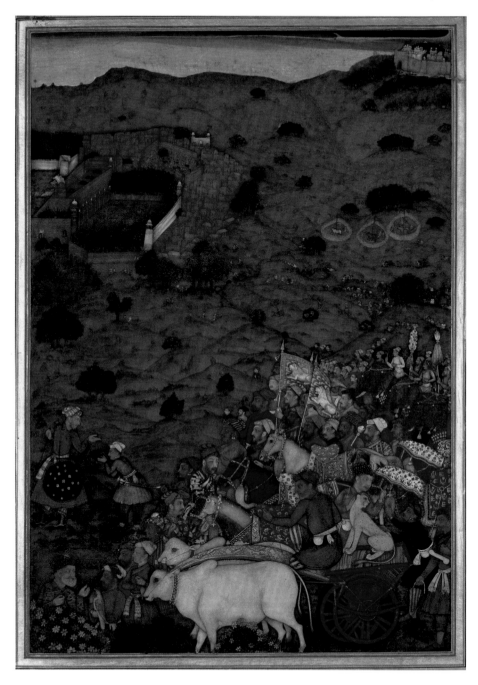

FIGURE 2.3: *A Royal Procession,* from the *Windsor Padshahnama,* fol. 166b. Attributed to the "Kashmiri Painter," *c.*1656–57, Mughal India. Opaque watercolor, ink and gold on paper, 33.1 × 22.9 cm. (Courtesy of The Royal Collection, Windsor, RCIN 1005025.ai, Royal Collection Trust / © Her Majesty Queen Elizabeth II 2020.)

the emperor was actively watching over his empire and, by extension, his subjects. The hunt was, in effect, a performative act of governance that was entwined with the administration of the empire. By carrying out hunting expeditions right up to the vicinity of Amanabad, Jahangir was exhibiting himself as a present, virile, potent ruler still actively engaged in ruling his domains even during the plague. It is also likely that, by hunting in the region of Amanabad, Jahangir was purposefully projecting another element of symbolic control specifically in relation to the ravages of plague on the landscape: through the hunt the emperor conveyed their control of nature and the bending of it to one's will.[15]

While isolation of the population at both the local and regional levels appears to have been employed to control the plague's spread, Jahangir notes that while he was at Fatehpur Sikri, an official who had been stationed to guard Agra came and paid homage,[16] as did Jahangir's elderly mother, Mariam Zamani, a second noblewoman,[17] and two courtiers.[18] Audiences with the emperor were fundamental to Mughal governance and ceremony, and visits by courtiers, administrators, and those who came to pay obeisance to Jahangir continued without interruption during this time.[19]

This was possible because wherever he was, Jahangir was accompanied by a fully functioning court administration. This included the accoutrements for giving daily audiences, equipment to continue with the artistic production of the court, and everything necessary for members of the harem traveling with the ruler.[20] Ceremonial activity and appearances were fundamental to the projection of Mughal governance and therefore necessary, even when the court was on the move, as seen in a Mughal painting showing Jahangir holding court in an outdoor setting (Figure 2.4). There, red tent panels are used to create a royal enclosure within which the audience takes place; a gold platform throne has been placed in the center, resting on luxurious carpets, and multiple canopies of rich textiles are raised above the emperor's head to denote royal space. All of these accoutrements, plus the book being gifted, illustrate items carried with the emperor whenever he traveled within his borders.

Conclusion

The importance of the role of government becomes clear during times of crisis, endemic illness, and social anxiety. The projection of competence and authority is paramount, as exemplified by Jahangir's ability to carry out activities of everyday governance, hold audiences, and undertake ritual, ceremonial activities, regardless of his location. As the head of the entrenched system of the provincial and local

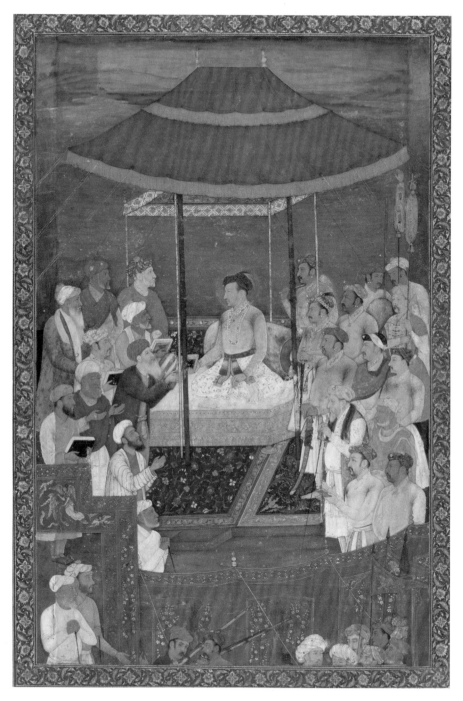

FIGURE 2.4: *Jahangir giving Books to Shaykhs*, from the *St. Petersburg Album*. Attributed to Lalchand, *c.*1620, Mughal India. Opaque watercolor, ink and gold on paper, 31.7 × 20.5 cm, full folio. (Courtesy of Freer Gallery of Art, F1931.20, Charles Lang Freer Endowment.)

administration, the emperor made all the important decisions for the empire and was kept apprised of important administrative matters.[21]

The Mughal Empire was divided and subdivided into provinces, *sarkars*, and *parganas*, each of which had an appointed official in charge of daily administrative details and revenue collection. Whether in a city, or traveling between sites, Jahangir was kept informed of occurrences of the plague and its severity as continuous movement of his administrators, messengers, and underlings occurred unabated throughout his empire. Such was Jahangir's authority that he could decide to move into any city at any time with his entire court and administration if the situation demanded it. The theater of the emperor and the court could continue therefore as normal, projecting strength, competency, and control and ensuring that governance continued in times of crisis. That this was widely known by the general population allowed for faith in governmental systems to continue.

NOTES

1. Jahangir described bubonic plague symptoms in his Nuruddin Muhammad Jahangir, *The Tuzuk-i Jahangiri*, trans. Alexander Rogers, ed. Henry Beveridge (Delhi: D.K. Fine Art Press, 1989 rpt., 2 volumes bound as 1), vol. 2, 65; and Nuruddin Muhammad Jahangir, *The Jahangirnama: Memoirs of Jahangir, Emperor of India*, trans. and ed., Wheeler M. Thackston (Washington, DC: Oxford University Press, 1999), 291. Without treatment, the bacteria moves to the blood and can progress to septicemic plague.

2. Agra is located on the Jumna/Yamuna river in North India, roughly 128 miles south of New Delhi.

3. Jahangir, *Jahangirnama*, 261.

4. K. K. Trivedi, "The Emergence of Agra as a Capital and a City: A Note on its Spatial and Historical background during the Sixteenth and Seventeenth Centuries," *Journal of the Economic and Social History of the Orient* 37, no. 2 (1994): 166.

5. Jahangir references the concentration of housing on the west side of the city and the density of the urban area, writing that "the congestion is so great that one can scarcely pass in the lanes and markets." Jahangir, *Jahangirnama*, 22. Agra's density was also noted by European visitors, including the Portuguese factor Francisco Pelsaert, in Agra between 1621 and 1627. Francisco Pelsaert, *Jahangir's India: The Remonstrantie of Francisco Persaert*, trans. W.H. Moreland and P. Geyl (Cambridge: W. Heffer & Sons, 1925), 1. The Englishman William Finch visited Agra in 1610 and commented on the narrow streets and large population. William Foster, ed., *Early Travels in India 1583–1619* (London: Oxford University Press, 1921), 182.

6. Jahangir, *Tuzuk*, vol. 2, 66; Jahangir, *Jahangirnama*, 291–92.

7. "2.5 *kos*" from Amanabad, or roughly 19 miles west of Agra. Jahangir, *Tuzuk*, vol. 2, 65; Jahangir, *Jahangirnama*, 291.

8. Enayatullah Khan, "Visitations of Plague in Mughal India," *Proceedings of the Indian History Congress* 74 (2013): 307; Beni Prasad, *History of Jahangir* (Allahabad: The Indian Press, 1930), 292.

9. William Foster, ed., *The Embassy of Sir Thomas Roe to the Court of the Great Mogul, 1615–1619*, vol. 2 (London: Hakluyt Society, 1899), 366.

10. Mu'tamad Khan's *Iqbal-nama Jahangiri* in Henry M. Elliott, *The History if India as Told by Its Own Historians: The Muhammadan Period*, vol. 6, ed. John Dowson (London: Trübner, 1875), 406. This preventative relocation was long practiced in the region. A breakout of the plague in a village in Jalandhar in the Punjab in 1897 was practically brought to a halt once the site was evacuated, and the last case from that particular village occurred 35 days after the evacuation took place. See Surgeon-Captain C. H. James, I.M.S., *Report on the Outbreak of Plague in the Jullundar and Hoshiarpur Districts of the Punjab, 1897-98* (Lahore: The Civil & Military Gazette Press, 1898), 5.

11. Attilio Petrucciolo, "Fathpur Sikri, Akbar's Capital and Construction Models for Mughal Towns," in *Akbar the Great Emperor of India*, ed. Gian Carlo Calza (Milan: Fondazione Roma and Skira Editore, 2012), 41.

12. The text accompanying this painting in the Windsor *Padshahnama* describes an imperial procession traveling between Lahore and Agra. See Milo Cleveland Beach and Ebba Koch, *King of the World: The Padshahnama, an Imperial Mughal Manuscript from the Royal Library, Windsor Castle* (London: Azimuth Editions, 1997), 86.

13. Jahangir notes that the winter 1616 plague began in the province of Lahore's outer districts before spreading to the city of Lahore, after which it spread east to reach Delhi and its surrounds. See Jahangir, *Tuzuk*, vol. 1, 330; Jahangir, *Jahangirnama*, 196–97.

14. Jahangir, *Tuzuk*, vol. 2, 70, 73; Jahangir, *Jahangirnama*, 293, 295. While isolation was a means of controlling the plague, those of elite status were clearly permitted to move freely between Fatehpur Sikri and Agra. Movement of other populations also still occurred to maintain the necessary delivery of goods and trade within the empire. A letter dated February 20, 1619, for example, lists the goods sent to Surat from Agra by the East India Company, highlighting that both people and material goods left the city while the plague was endemic there. See William Foster, ed., *The English Factories in India 1618–1621* (Oxford: Clarendon Press, 1906), 73.

15. On this topic, see Shaha Parpia, "Reordering Nature: Power Politics in the Mughal *Shikargah*," *International Journal of Islamic Architecture* 7, no. 1 (2018): 39–66.

16. Jahangir, *Jahangirnama*, 292.

17. During her audience with the emperor, the visiting noblewoman implies that those who have fallen ill with the plague have been quarantined to limit the potential to spread the disease to others in their family. Jahangir, *Tuzuk*, vol. 2, 66; Jahangir, *Jahangirnama*, 291–92.

18. Jahangir, *Tuzuk*, vol. 2, 66, 68–69; Jahangir, *Jahangirnama*, 291–93.

19. Within a few days of entering Fatehpur Sikri, for example, Jahangir presented robes of honor; distributed vast amounts of material wealth in the form of coins; sent a copy of the

Jahangirnama and a "royal topchaq horse" to his son, Sultan Parvez; and gifted a horse, an elephant, a robe of honor, and jeweled objects to a courtier (Jahangir, *Jahangirnama*, 292–93). Such items were available as they were part of the court trappings and treasuries that moved with the emperor wherever he roamed (see Figure 2.4, for example, the gifting of a book).

20. On the continued artistic production see Susan Stronge, "Jahangir's Itinerant Masters," in *Indian Painting: Themes, Histories, Interpretations: Essays in Honour of B.N. Goswamy*, ed. M. Sharma and P. Kaimal (Ahmedabad: Mapin, 2013), 125–35.

21. Jahangir, *Jahangirnama*, xviii.

3

Urban Governance, Economic Intervention, and the Plague in Bristol, England, 1665–66

Andrew Wells

The last outbreak of bubonic plague to hit the city of Bristol in southwest England struck in the second half of 1665. It was an inopportune moment. The city was struggling to come to terms with the deep divisions left by the Civil War, when it had been besieged and occupied by both Royalist and Parliamentarian forces, and by the unsettled years of the 1650s. The restoration of the monarchy in 1660 had resolved little and the city's large population remained divided, principally over religion: Bristol was home to a substantial number of Protestant Dissenters, who felt keenly the efforts of Parliament after 1661 to restore a religious uniformity that had never actually existed. Bristolians were politically active and well informed but could find no outlet in their small, oligarchic corporation (city, or Common, council), so they instead focused on the politics of the guild, parish, and Parliament. Each freeman possessed the franchise, which was just one of a number of jealously guarded privileges: Bristol's citizens were notoriously hostile to outsiders trading in their midst (which earned the city a stinging rebuke from the writer Daniel Defoe) due to fierce competition for business and space in what was fast becoming England's principal provincial trading city.[1]

These pressures were poorly managed in the years before 1665. The show of local solidarity in the immediate aftermath of the Restoration—when the Corporation only half-heartedly purged supporters of the revolutionary regime—gave way in 1663 to an enthusiastic persecution of religious minorities, particularly Quakers and Baptists, orchestrated by Bristol's mayor. This was fueled as much by religious bigotry as it was by fear of disaffection, something that preoccupied the authorities in London. By 1665 religious and political strife was compounded with the disrupted trade and widespread naval impressment produced by the Second Anglo-Dutch War (1665–67). The government was concerned that Bristol was ripe for rebellion, so the Duke of Ormond, Lord Lieutenant of Ireland, was sent to bolster the city's civic authorities and organize its militia. Notwithstanding the pomp and ceremony of his visit, he worryingly reported that further efforts were necessary to ensure that Bristol remained friendly to the King.[2]

He need not have been so concerned. With the election of a more tolerant mayor in 1665, religious persecution momentarily subsided, lowering the political temperature. This was the lens through which one local Baptist clergyman viewed the comparatively light outbreak of the plague in 1665–66. "This Citty of Bristoll was visited with that Judgment of ye Lord, ye Plague," he wrote, "which struck Terror in ye Magistrats," but thanks to the moderate course steered by the new mayor, "who began a stop to Persecution … ye Lord dealt very mercifull and gracious with ye Citty, that ye Plague abated and stopt."[3] The outbreak was indeed lighter than previous visitations, claiming probably fewer than a hundred lives, and took almost a year to arrive in the city after the first reports of the illness in London. By the end of 1665, plague was present in the nearby village of Bedminster, to the south, and in the suburb outside Lawford's Gate, which was in the east, where the main roads to London and Gloucester converged on the city.

Case study: Bubonic plague in Bristol, 1665–66

Bristol responded to the plague long before it arrived at the city's gates. Once it was clear that the disease had taken hold in London, where by early June 1665 fatalities trebled with every passing week, the most urgent measure was to prevent traders from the capital and elsewhere gathering in Bristol for St. James's Fair, due to be held in late July. In June, the Corporation spent a considerable sum of money—almost £24—to obtain a proclamation from the Privy Council prohibiting the fair (Figure 3.1).[4] Such expense, and the readiness to incur it, was likely due to the urgency of the matter, as already on June 13 it was reported that "Londoners w[i]th their goods are dayly resorting hither."[5]

This urgency also explains why Bristol's authorities began to issue orders on the basis of the proclamation even before the King and Council had agreed to it.[6] Ten days before its publication, the city's magistrates ordered that goods from London, as potential bearers of contagion, were not to enter Bristol without first being aired outside the city's walls for a period of thirty days. Strangers were suspect—constables were to search the city every night and report on them twice weekly to the mayor and aldermen—but they were not yet excluded.[7] This came almost a week later (and fully four days before the proclamation was issued), when the mayor and aldermen permitted entry only to those Londoners bearing a certificate of health from the Lord Mayor of London. Defoe later recorded that these certificates were easy to obtain in May and June, although the reason he gave—"there

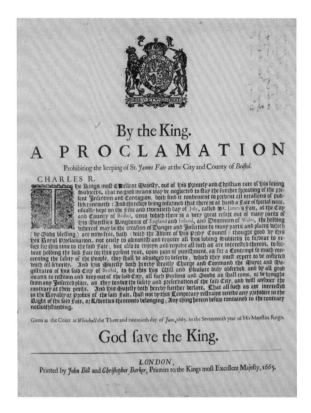

FIGURE 3.1: Proclamation prohibiting the keeping of St. James Fair at the City and County of Bristol, June 23, 1665. (Courtesy of The National Archives of the UK, SP 45/11 (192).)

had none died in the City for all this time"—was obviously false, even to those in a city a hundred miles distant.[8] Such restrictions on the admission of people and goods were not toothless but were accompanied by the establishment of a civic watch in which all citizens took part to guard against unlawful entry.[9]

These early regulations were specific interventions based on local (primarily commercial) circumstances. But when the plague finally hit Bristol later in the year, the city's response largely accorded with a set of national rules, dating originally from 1578 and strengthened by statute in 1604. Among other things, these rules provided for the appointment of searchers to ascertain whether the recently deceased had died of the plague, for orderly burial, for quarantine and the isolation of infected dwellings, for the establishment of pesthouses, and for levying local taxation to pay for their construction, for the wages of searchers and other officials, and for the support of those isolated in their own homes or in pesthouses. A lively debate on this "Book of Orders" took place across the late 16th and early

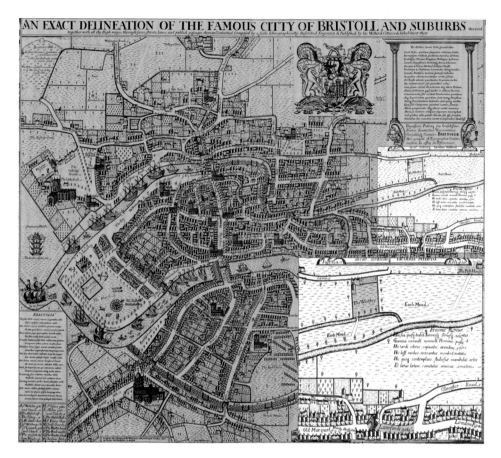

FIGURE 3.2: James Millerd, *An Exact Delineation of the Famout Citty of Bristoll and Suburbs Thereof* (Bristol, 1673), with detail showing (clockwise from top left) "The Whitstry," "The Pest House," and Lawford's Gate. © Bristol Culture. (Courtesy of Bristol Museum and Art Gallery, Object Number R0020.)

17th centuries, especially concerning the hardships inflicted on those confined to their homes, and it was finally revised only in 1666, once the danger for Bristol had passed.[10]

In the meantime, Bristol's response was guided principally by these rules. Pesthouses were set up at considerable cost in December 1665 outside the city in an area inaptly known as the Forlorn Hope (Figure 3.2).[11] Possibly because of the anticipated severity of the epidemic, these structures were more permanent than the tents and huts—labeled "hovels" by Bristolians—set up in parkland to the north of the city during earlier plague outbreaks.[12] The closest urban parish to the new establishments was St. Philip's, one of the poorest in the city and the worst

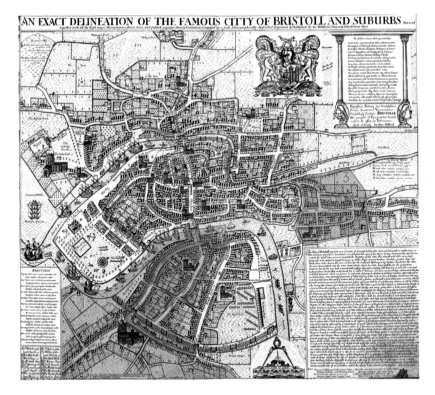

FIGURE 3.3: Parishes of Bristol (1: St Mary Redcliff, 2: St Thomas, 3: St Philip) and individual streets with 1665–66 plague cases. Plague was endemic in St. Philip's Parish. From James Millerd, *An Exact Delineation of the Famout Citty of Bristoll and Suburbs Thereof* (Bristol, 1673).

hit in the outbreak. Isolated cases occurred in wealthier (St. Thomas) or more mixed (St. Mary Redcliff) parishes to the west and south of the city (Figure 3.3).[13] Many cases were sent to the pesthouses, but for others the older regulations were upheld and infected families were isolated in their homes. Local taxes were raised to pay these expenses, and the hardships suffered by the poor led to further levies in April and August 1666.[14]

These measures were met with sporadic resistance from a variety of groups, often with financial motives. Many fled in the face of plague, which not only was widely accepted but also was sound medical advice recommended by, among many others, the Bristol-born William Kemp in his *Brief Treatise … of the Pestilence* (1665).[15] But in April 1666 the Common Council clamped down on any who sought thereby to avoid their financial obligations: the wealthy were not permitted to leave Bristol without first providing securities that they would meet any tax liability that might arise from the need to support the sick and poor.[16] Three weeks later, local magistrates ordered the confiscation of goods belonging to those who refused to pay for the relief of impoverished plague victims. This order was repeated in June, suggesting a stubborn or widespread refusal to pay (or both).[17] Whether to pursue business or from other motives, outsiders sought to slip or force their way into the city, and some refused to accept the finality even of royal orders.[18] For example, a second proclamation was obtained in December 1665 to prevent St. Paul's Fair from taking place in January, despite awareness that "the Contagion be now in a very great measure ceased through Gods mercy."[19] Perhaps it was this abatement that encouraged a crowd of traders to gather outside Lawford's Gate in early 1666 in the hope that the fair would take place after all. Lacking jurisdiction beyond the city, Bristol's authorities had to ask colleagues in Gloucestershire to order the dispersal of these would-be fairgoers.[20]

Such resistance is perhaps understandable given the intensity of economic competition not only within Bristol but also from nearby towns, distant ports, and foreign nations, especially during wartime. Already in November 1665, the city's merchants asked both the King and the Portuguese ambassador to have Bristol declared free of infection so that trade with Lisbon could resume.[21] Citizens who suffered economic loss from the cancellation of the fairs petitioned for compensation from the Common Council with mixed results.[22] And Bristol had to defend itself against the machinations of the nearby city of Bath, which spread rumors in the summer of 1666 that the plague continued at Bristol, in order that St. James's Fair be relocated to Bath.[23] These examples demonstrate the economic hardship and commercial dislocation produced by even a limited outbreak of plague.

The lasting impact of the outbreak on Bristol's built environment was negligible in comparison to its symbolic import. The "Pest-House" was still standing when the Bristolian James Millerd produced his plan of Bristol in 1673, and it featured in all subsequent versions of this plan (the last was produced *c.*1730) but had disappeared by the time of the next major survey of the city in 1742 (Figure 3.4). The building may have vanished, but its name endured and was associated with the nearby "Whitstry." This unfortunate association lingered into the 19th century, well after the demolition of the Whitstry in the wake of the city's expansion.[24] It ensured that Bristol's last outbreak of bubonic plague persisted topographically in local memory even once its other aspects had long faded from view.

Conclusion

The most long-lasting consequences of Bristol's experience of plague in 1665–66 were economic. By the spring of 1666, the immediate danger to life had passed, so the city's watch was reduced, as was the length of time goods were quarantined

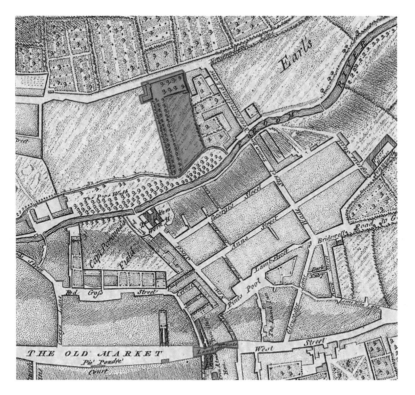

FIGURE 3.4: The Whitstry and Lawford's Gate. Detail from John Rocque, *A Survey of the City and Suburbs of Bristol* (1750). © Bristol Culture. (Courtesy of Bristol Museum and Art Gallery, Object Number Mb374.)

before being allowed to enter.[25] Fear that the epidemic might yet increase persisted into June, but by the end of the month the Corporation, in its defense against Bath, assured the Privy Council that there had been no new cases in the past ten days.[26] Yet the damage to the fragile livelihoods of the poor continued to be severe, hence the special levies of April and August, the regulations governing financial provision for those leaving the city, and the confiscations from those unwilling to pay, all of which occurred as the outbreak was petering out.

Making ends meet was not made any easier by the habit of the Corporation to be tardy in paying its bills, even of those who had built and provisioned its pesthouses. Several of these remained unpaid as late as 1667, long after wealthy merchants such as Richard Streamer, a common councilman and one of the two wardens of Bristol's Society of Merchant Venturers, had received generous compensation for the cancellation of St. James's Fair.[27] Naked profiteering from the crisis was prevented by Bristol's strong trading regulations and the evident readiness of its authorities to police the city's boundaries and confiscate property for the relief of poor plague sufferers. Yet by prioritizing the discretionary compensation of its own members, such as Streamer, above fair payment for goods and services, the Corporation clearly demonstrated the oligarchic limits of early modern urban governance when responding to a universal public health crisis.

NOTES

1. John Miller, *Cities Divided* (Oxford: Oxford University Press, 2007), 198–99; Daniel Defoe, *Tour through the Whole Island of Great Britain*, ed. Pat Rogers (London: Penguin, 1971), 362.

2. Clarendon to Ormond, August 31, 1665. Oxford, Bodleian Library, Carte MS 47, fol. 98.

3. *Records of a Church of Christ in Bristol, 1640-1687*, ed. Roger Hayden, Bristol Record Society, 27 (Bristol: Bristol Record Society, 1974), 121.

4. Great Audit Book (1664–65), p. 51, Bristol Archives (BA), F/Au/1/34.

5. Court of Quarter Sessions (CQS) Minutes (1653–1671), fol. 64r (June 13, 1665), BA, JQS/M/4.

6. The first regulations were issued in the Court of Quarter Sessions on June 13. The proclamation was approved on June 21 and published on June 23. Privy Council (PC) Register (1665–66), The National Archives of the UK (TNA), PC2/58, fol. 94v; "A Proclamation Prohibiting the keeping of St. James Fair at the City and County of Bristol," June 23, 1665, TNA, SP45/11.

7. CQS Minutes, fol. 64r (June 13, 1665).

8. Daniel Defoe, *Journal of the Plague Year*, ed. Louis Landa (Oxford: Oxford University Press, 2010), 8.

9. Orders of the Mayor and Aldermen (OMA) (1660–66), June 19, 1665, BA, M/BCC/MAY/1/2.

10. *Orders thought meete by her Majestie, and her priuie Councell* (1578; STC 9187.9); Paul Slack, *The Impact of Plague in Tudor and Stuart England* (Oxford: Oxford University Press, 1990), ch. 9; "Rules and Orders ... for prevention of ... the Plague" (1666), TNA, SP46/131/64; CQS Minutes, fol. 73r (June 25, 1666).

11. Common Council Proceedings (CCP) (1659–75), November 7 and December 5, 1665, January 15, 1666/67, BA M/BCC/CCP/1/6.

12. John Latimer, *The Annals of Bristol in the Seventeenth Century* (Bristol: William George's Sons, 1900), 195–96, 228; Slack, *Impact*, 277.

13. These estimates of comparative wealth are based on Bristol's hearth tax returns of the 1660s and 1670s. See Roger Leech et al. (eds.), *The Bristol Hearth Tax, 1662–1673*, Bristol Record Society, 70 (Bristol: Bristol Record Society, 2018), esp. 66–72 and tables 5–7.

14. Slack, *Impact*, 225; Latimer, *Annals*, 333–34; CCP, April 3 and August 7, 1666.

15. William Kemp, *Brief Treatise ... of the Pestilence* (London: D. Kemp, 1665).

16. CCP, April 3, 1666.

17. CQS Minutes, fols. 72v–73r (April 24 and June 25, 1666).

18. OMA, July 13, 1665; CQS Minutes, fol. 64v (August 1, 1665).

19. "A Proclamation, Prohibiting the keeping of the Fair at Bristol, commonly called St. Paul's Fair," December 21, 1665, TNA, SP45/11.

20. OMA, January 13, 1665/6.

21. Colston to Williamson, November 29, 1665, in Mary Ann Everett Green (ed.), *Calendar of State Papers, Domestic Series … 1665–66* (London: Longman, 1864), 77.

22. CCP, February 6, 1665/66, August 7, 1666.

23. Latimer, *Annals*, 341; PC Register (1666–67), TNA PC2/59, fol. 39v.

24. Samuel Seyer, *Memoirs, Historical and Topographical, of Bristol*, 2 vols. (Bristol: John Mathew Gutch, 1821–3), vol. 2, 305; John Evans, *A Chronological Outline of the History of Bristol* (Bristol: John Evans, 1824), 225.

25. CCP, February 6, 1665/66.

26. CCP, June 19, 1666; PC Register (1666–67), fol. 39v.

27. CCP, January 15 and February 26, 1666/67, August 7, 1666.

4

Smallpox and the Specter of Mexican Citizenship, 1826

Farren Yero

On April 9, 1825, the ship *Sally* arrived from the United States, landing in the Yucatán port of Sisal. In the months that followed, urban authorities received urgent messages from Maya villages throughout the Yucatán requesting that supplies for vaccinations—a technology introduced two decades earlier—be sent at once.[1] As the newspaper the *Aguila Mexicana* would later report, smallpox spread from the *Sally* and slowly crisscrossed the peninsula over the course of the summer. In November, outbreaks finally erupted in the regional capital of Mérida (Figure 4.1).[2] Local authorities attempted to cordon off the disease, keeping news of the epidemic to themselves for over a year. But in the spring of 1826, word finally reached Mexico City. By then, smallpox had laid claim to the cities of New Orleans, Tampico, and Tabasco, catalyzing a series of quarantines up and down the coast.

The authorities who responded to this epidemic now did so as representatives of the Federal Republic of Mexico. Beginning in 1810, groups of insurgents waged a decade-long war against Spanish loyalists and colonial rule. The victors claimed independence on September 27, 1821, ushering in a series of reforms aimed at rebuilding the new country, including the opening of global trade. Consequently, the ports of Sisal, Campeche, and Veracruz on the Gulf of Mexico witnessed a flood of littoral traffic, especially from the United States, as ships introduced merchants and foreigners whose entry the Spanish Crown had previously prohibited.[3] With these visitors came additional outbreaks of smallpox, first introduced to what would become Mexico by the conquistador Hernán Cortés in 1520, as depicted in a folio of a 16th-century text known as the Florentine Codex (Figure 4.2). The 1826 epidemic, however, was the first that Mexico faced as an independent nation, and its leaders were met with fundamental questions about the state's obligation to ensure public health, as well as who the "public" truly entailed. In short, the

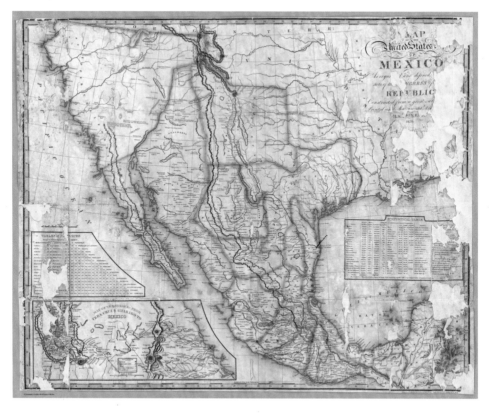

FIGURE 4.1: A map of the United States of Mexico: as organized and defined by the several acts of the Congress of that Republic. H. S. Tanner. Philadelphia, 1826. (Courtesy of the United States Library of Congress, Control Number 2010593159.)

nascent Mexican state was forced to confront the contradictions of its so-called racial democracy built on three hundred years of slavery and colonialism.

Case study: "A thing they call witchcraft": Vaccination in 1826

Mexico's internal political questions and social conflicts came to a head in Veracruz. The state was home to thousands of mixed-race men with Spanish, African, and Indigenous ancestry, whose citizenship, despite the protections written into the new federal constitution, remained uncertain.[4] The 1826 smallpox epidemic would bring the precarity of their legal status to light. According to federal law, each state in Mexico retained the power to make its own public health policy, and on June 1, congressional representatives met in Jalapa, the state capital of Veracruz, to plot

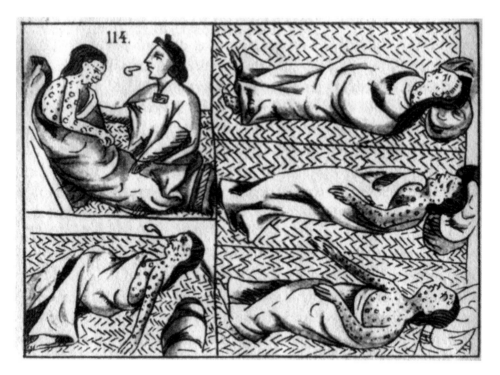

FIGURE 4.2: Depiction of smallpox, Fray Bernardino de Sahagún, of *General History of the Things of New Spain* Book XII (Florentine Codex), Mexico, 1577. Plate 114, fol. 54. Florence, Biblioteca Medicea Laurenziana. Ms. Med. Palat. 220. (Courtesy of MiBACT. Any further reproduction by any means is prohibited.)

their course of action.[5] Tucked into the Sierra Madre Oriental mountain range, Jalapa became a major site of global trade beginning in the 18th century, when merchants gathered to conduct business within its cool clime. Spanish families, attracted by the prospect of wealth, settled in the area. It was their children who would make decisions on behalf of the largely Indigenous and African-descended families whose ancestors had lived in the region for generations (Figure 4.3).[6]

The congress of Veracruz unanimously agreed to fund a smallpox vaccination campaign during the epidemic of 1826. Prickly questions came to the fore, however, when the congress revisited a law they had passed two years prior, which dictated how they should proceed.[7] Among other things, the code included an article that ordered spiritual leaders to persuade parents of the virtues of vaccination. Without stating it outright, the article effectively protected the right to medical consent for parents, a point that prompted one statesman, Pedro José Echeverría, to issue a vote in favor of its redaction. As he argued to his fellow lawmakers, "all should be obligated [to vaccinate], by force if necessary."[8]

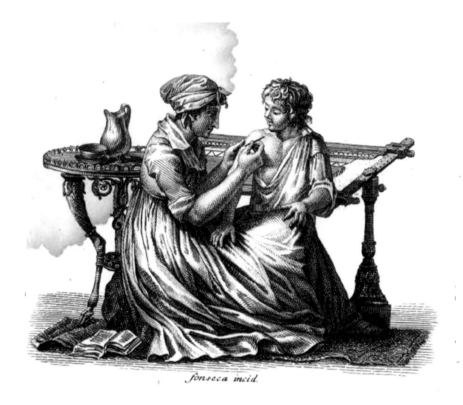

FIGURE 4.3: Illustration of a woman vaccinating her son, *Origen y descubrimiento de la vaccina /traducida del francés con arreglo a las últimas observaciones hechas hasta el mes de mayo del presente año, y enriquecido con varias notas por Pedro Hernández [Origin and Discovery of the Vaccine/translated from French, according to the last observations made until May of this year and enriched with several notes by Pedro Hernández]*. Madrid, 1801, p. 83. (Courtesy of the Universidad Complutense de Madrid.)

Few in office questioned the efficacy or utility of a state vaccination program, but issues arose regarding whether citizens had a legal right to refuse smallpox vaccination. And if citizens did refuse, could the state simultaneously protect the civil liberties that were so recently won with independence and prevent a potentially devastating epidemic? Mired in uncertainty, statesmen in Veracruz looked to both the constitution and colonial precedents for answers. Under Spanish rule, parents had retained the legal right to refuse under a policy instituted by King Carlos IV (1748–1819). The king preferred persuasion over punishment to ensure his subjects' compliance, and the vaccine was proffered as a divine gift that would bind families to the Crown through a ritualized blood pact and act of salvation. Through sermons and public spectacles, state, religious, and health authorities together advocated for the vaccine, embedding this technology into both the public health and religious landscape of the empire (Figure 4.4).[9] After independence, Mexican officials returned to these same methods (and to many of the same priests) to engender trust within communities still recovering from a decade of war.

The issue of voluntary vaccination faced ongoing public opposition, which was increasingly figured in terms of class and ethnicity by those in power. The Mexican minister of foreign affairs, Sebastian Camacho, employed class-conscious language in an order communicated on behalf of President Guadalupe Victoria (1825–29), in which he insisted that the country needed to take immediate preventative measures, "which in this case" meant "coming to an understanding with the poorer classes."[10] Newspapers covering the epidemic echoed this rhetoric, reporting that the lower classes were not only more heavily affected by the disease but also responsible for its spread. The *Aguila Mexicana* reprinted an anonymous

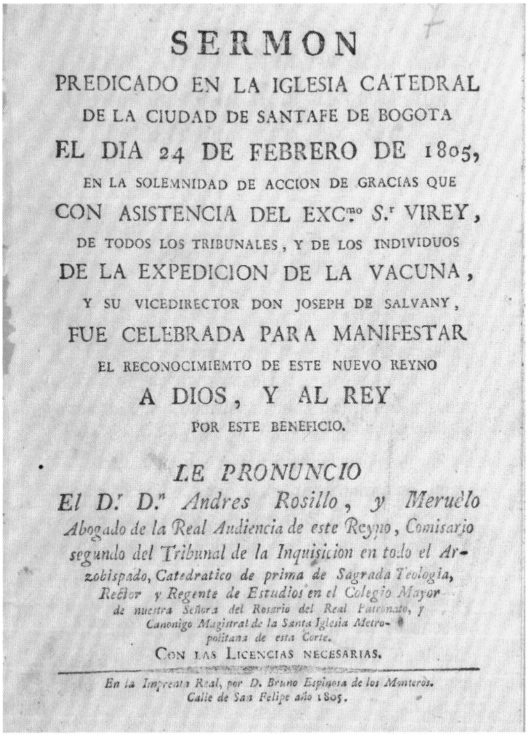

SERMON
PREDICADO EN LA IGLESIA CATEDRAL
DE LA CIUDAD DE SANTAFE DE BOGOTA
EL DIA 24 DE FEBRERO DE 1805,
EN LA SOLEMNIDAD DE ACCION DE GRACIAS QUE
CON ASISTENCIA DEL EXC.mo S.r VIREY,
DE TODOS LOS TRIBUNALES, Y DE LOS INDIVIDUOS
DE LA EXPEDICION DE LA VACUNA,
Y SU VICEDIRECTOR DON JOSEPH DE SALVANY,
FUE CELEBRADA PARA MANIFESTAR
EL RECONOCIMIEMTO DE ESTE NUEVO REYNO
A DIOS, Y AL REY
POR ESTE BENEFICIO.

LE PRONUNCIO
El D.r D.n Andres Rosillo, y Meruèlo
Abogado de la Real Audiencia de este Reyno, Comisario segundo del Tribunal de la Inquisicion en todo el Arzobispado, Catedratico de prima de Sagrada Teologia, Rector y Regente de Estudios en el Colegio Mayor de nuestra Señora del Rosario del Real Patronato, y Canonigo Magistral de la Santa Iglesia Metropolitana de esta Corte.
CON LAS LICENCIAS NECESARIAS.

En la Imprenta Real, por D. Bruno Espinosa de los Monteros.
Calle de San Felipe año 1805.

FIGURE 4.4: Andrés Rosillo y Meruelo, *Sermon...fue celebrada para manifestar el reconocimiemto de este nuevo reyno a Dios, y al rey por este beneficio [Sermon...preached in the cathedral church of the city of Santa Fé de Bogota]*. En la Imprenta Real: por D. Bruno Espinosa de los Monteros. Calle de San Felipe, 1805. (Courtesy of the John Carter Brown Library. Attribution 4.0 International CCBY 4.0.)

rebuke against the absentee governor, Antonio López de Santa Anna. The newspaper chided that after letting the Yucatán fester for months, the governor had left his post for Mexico City, with the result that a slew of Indigenous towns suffered. This censure fashioned Maya communities like Junucmá and Izamal into pitiable victims of government neglect, vulnerable to disease and their own backwardness.

Congressmen in Jalapa consumed the newspaper's paternalism and harnessed language that reflected their views of their own superiority in the debate over compulsory vaccination. In doing so, they cast Indigenous parents as superstitious innocents wary of modern medicine. Congressman Juan Francisco Bárcena suggested that "as soon as they are warned that [vaccination] will be forced, a thing that they call witchcraft, they will run to the forests, all of them worried and gullible."[11] Bárcena and his colleagues knew very well that Maya parents in the region had willingly taken up vaccination less than a decade earlier, as indicated by letters from local priests like Father Jacinto Rodríguez, who wrote to the capital to request payment for his efforts in disseminating the vaccine.[12] Municipal authorities had distributed money to parents for each vaccinated child, and vaccination rosters written in both Spanish and Yucatec Maya attested to this practice and provided the names and ages of those vaccinated; this included families in the pueblo of Izamal.[13] Yet, despite their early, documented adoption of vaccination and their new status as citizens, Indigenous people remained incapable of making reasoned medical decisions for themselves and their families in the eyes of the elite.

This systemic infantilization stemmed from long-standing debates about the nature of Indigenous people and their capacity to be converted to Christianity (and thus become governable Catholic subjects).[14] Statesman Echeverría redeployed colonizing logic under the rubric of the constitution at the time of the epidemic in order to make an argument about the state's responsibility to manage public health. He cited constitutional article 33 to insist that federal law obligated elected officials to "procure the prosperity of the state," which for him meant "that the first, most indispensable object, is public health."[15] Any public opposition, real or imagined, was for him a national threat best met with violence. He argued,

> We are in the position of fighting the commoners and their opposition to vaccination, but the laws of a well-regulated police and public health know no exception. They cannot say that with this forced measure, freedom is restricted. Nothing of the sort. In that which interests the whole of society, there is no course so detrimental to its wellbeing. And because of this, if one resists, one should be obligated, even with the use of militarized force, because it is that important to the health of the public.[16]

In the end, the delegation voted against Echeverría's proposed measure of militarized force for the state's vaccination program, refusing to impose the strict orders he hoped to mandate. The congress ultimately left the matter in the hands of municipal authorities and local clergymen, but the decision to do so reflected the unease and instability of the new nation. Mexico's foundation on a theory of universal rights served as a thin disguise for the same racism that had sustained colonial rule. Although revisions to the 1824 constitution theoretically allowed the residents of Veracruz to refuse vaccination, law and policy left the use of state violence open for debate. Congress explicitly engaged both the ambiguity and the debate with Indigenous families in mind.

Congressman Carvajal underscored how irrational he assumed Indigenous fathers to be by insisting that priests were essential mediators in "in populations where they are the only ones who can be called reasonable, and who have immediate contact with their parishes" and "who know how to reconcile, with their diligence and paternal care."[17] Congressman Moreno shared this view and believed that the congress need not formally mandate compulsory vaccination for them to be carried out. He reflected that enforcement might actually undermine their goal, reflecting that "whatever is not derived from the charitable and efficacious insinuations of the parish priests will be futile, as force does not compel the conviction of people who resist something so obviously beneficial."[18] Confident in the power of the vaccine, Moreno drew on established practices of quarantine and seemingly his own involvement in prior vaccination campaigns to deliver his argument just as the session came to a close:

> The laws of the *policía* [health and sanitation officers] are very old and mandate that one suffering from leprosy should be separated from the population: they do not say to do it by force, but that is how it is done. [...] It is therefore unnecessary to tell the government to use force; they will do so, because it is in their power.[19]

Officials rarely allowed patients to resist quarantine when the threat of contagion was imminent. Vaccination policies and Mexican constitutional law theoretically changed this arrangement, as officials could no longer rely on the immediacy of an epidemic as a tool to curtail individual rights. Yet Moreno's comments revealed his assumption that Indigenous parents were incapable of the reasoned decision-making that legislators anticipated from Mexican citizens; because of this, the government had a duty to intervene in whichever way it saw fit. When the state deemed parents to be incompetent, vaccine refusal was no longer an option.[20]

Conclusion

Mexican states continued to adopt policies that precipitated a startling use of public health measures and epidemic threats to selectively surveil and contain bodies that authorities deemed dangerous to the body politic.[21] These interventions disproportionately affected Indigenous and mixed-race individuals, despite Mexico's constitutional dissolution of these ethnic categories. Citizenship glossed over racialized distinctions, but the colonial logic and assumptions that categorized the rights and decision-making abilities of people based on culture, religious belief, and bodily difference did not disappear in this new era of liberty. An ideology of paternalism remained. Congressmen, like Spanish colonizers before them, claimed that it was their duty to override the choices and preferences of Indigenous people to "save" them from themselves.

Vaccination and its enforcement, as historian Nadja Durbach argues, was always a political act, because "who wielded the needle or the lancet and whose body was marked governed how vaccination was experienced and the meaning attached to it."[22] The Mexican vaccination program may have hastened the end of the 1826 smallpox epidemic, but deployment policies dangerously encoded racist assumptions about Indigenous families and their culture even as politicians passed laws to uphold the virtues of individual liberty, revealing the asymmetry of Mexican citizenship, along with the potential inequity of voluntary vaccination. This health policy, despite its ostensible protection of individual rights, skewed toward those in power, who mobilized vaccination to maintain divisions that had ordered colonial society. The deployment of vaccination during an epidemic, as this case study suggests, demands the anticipation of the political afterlife of vaccine policy once the crisis has passed.

NOTES

1. José Tiburcio López, Correspondencia del Gobierno dirigida al R. A. y a la Junta General de Sanidad (La Biblioteca Virtual de Yucatán, CAIHY, MS. 357, 1825). On the introduction of the vaccine, see Francisco Fernández del Castillo, *Los viajes de Don Francisco Xavier de Balmis; notas para la historia de la expedición vacunal de España a America y Filipinas (1803-1806)* (México: Galas de México, 1960); Michael M. Smith, "The 'Real Expedición Marítima de La Vacuna' in New Spain and Guatemala," *Transactions of the American Philosophical Society* 64, no. 1 (1974): 1–74; José G. Rigau-Pérez, "The Introduction of Smallpox Vaccine in 1803 and the Adoption of Immunization as a Government Function in Puerto Rico," *The Hispanic American Historical Review* 69, no. 3 (1989): 393–423; Martha Few, "Circulating Smallpox Knowledge: Guatemalan Doctors, Maya Indians and Designing Spain's Smallpox Vaccination Expedition, 1780-1803," *British Journal for the History of Science*, 43, no. 159 (December 2010): 519–37; Farren Yero, "Laboratories of Consent: Vaccine Science in the Spanish Atlantic World, 1779-1840" (Ph.D. diss., Duke University, 2020).

2. *Aguila Mexicana*, no. 31, May 31, 1826. Report by José María Perez, president of the Veracruz Junta de Sanidad.

3.   Archivo Nacional de Cuba (ANC), Gobierno Superior Civil, Leg. 1528, No. 70620. Geronimo Ferrer y Valle, Spanish Commercial Agent in the Yucatan, to the Captain General de la Isla de Cuba. Campeche. February 17, 1842. Notice of smallpox (*viruela negra*) in Tabasco and sanitary measures taken in Campeche.

4.   *Constitución federal de los Estados Unidos Mexicanos sancionada por el Congreso General Constituyente el 4 de Octubre de 1824* (Guadalajara: Poderes de Jalisco, 1973). Women would remain barred from full citizenship and the rights it theoretically granted until well after the Mexican Revolution (1910–20).

5.   Luz María Hernández-Sáenz, *Carving a Niche: The Medical Profession in Mexico, 1800–1870* (Montreal: McGill-Queen's University Press, 2018), 38–39.

6.   This region was notably home to a significant population of afro-descendants. Patrick J. Carroll, *Blacks in Colonial Veracruz: Race, Ethnicity, and Regional Development* (Austin: University of Texas Press, 2001).

7.   This code was passed in 1824 and printed in *Colección de Decretos y Ordenes* (Jalapa: Imprenta del Gobierno, 1826).

8.   *El Oriente de Jalapa*, no. 680, August 1, 1826, fol. 2808.

9.   See Paul F. Ramírez, *Enlightened Immunity: Mexico's Experiments with Disease Prevention in the Age of Reason* (Stanford: Stanford University Press, 2018).

10.   *Gaceta del Gobierno Supremo de la Federación Mexicana*, vol. 1, no. 19, June 11, 1826, s/f. The order concerned the state's responsibility to extend vaccine propagation across the republic. Camacho originally delivered this statement to the chamber of congress in Mexico City on June 14.

11.   *El Oriente de Jalapa*, no. 680, August 1, 1826, f. 2808–9.

12.   Archivo General de la Nación (AGN), Indiferente Virreinal, Caja 1997, Exp. 2, f. 1–41. Jacinto Rodríguez, Iglesia de Tekanto, 1817. Earlier records indicate that these campaigns were ongoing. See: AGN, Indiferente Virreinal, Caja 6249, Exp. 28, f. 1–27. Manuel Palomeque, by order of the señor intendant, Don Benito Pérez, and the physician, Don Martín de Larralde. Mérida. 1811; AGN, Indiferente Virrenial, Epidemias, Caja 4848, Exp. 25, f. 1–16. Miguel de Castro Araez to Virrey Apodaca. March, 17, 1817. Delayed reports signed by Ciprian Blanco from Campeche on July 1, 1815, referring to those vaccinated in the year prior during the epidemic.

13.   AGN, Indiferente Virreinal, Epidemias, Caja 1997, Exp. 3, f. 1–52. Reports from José Sebastián María Gonzáles, commissioned vaccinator. 1818. These records also include children vaccinated in Tixkobo, Citilcum, Kimbilá, Ixil, Bokobá, Tepakán, Teya, and Tikul, among others.

14.   Pope Paul III theoretically resolved this issue in 1537 when he issued a bull declaring that "the Indians are truly men and that they are not only capable of understanding the Catholic Faith but, according to our information, they desire exceedingly to receive it." Paul III, "Sublimus Dei." Quoted in Rebecca Earle, *The Body of the Conquistador: Food, Race, and*

the Colonial Experience in Spanish America, 1492–1700 (Cambridge: Cambridge University Press, 2012), 153.

15. *El Oriente de Jalapa*, no. 681, August 2, 1826, f. 2811. Camacho made similar statements in Mexico City, arguing, "To care for the public's health and foster population growth, are not only the first responsibilities of a man of the public, but the noblest attributes of his authority, in whose performance can most honorably employ the patrimony of the people." *Gaceta del Gobierno Supremo de la Federación Mexicana*, vol. 1, no. 19, June 11, 1826, s/f.

16. *El Oriente de Jalapa*, no. 680, August 1, 1826, f. 2808.

17. Ibid.

18. *El Oriente de Jalapa*, no. 681, August 2, 1826, f. 2811.

19. Ibid., 2811–12.

20. This decision was informed by elite assumptions about competence and reason. See Shannon Speed, *Rights in Rebellion: Indigenous Struggle and Human Rights in Chiapas* (Stanford, CA: Stanford University Press, 2008); Autumn Quezada-Grant, "Indians, Ladinos, and the Resurrection of the Protector de Indios, San Cristobal de Las Casas, Chiapas, 1870–85," *Ethnohistory* 60, no. 2 (2013): 295–318.

21. See Katherine Bliss, *Compromised Position: Prostitution, Public Health, and Gender Politics in Revolutionary Mexico City* (University Park: Pennsylvania State University Press, 2001); Nancy Stepan, *The Hour of Eugenics: Race, Gender, and Nation in Latin America* (Ithaca, NY: Cornell University Press, 1991).

22. Nadja Durbach, *Bodily Matters: The Anti-Vaccination Movement in England, 1853–1907* (Durham, NC: Duke University Press, 2005), 5.

5

Complacency, Confusion, and the Mismanagement of Cholera in York, England, 1832

Ann-Marie Akehurst

As an archipelago of over six thousand islands located off the northwestern coast of continental Europe, the British Isles were historically conferred some geographical protection from epidemic disease. When the bubonic plague (*Yersinia pestis*) killed 100,000 people in Marseille, France, in 1720, British authorities passed a Quarantine Act, and publishers proliferated self-help literature. After the alarm was raised, the plague did not manage to cross to the Isles from Europe and the country escaped. Despite originating in what was regarded as British overseas territory, the first Asiatic cholera (*Vibrio cholerae*) pandemic (1817–24) did not reach Europe. Britain had not suffered pandemic disease since the 17th-century Great Plague by the time the much more widespread second Asiatic cholera pandemic reached British shores in the 1830s.

Located in northeastern England midway between London and Edinburgh, the ancient, provincial city of York was a market town of 26,000 people that served the professional urban elite and visiting nobility. York's slow response to the 1832 cholera epidemic was the result of complacency, confusion regarding authority and resources, and conspiracy theories regarding those authorities. A kind of cultural amnesia combined with outdated financial and administrative systems stress-tested Britain's urban governance with a challenge that originated in the dominion of the British East India Company.

In the 1830s, England succumbed to the second Asiatic cholera pandemic originating in "British India." In September 1831, the disease entered northern England at Sunderland and dispersed slowly (Figure 5.1). By June 1832, cholera had spread to York. Cholera differed from plague, as it was transmitted through feces-contaminated foods and river water. The primary symptoms of cholera—profuse vomiting and diarrhea—typically killed 50 percent of untreated

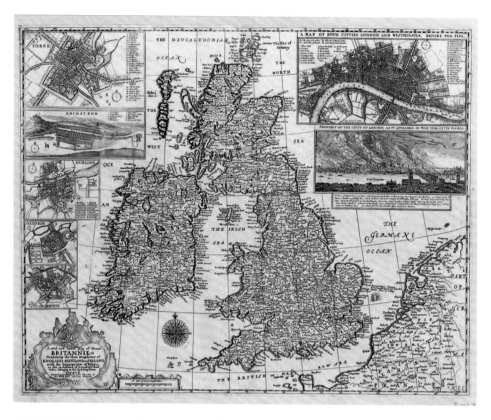

FIGURE 5.1: "A new and exact map of Great Britannie &c.," highlighting York, Wenceslaus Hollar, 1667. (Courtesy of The Trustees of the British Museum Q, 8.227, public domain.)

individuals. York's epidemic management was documented by a local doctor from the York Dispensary.[1] York's reputation as a medical center was built on the Dispensary, the County Hospital, two asylums, and many physicians and surgeons, yet the city lacked clear medical leadership. This rendered York's medical center ineffective at stemming the cholera outbreak, and 185 people died.

In preparation for the arrival of the disease, lectures were delivered by York's Medical Society, but cholera's cause and progress were not yet well understood, complicating strategic planning.[2] British authorities followed the ancient miasma theory that argued that disease was transmitted by airborne particles from foul smelling, decomposing matter. It is clear from the contemporary account of Dr. J. P. Needham, written in 1833, that clinicians recognized a relationship between poverty and overcrowding, and that they were aware that certain areas were healthier than others and that cholera was contagious, but these experts misconstrued the vectors of transmission.[3] Needham's report included an account by the eminent French statistician Alexandre Moreau de Jonnès (1778–1870) who, based on his study of

Paris, argued for the contagion theory. Needham, reviewing his York experience, concurred that cholera's spread was "fairly attributed to contagion."[4] The conflict between theories concerning cholera's etiology and transmission was simply one confusing element of several, but this helps to inform our understanding of why York's response was ineffective despite its position as a known center of medicine.

Case study: Cholera in York, 1832

Complacency characterized the York authorities' dilatory responses in addressing the impending cholera situation. Though the first case appeared in September 1831, only after cholera reached London in February 1832 was the general alarm sounded. This moment is captured in the cartoon "John Bull Catching the Cholera," published in 1831 (Figure 5.2). The cadaverous, blue personification of cholera—wearing a turban denoting Indian dress surmounted by a death's-head skull—characterizes the disease confronted by an aggressive John Bull—the robust personification of national character—who throttles cholera with a club of "hearts of oak." The illustration represents the tensions surrounding national identity and Britain's burgeoning trading empire. These tensions were crystallized centuries before by William Shakespeare, who wrote that the "sceptered isle" was a "fortress built by Nature for herself/Against infection and the hand of war."[5] The image reflects the misplaced belief that the "wooden walls of Old England"—a patriotic trope regarding the imperial fleet—were being assailed by colonial subjects as England was being protected by Boards of Health.[6] This belligerent othering of the disease, based on the assumption that the "sceptered isle" was protected by the English sea, navy, and stout national character, reflects the complacency of late 1831 when authorities' attentions were distracted with major political affairs.

The print also reflects domestic politics. Cholera lunges for a rolled-up paper titled "Reform Bill," but John Bull defensively stands astride the document. The passage of the Reform Bill into law on June 7, 1832, as the Representation of the People Act was a significant moment in British constitutional history that extended the political franchise and enlarged units of authority from the previously tiny 16th-century parishes.[7] Britain's outdated legal, administrative, and financial apparatus was inappropriate: power devolved from the Privy Council, a formal body of senior politicians acting as advisers to the Sovereign. Locally, York's economy was administered by a cash-strapped Corporation of Anglican freemen who administered corporate property, public spaces, and charities; a subcommittee neglected the rivers it was tasked with controlling and overlooked the needs of a growing population. On the micro scale, the parish was the ancient unit of secular and ecclesiastical administration, managed by parish vestries—comprising

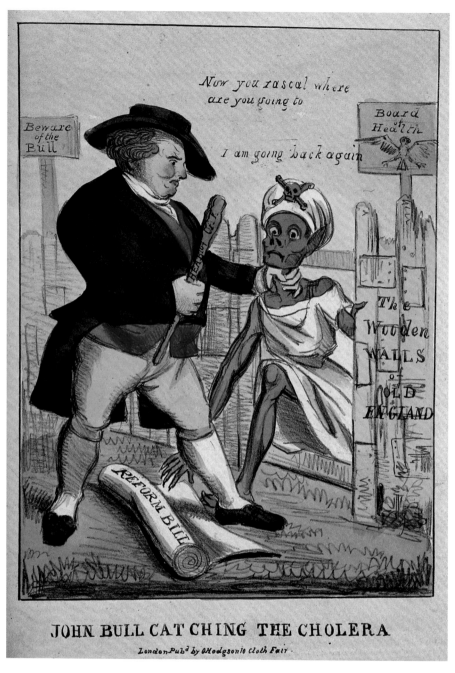

FIGURE 5.2: "John Bull Catching the Cholera," London: Orlando Hodgson, 1831, lithograph, with watercolor. (Courtesy of the Wellcome Collection, Wellcome Library no. 12236i, public domain.)

clergymen, medical men, churchwardens, Overseers of the Poor, and principal inhabitants—that were directed by district boards for each ward—or district—of the city. York consequently took a short-term, literally parochial view of public health. This complex hierarchy, combined with inflexible legal and financial frameworks, failed to accommodate overlapping national and local knowledge and priorities. It was the antithesis of the responsive system necessary for epidemic management. Misplaced belief in Britain's invulnerability, government resistance to empowering local authorities, and legal and epidemiological confusion wasted vital preparation time, as illustrated by the timeline of the epidemic.

In October 1831, the York Corporation was ordered by the Privy Council to establish a local Board of Health comprising magistrates, clergy, and two or three doctors. Following miasma theory, these doctors were directed to establish an isolated house for victims and to burn old paper, rugs, and clothes.[8] Drains and sinks were to be cleaned, walls and roofs limewashed. York's poorer districts retained much medieval housing and infrastructure. Its rivers were silted up with sewage and polluted with factory effluent, but in November 1831, rather than address drainage improvement, parochial committees complacently visited each house in order to compile a status report that was sent to London, 200 miles away (Figure 5.3). Though witnessing much poverty, York was judged well placed regarding the city's health and cleanliness.[9]

Improvement Commissioners independently levied rates for lighting and detritus removal. Their powers were limited, yet the Privy Council subsequently advised the Board of Health not to act on its own authority since it could only direct the details of those actions that Parliament had already decreed.[10] The Board was thus unable even to support its own expenses and was entirely dependent on Improvement Commissioners' and subscribers' generosity, though those contributions were restricted to corporate or parochial uses. Civic cleanliness was paramount, yet despite York's inefficient drainage and lack of common sewers, funds raised to combat cholera could not legally be used to improve sewage infrastructure. Authorities could only borrow £700 towards the projected £4,000 cost, so the money was spent clothing impoverished people instead. The drains laid after the epidemic were deemed cheap and insufficient.

In February 1832, the Cholera Morbus Prevention Act was passed, but the Privy Council withheld effective local power until the Board of Health was reconstituted under the provisions of the Act in April. This finally invested the Board with the power to compel vestries to pay for improvements when cholera was locally confirmed.[11] The dilatory nature of the centralized administration undermined trust in its authority because their actions were viewed as too little too late. Finally, the local Board of Health could compel reluctant vestries to levy a parochial rate for a temporary cholera hospital, though that hospital became quickly overwhelmed.[12]

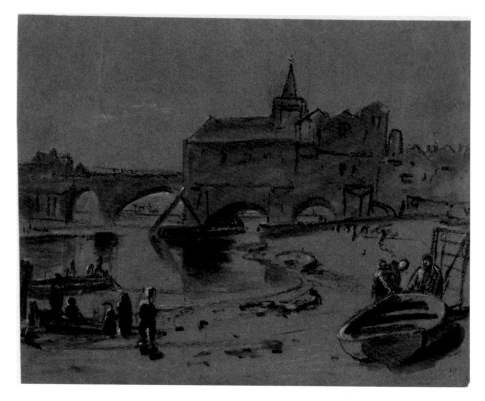

FIGURE 5.3: *The Ouse Bridge, York*, John Varley, first half of the 1800s, chalk, charcoal and gouache on paper. (Courtesy of Tate T09396, public domain.)

Financial and administrative confusion was compounded by local disagreements. Despite the eventual empowerment of elites, their partisanship stymied decision-making.[13] Though the Board of Health was equally divided between two political parties—the Whigs and the Tories—the Lord Mayor was accused of party favoritism. There was division between the Board of Health and the Whig-dominated Corporation. Burials became a lightning rod for controversy and authorities disagreed on the selection of a cemetery ground for cholera victims. People were entitled to be buried in the churchyards of their local parish church, causing problems: following such a burial, churches had to be closed for fumigation, and interment in overfull, ancient churchyards disturbed existing burials. York's influential Quaker community objected to one proposed new site because it fronted their school.[14] The Corporation objected to using the ramparts of the city walls. The dedication of an extramural plot by the Corporation generated disagreements concerning its capacity to alienate lands indefinitely, meaning burials were only guaranteed to lie undisturbed for twenty years.[15] In response, the railway magnate George Hudson, Quaker philanthropist and mental health reformer Samuel Tuke, and chocolatier businessman Joseph Rowntree argued for the site's enduring sanctity. The Corporation offered the plot to Archbishop of York Edward Venables-Vernon-Harcourt, whose intention to consecrate the ground for 60 years was overturned in London. Rowntree's failed proposal to raise a further rate for whitewashing and medicines resulted in his resignation from the Corporation.

Disagreements were not restricted to elites. Though the Reform Act removed some exploitations and extended the franchise to new industrial cities, the build-up polarized England along class lines. This polarization resulted in a mistrust by lower socio-economic classes of authorities from both the traditional aristocratic governing classes and the new free-enterprise laissez-faire manufacturers. This was clearly demonstrated in York, where the epidemic took place in the context of major class unrest and suspicion.[16]

In May 1832, a month before York's first cholera death, Reform rioting broke out. An effigy of the archbishop was burned and the house of a well-known Tory was attacked, which resulted in arrests by the military for riotous assembly.[17] The anxious atmosphere persisted during the epidemic when fear of group assembly continued and conspiracy theories focused on the elite developed. During the epidemic, wealthy citizens retreated to rural safety.[18] Local newspapers exaggerated the scale of the exodus and criticized the abnegation of civic responsibility and the engendering of alarm. Since York's primary trade was servicing the elites, social and economic inequalities were emphasized by concomitant reductions in business, particularly among those selling fresh produce. Political tensions peaked when the Reform Act was passed in June 1832.

The tension concatenated with the preexisting suspicion of doctors by the lower classes in relation to cadavers. New medical schools required corpses to anatomize, but there were strict limitations on the provision of executed felons. It was a live topic: high-profile cases captured the public's attention as with the execution in 1829 of serial-killer William Burke (1792–1829), who, together with William Hare (1792/1804–after c.1858), murdered people to supply cadavers to anatomists.[19] This climate of national hysteria was amplified in August by the passing of the Anatomy Act of 1832, which permitted the use of unclaimed bodies from hospitals and workhouses for dissection. Anti-doctor riots occurred in cities including nearby Leeds, where a mob attacked the cholera hospital. In York, doctors were suspected of pecuniary interest in promoting the epidemic, and the authorities of working with them, by targeting poor people and harvesting corpses for dissection.[20]

Such sentiments were not limited to York and were reflected in prints such as Henry Heath's "A Sketch from the Central Board of Health or the Real Ass-i-antic Cholera!!," in which corpulent doctors brandish a blue cholera scarecrow at a

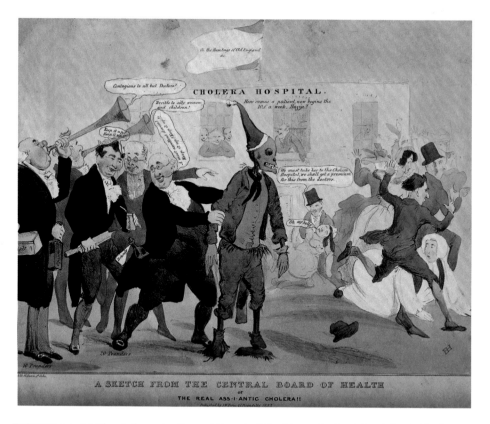

FIGURE 5.4: "A Sketch from the Central Board of Health, or the Real Ass-i-Antic Cholera!!," Henry Heath (London: S.W. Fores, 1832), lithograph. (Courtesy of the Wellcome Collection, Wellcome Library no. 11405i, public domain.)

bewigged cleric and well-dressed valetudinarians (Figure 5.4). Cynically motivated physicians claim cholera is "[c]ontagious to all but doctors!" and "terrible to silly women and children!" A man regards a collapsed woman as a potential bonus, rejoicing that "we must take her to the cholera hospital, we shall get a premium for this from the doctors." A flag above the hospital parodies the popular song "The Roast Beef of Old England" while inside a doctor gloats: "Here comes a patient, now begins the 10 pounds a week. Huzza!"

Conclusion

Despite a reputation to the contrary, doctors had actively addressed the epidemic in York. The disappearance of plague from England over a century before together with emerging theories to manage endemic diseases resulted in clinical confusion.

Britain's legal and financial apparatus was chronically outdated. Policy-makers complacently lacked political will and urgency: nationally they were preoccupied with constitutional reform, but locally they lost direction and succumbed to infighting because they were protected from the immediate effects of contagion associated with poor people and insanitary housing. Indeed, it was only a generation later in 1858 during the third cholera pandemic that public health management became imperative, when the politicians in Parliament were assailed by London's "Great Stink." By then, the Municipal Corporation Act of 1835 enabled larger-scale, longer-term thinking that was motivated by utilitarian Edwin Chadwick's demonstration of the link between economic productivity and epidemic disease and his arguments for improvements in housing and urban layouts.

Though suspicion of the medical profession remained endemic, radical doctors demonstrated concern for public health by tracking cholera transmission with the support of mapping and statistics. Public health management requires resilient, long-term, cathedral thinking that risks energy, time, and money to protect future generations. The cholera epidemic in 19th-century York ran its course in a complex, sociopolitical context that shaped and distorted urban health control. During York's time of pestilence, public confidence in the authorities who brokered information and directed strategies and resources for infection management and control was essential. During such emergencies, clear command and control management instills trust and makes the conditions for developing effective strategies for navigating the chaos of epidemic urbanism.

NOTES

1. Michael Durey, *The First Spasmodic Cholera Epidemic in York, 1832* (York: St Anthony's Press, 1974), 2. Durey laid out the facts, figures, and controversies as recorded in local archives. J. P. Needham, *Facts and Observations Relative to the Disease Commonly Called Cholera as It Has Recently Prevailed in the City of York* (London: Longman, Rees, Orme, Brown, Green, 1833).

2. Durey, *Spasmodic Cholera*, 5–6.

3. Needham, *Facts and Observations*, Appendix.

4. Ibid.

5. William Shakespeare, *King Richard II*, Act II, Scene i, 43–44.

6. Henry Green, "The Wooden Walls of England," *Morning Chronicle and London Advertiser*, June 25, 1773; Green, "The Wooden Walls of Old England" (Manchester: William and John Shelmerdine, 1830).

7. "About Parliament: The Reform Act 1832," UK Parliament website, https://www.parliament.uk/about/living-heritage/evolutionofparliament/houseofcommons/reformacts/overview/reformact1832/ (accessed October 11, 2020).

8. Durey, *Spasmodic Cholera*, 3–4.

9. Ibid., 5.

10. Ibid.

11. "About Parliament: Cholera in Sunderland," UK Parliament website, https://www.parliament.uk/about/living-heritage/transformingsociety/towncountry/towns/tyne-and-wear-case-study/introduction/Cholera-in-sunderland/ (accessed October 11, 2020).

12. Durey, *Spasmodic Cholera*, 6, 14.

13. Ibid., 21.

14. Ibid., 6.

15. Ibid., 21.

16. Edward Royle, *Modern Britain: A Social History 1750–1997* (London: Arnold, 1997), 124–26.

17. Ibid., 23.

18. Ibid., 25.

19. J. Gilliland, "Burke, William (1792–1829), murderer," *Oxford Dictionary of National Biography*, https://www.oxforddnb.com/view/10.1093/ref:odnb/9780198614128.001.0001/odnb-9780198614128-e-4031 (accessed November 11, 2020).

20. Durey, *Spasmodic Cholera*, 23–24.

6

Cholera, the Roman Aqueduct, and Urban Renewal in Naples, Italy, 1860–1914

Sofia Greaves

The southern Italian coastal city of Naples suffered from frequent and devastating cholera epidemics during the 19th century. Primarily cholera entered through the busy port and spread among the poor residents living in high-density housing built upon waterlogged soil. As studied in depth by historian Frank Snowden, the public lacked a crucial education in proper hygiene, therefore cholera spread easily, particularly because Neapolitans drew water from wells and fountains infected by sewage.[1] They reused their water for cooking and washing several times.[2] In addition, water was sold by thousands of *acquaioli* (water vendors), who unwittingly helped to spread disease across the city. The worst epidemic occurred in 1884 and triggered the state's first sanitation campaign: the *Risanamento*.

Neapolitan reformers attempted to combat cholera outbreaks through redevelopments that were freshly essential for successful urban governance in the 19th century.[3] Reform pursued two primary changes: urban layout infrastructures and clean water systems, beginning with new drinking water, provided by an aqueduct, which was modeled on the city's ancient Roman example.[4] Both changes related to cholera transmission, which was understood according to a mixture of theories; in 1854, British physician John Snow correctly argued that water containing human feces was the essential disease vector. The years 1860–1914 were characterized by a slow switch to "germ theory" in Italy.[5]

The Neapolitan government remained ill-prepared to combat the cholera epidemics, because the city lacked adequate infrastructure, despite being the largest urban center in Italy. While the water supply continued to dwindle, sanitary reform remained subordinate to solving the administrative pressures of Italian unification, which began in 1861. Italy was saddled with heavy Risorgimento debts and in Naples there was general disorder.[6] In addition, the failure of the Liberal government to provide effectively coordinated social welfare allowed the Camorra, a criminal organization, to declare itself the protector of the poor.[7] The Camorra's power was consolidated by the political factions that engaged its services to compete, rather than to address, public health concerns.[8]

Case study: The Neapolitan aqueduct

Neapolitan reformers framed their proposals to obtain clean drinking water and to regenerate the city with a story about the Greco-Roman past. Politicians and sanitarians argued that a new aqueduct would cure Naples of cholera and return it to the glory of the Roman period, when "Neapolis" had been clean and prosperous.[9] In Neapolis the aqueduct and baths, fed by the waters from the Serino springs, indicated a sophisticated and healthy water culture which had since been "lost." This Roman past (rather than the Greek) was prestigious and relevant for a city looking to carve itself a place within the emerging nation because it tied Naples to contemporary Rome, the new capital.[10] Moreover, over the past century, cities modernizing across Europe had taken Imperial Rome as a model—for them Rome stood at the pinnacle of a false hierarchy between civilizations, a status confirmed by its construction techniques, particularly straight streets and water infrastructures. Reform occurred because cities competed to be Rome—as they imagined it. Paris built aqueducts to indicate its good governance and industrial prowess, and the French capital had long acted as a model for Naples.[11] Thus, in this context, it was advantageous and necessary for Naples to exhibit "Roman" urban characteristics, which could symbolize its civility and modernity, at home and abroad.

Naples did not have clean water, which contributed to the impression that the city was badly governed and its inhabitants were uncivilized. The city had long been placed within an imaginary geography of "the south," where the site and local climate were assumed to have made Neapolitans "barbarians" by nature.[12] This stereotype was reinforced by both water practices and disease cartography, which stigmatized the city as a kind of "bacterial growth upon Italian soil" (Figure 6.1). The Neapolitan government sought solve cholera and so to contest the idea that Naples was backwards and barbarian, by emphasizing its Roman past, a marker of civility.

The idea of Roman Naples offered reformers with powerful means to advance their reforms. This is seen in the proposals made by Marino Turchi (1808–1890), a nationalist anti-Bourbon Liberal who founded the Neapolitan Institute of Hygiene in 1860. Turchi pioneered renewal, and his proposals argued that Neapolis was a suitable model because it met both aesthetic and hygienic standards. To prove his point, he imagined the actions of Emperor Nero (d. 68 CE), arguing that "Nero would not have specially selected Naples as location for his artistic glory" if it had

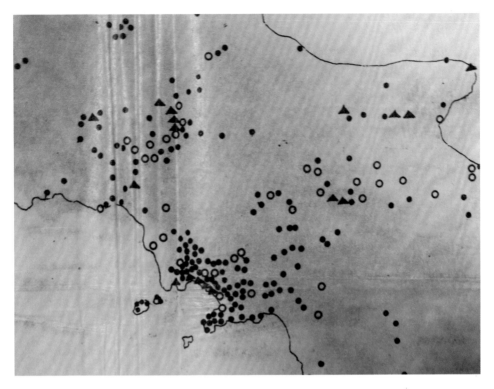

FIGURE 6.1: Detail of cholera map, "Carta delle Epidemie di Colera, 1884–1887," in Luigi Pagliani, *Trattato di Igiene e di Sanità Pubblica colle Applicazioni alla Ingegneria e alla Vigilanza Sanitaria [Treatise of Hygiene and Public Health applied to Engineering and Sanitary Vigilance]. Vol. II. Degli Ambienti Liberi e Confinati in rapporto colla Igiene e colla Sanità pubblica [Internal and External Environments in Relation to Hygiene and Public Health]*, Milan: Francesco Vallardi, 1912.

been an unhealthy city at that time. He posited that Nero, infamously culpable for the devastating fire of Rome in 64 CE, would naturally have burned Naples to the ground had he seen the disastrous 19th-century urban layout. According to Turchi, Naples now resembled ancient Rome, with "the great deformity of old and very tall buildings [...] the roads narrow and willowy [...] and such insalubrious and dirty conditions."[13]

Thus, the fire of Rome was recast as an urban planning initiative that Nero executed with "a certain taste for the arts, a sense of aesthetics" and an underlying "need to render the city cleaner and healthier."[14] The ancient Roman historian Suetonius described the fire as an act of tyranny that annihilated the cultural identity of Rome to make place for the Domus Aurea (Golden Palace), his Imperial vanity project on the Oppian Hill. The Roman people took refuge and watched

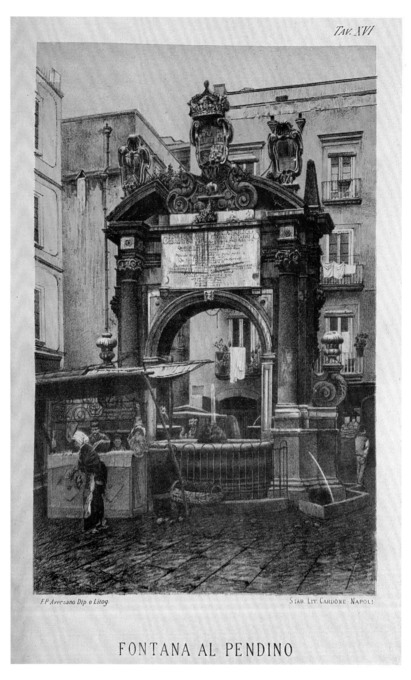

F.P. Aversano Dip. e Litog.   Stab. Lit. Cardone - Napoli

FONTANA AL PENDINO

FIGURE 6.2: Fontana al Pendino (demolished). Raffaele D'Ambra, *Napoli Antica Illustrata con 118 Tavole in Cromo-Litografia [Historic Naples Illustrated with 118 Tables in Color]*, Naples: Reale Stabilimento Litografico Cardone, 1885. Tav. XVI.

as the memories kept in "the houses of leaders of old" burned.[15] In stark contrast, Turchi used the fire of Rome to provide a precedent for the demolitions he believed would be a sanitary act.[16] In the years that followed, the Neapolitan Risanamento, the state-financed sanitation campaign, led to the demolition and reconstruction of the unsanitary areas of the city, including many of its fountains (Figure 6.2).[17] The *Illustrazione Italiana*, a northern-based, nationalist publication, cried, "*delenda Carthago* [Carthage must be destroyed]! Naples will never be civilized, tamed or great with these filthy areas in which [...] the germs of crime, social plague and ignorance have their hideouts."[18] This process intended to move Naples closer toward a Roman urban image that was synonymous with modernity.

The Neapolitan aqueduct was inaugurated in 1885, "restoring" the Serino water source to the city.[19] The structure was monumental, glorious, and effective: following a disastrous cholera epidemic in 1884, disease mortality fell with the city's access to clean water. Songs celebrated the fact that, with this truly Roman water, cholera had been conquered (Figure 6.3). However, the Romanness of this system was a myth used to emphasize Naples' new invincible and cholera-free status. Problems emerged, because leaky pipes caused houses to collapse and sink. Once, the Serino failed to supply the city for several days, and Neapolitans, angered by having to pay high prices for this new water, began to break into the

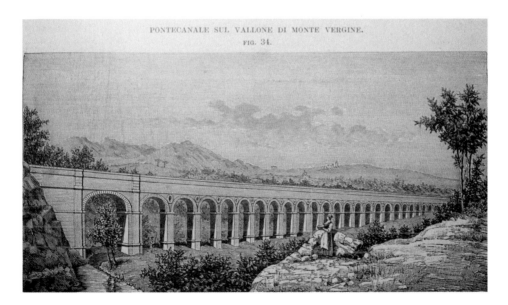

FIGURE 6.3: The Neapolitan aqueduct, illustrated in the monograph that commemorated its construction. *La Società Veneta per Imprese e Costruzioni Pubbliche. L'Acquedotto di Napoli* [*La Società Veneta, Building and Public Construction. The Aqueduct in Naples*], Bassano, 1883. (Courtesy of the British School at Rome, Special Collections.)

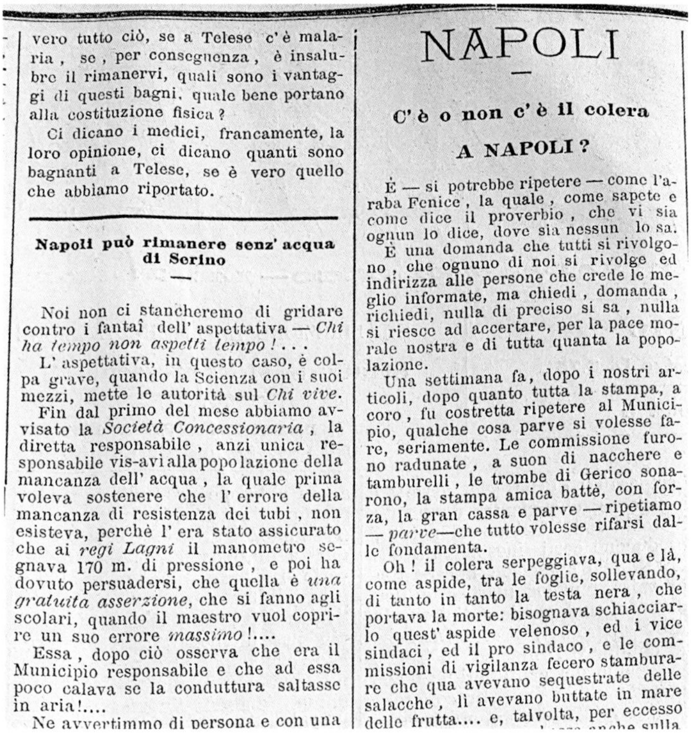

vero tutto ciò, se a Telese c'è malaria, se, per conseguenza, è insalu-
bre il rimanervi, quali sono i vantag-
gi di questi bagni, quale bene portano
alla costituzione fisica?

Ci dicano i medici, francamente, la
loro opinione, ci dicano quanti sono
bagnanti a Telese, se è vero quello
che abbiamo riportato.

**Napoli può rimanere senz' acqua
di Serino**
—

Noi non ci stancheremo di gridare
contro i fantaî dell' aspettativa — *Chi
ha tempo non aspetti tempo!*...

L' aspettativa, in questo caso, è col-
pa grave, quando la Scienza con i suoi
mezzi, mette le autorità sul *Chi vive*.

Fin dal primo del mese abbiamo av-
visato la *Società Concessionaria*, la
diretta responsabile, anzi unica responsabile vis-avì alla popolazione della
mancanza dell' acqua, la quale prima
voleva sostenere che l' errore della
mancanza di resistenza dei tubi, non
esisteva, perchè l' era stato assicurato
che ai *regi Lagni* il manometro se-
gnava 170 m. di pressione, e poi ha
dovuto persuadersi, che quella è *una
gratuita asserzione*, che si fanno agli
scolari, quando il maestro vuol copri-
re un suo errore *massimo*!....

Essa, dopo ciò osserva che era il
Municipio responsabile e che ad essa
poco calava se la conduttura saltasse
in aria!....

Ne avvertimmo di persona e con una

NAPOLI
—

C'è o non c'è il colera

A NAPOLI ?

È — si potrebbe ripetere — come l'a-
raba Fenice, la quale, come sapete e
come dice il proverbio, che vi sia
ognun lo dice, dove sia nessun lo sa:
È una domanda che tutti si rivolgo-
no, che ognuno di noi si rivolge ed
indirizza alle persone che crede le me-
glio informate, ma chiedi, domanda,
richiedi, nulla di preciso si sa, nulla
si riesce ad accertare, per la pace mo-
rale nostra e di tutta quanta la popolazione.

Una settimana fa, dopo i nostri ar-
ticoli, dopo quanto tutta la stampa, a
coro, fu costretta ripetere al Municipio, qualche cosa parve si volesse fa-
re, seriamente. Le commissione furo-
no radunate, a suon di nacchere e
tamburelli, le trombe di Gerico sona-
rono, la stampa amica battè, con for-
za, la gran cassa e parve — ripetiamo
— *parve*—che tutto volesse rifarsi dal-
le fondamenta.

Oh! il colera serpeggiava, qua e là,
come aspide, tra le foglie, sollevando,
di tanto in tanto la testa nera, che
portava la morte: bisognava schiacciar-
lo quest'aspide velenoso, ed i vice
sindaci, ed il pro sindaco, e le com-
missioni di vigilanza fecero stambura-
re che qua avevano sequestrate delle
salacche, lì avevano buttate in mare
delle frutta.... e, talvolta, per eccesso
.... anche sulla

FIGURE 6.4: "Is There, or Is There Not Cholera? / Serino Water Poisoned," *Il Napoli News-paper,* August 21, 1887.

old fountains.[20] An adequate understanding of disease was still lacking and rumors spread that the Serino itself was poisoned (Figure 6.4). A Risanamento inquest found that very little had been done to improve conditions for the neediest. The poor had been squashed behind facades to create a Parisian style shopping promenade for the middle class, and in the same year that Naples was declared the city with most urgent health needs in the Kingdom, the town hall spent just 1 percent of the total urban budget on sanitation and hygiene.[21]

There was no greater proof that the underlying issues affecting disease had not been fully addressed than the cholera epidemic of 1910, labeled by Snowden as "The epidemic that disappeared."[22] The government denied that cholera had returned to protect trade interests and guarantee its own stability. As part of the cover-up, hygiene minister Orazio Caro asserted that Naples had avoided cholera because its Roman infrastructure, built by the modern Neapolitans, relied upon "a powerful and magnificent mindset," a "marvelous wisdom and technique," and a "truly Latin firmness," and was executed "in a manner worthy of ancient men."[23]

Caro concluded with the "guarantee that the Serino, which saved the ancient city of the siren from so many epidemics," was to do so again.[24]

Conclusion

The implementation of infrastructure and practices can demonstrate good governance, but the Neapolitan effort to acquire and display successful urban planning measures presented a series of problems. A monumental display of technology, in Naples' case a Roman aqueduct, was not a catch-all solution for disease prevention. Disease is caused by a myriad of complex and interlinking factors that require sensitive analysis and small-scale interventions. In Naples, the demolition of unhealthy water systems and the displacement of low-income populations was no remedy for the underlying poverty and lack of hygiene education.

Trust in good governance cannot be achieved through vanity projects and immediate gratification at the expense of vulnerable populations. It is rather dependent upon the formation of bridges between citizens and health authorities who communicate well and honestly. This is key to ensuring good practices and preventing the recurrence of disease. In Naples, the reformers emphasized the Romanness of their modern infrastructure to guarantee its efficacy, which ultimately undermined the citizens' trust in their government. This lack of trust proved to be destabilizing and detrimental to urban health in the longer term, as demonstrated by the recurrence of cholera in Naples in the early 20th century. Elites with aesthetic and economic interests continued to underwrite destabilizing initiatives such as relocations of impoverished residents when change did not go to plan. The response to cholera in Naples reinforced a class divide and left major, underlying urban health issues unresolved.

NOTES

1. Frank M. Snowden, *Naples in the Time of Cholera, 1884–1911* (Cambridge: Cambridge University Press, 2002).

2. Felice Abate, *Per Provvedere di Acque Potabili la Città di Napoli ed 89 Comuni de' suoi Dintorni* (Naples: tip. del Giornale di Napoli, 1868), 15.

3. See Thomas Osborne, "Security and Vitality: Drains, Liberalism and Power in the Nineteenth Century," in *Foucault and Political Reason. Liberalism, Neo-liberalism and Rationalities of Government*, ed. A. Barry, T. Osborne, and N. Rose (London: UCL Press, 1996), 99–123.

4. For the aqueduct, see Clemente Esposito, *Il Sottosuolo di Napoli: Acquedotti e Cavità in Duemila Anni di Scavi* (Naples: Intra Moenia, 2018).

5. German physicist Max von Pettenkofer (1818–1901) also proposed the "ground water theory" in 1854, in which he argued that microorganisms in the soil released infectious material into the air when provided with humid conditions and warm temperatures. In Italy, germ theory was definitively accepted in 1897, after studies of the epidemics in Naples, Cassino, and Palermo.

6. For Italy's welfare state, economic debt, and liberal reform programs, see Maria Quine, *Italy's Social Revolution* (New York: Springer, 2002), 32.

7. For the formation of Italy's sanitary administration, see Gianfranco Donelli and Valeria Di Carlo, *I Laboratori della Sanità Pubblica. L'Amministrazione Sanitaria Italiana tra il 1887 e il 1912* (Rome: Laterza, 2002).

8. Snowden, *Naples in the Time of Cholera*, 255.

9. For the history of classical reception in Naples, see Jessica Hughes and Claudio Buongiovanni, *Remembering Parthenope: The Reception of Classical Naples from Antiquity to the Present* (Oxford: Oxford University Press, 2015).

10. On the formation of Italy and Rome, see Denis Mack-Smith, *The Making of Italy, 1796–1866* (London: Palgrave Macmillan, 1988).

11. David H. Pinkney, *Napoleon and the Rebuilding of Paris* (Princeton, NJ: New Haven, 1958).

12. Nelson Moe, *The View from Vesuvius: Italian Culture and the Southern Question* (London: University of California Press, 2006).

13. Marino Turchi, *L'Italia Igienica (1876)* (Naples: Giannini & Figli, 1891), 78.

14. Ibid.

15. Suetonius, *The Life of Nero*, 38.2, in *Suetonius, Lives of the Caesars, Vol. 1*, trans. J. C. Rolfe (Cambridge, MA: Harvard University Press, 1914).

16. Marino Turchi, *Sulla Igiene pubblica della città di Napoli: Osservazioni e Proposte di Marino Turchi* (Naples: Figli Morano, 1862).

17. Giancarlo Alisio, *Napoli e il Risanamento. Recupero di una Struttura Urbana* (Naples: Edizioni Scientifiche Italiane, 1980).

18. Note that Carthage was a Greek city destroyed by the Romans. Carlo del Balzo, "Napoli i quartieri bassi," *Illustrazione Italiana* (May 30, 1880): 22.

19. On the Roman and the modern aqueduct, see Esposito, *Il Sottosuolo di Napoli*.

20. Salvatore Fusco, *Sul risanamento di Napoli: Relazione letta nell'Adunanza Generale dell'Associazione Politica la Sinistra Meridionale, il dì 3 Novembre 1884* (Naples: Giannini e Figli, 1884).

21. Snowden, *Naples in the Time of Cholera*, 46.

22. Ibid., 247.

23. Orazio Caro, *L'Evoluzione Igienica di Napoli (Cenni storici – Osservazioni e Proposte – Dati Statistici* (Naples: Francesco Giannini & Figli, 1914), 76.

24. Ibid.

7

The Contested Governance of Border Railways and the Plague of Northeast China, 1910–11

Yongming Chen and Yishen Chen

The railway system carrying cross-border laborers and goods between Russia and northeastern China became infrastructure crucial to the spread of the Manchurian plague in 1910–11. Northeast China was the setting for the contested governance of the epidemic. The marmot, a large rodent that lived extensively in the Hulunbuir grasslands of Mongolia and the surrounding Siberian steppes, was considered to be the natural host for the plague. Consequently, the cross-border laborers who were active in hunting marmots in China and Russia became the source of human-to-human transmission of the epidemic.

Originating in the Siberian steppes, the outbreak first started in Manchuria and then spread eastward to Tsitsihar, the provincial capital of Heilongjiang. Harbin, with its convenient railway transportation, became the epicenter of the second wave. Finally, the plague spread southward to the critical cities along the railways, including Changchun, Jilin, Mekden, Dalian, and Shanhaiguan. The rapid spread of the epidemic in the northeast was mainly due to the developed network of railways in the region. Following the construction of the first railway in 1897, known as the Dongqing line, a railway system of 3,124 kilometers was completed in Northeast China by 1910.[1] Frozen rivers also acted as a highway system during the harsh winter and helped to spread the plague. The plague lasted more than seven months and killed more than sixty thousand people.[2] As a result, the plague outbreak in Northeast China was not only a local epidemic but also a cross-border disaster throughout northeastern Asia, with a large number of laborers becoming infected along the railway lines.

The development of transportation networks was conducive to the spread of the plague, so finding ways to cut off the transmission of the disease became the focus of epidemic governance in the region. After the plague outbreak was identified, the

Qing Dynasty (1636–1912) government carried out various epidemic prevention campaigns from the national to the local level. Dr. Wu Lien-teh (1879–1960), an Overseas Chinese from Malaya, was invited to Northeast China to fight against the plague. However, due to the geopolitical dynamics in Northeast China, the governance process was full of complexity. Following the outbreak of the Russo-Japanese War in 1904, Northeast China was governed jointly by Russia and Japan. This meant that, although China had nominal sovereignty over northeastern Asia at that time, Russia and Japan were the main powers in the region. The most direct manifestation was their control of the railways: Russia began to build the Chinese Far East Railway from Manchuria to Dalian in the northeast to connect Baikal Oblast with the Pacific Ocean in 1897, and Japan built the Andong-Sujiatun Railway during the war in 1904. After the war, Japan occupied the Changchun-Dalian section of the Far East Railway, which was later owned by the South Manchuria Railway Company.[3] In total, nearly two-thirds of the railways in Northeast China were under the control of Russia and Japan, while the Chinese government only controlled the Peking-Mukden Railway (Figure 7.1).

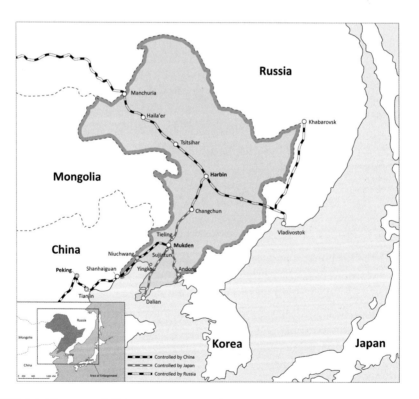

FIGURE 7.1: The map of Chinese, Russian, and Japanese railway control areas, 1901–11. (Courtesy of Yongming Chen and Yishen Chen.)

Case study: The railway and response to the plague in 1910–11

Northern Manchuria was largely Russian-controlled in the 1910s, with about ten thousand Russians living in Manchuria and Harbin along the Chinese Far East Railway line. As the epidemic began to erupt in Manchuria, the Russians initiated an epidemic prevention program, assuming that the railway formed a line of transmission. Russia sent doctors and soldiers to intercept suspected patients at Manchuria Station and transferred them out of the country. They also established health and quarantine stations in several cities along the Chinese Far East Railway and issued strict regulations restricting Chinese workers from riding on trains (Figure 7.2).[4] Chinese workers traveling to Baikal Oblast in Russia underwent a mandatory five-day quarantine before leaving. Right after these actions, a large-scale epidemic broke out in Fujiandian, Harbin, in the autumn of 1910, in which three out of ten people died directly from the plague, and as a result, Russian anxiety increased.[5] The Russian authorities immediately set up an isolation and observation hospital and established an epidemic prevention office dominated by the police and doctors. The authorities divided Harbin into eight surveillance areas, conducted strict inspection, enforced quarantine on Chinese who entered the city, and even published anti-epidemic propaganda materials in Chinese.

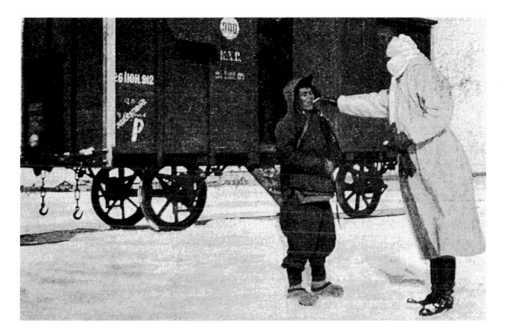

FIGURE 7.2: The examination of a Chinese laborer suspected to be plague-stricken in front of a quarantine wagon, January 1911. (Courtesy of Photo 12/Universal Images Group.)

Japan's sphere of influence was mainly in southern Manchuria, and its population was primarily distributed in Mukden and Dalian, with approximately ten thousand Japanese residents. The epidemic prevention awareness and measures of the Japanese authorities were relatively advanced at that time. When the epidemic was still isolated to northern Manchuria, the Japanese already paid close attention to railway control and initiated a series of protocols. After the Japanese authorities checked all passengers entering the South Manchurian Railway from the north, all the suspected cases and close contacts were sent to the isolation observation station. Epidemic prevention headquarters staff including senior officials of the colonial government, railway leaders, medical workers, and military personnel had responsibility for the coordination of the plague governance. Japanese authorities organized quarantine personnel along the railways in Changchun, Tieling, Liaoyang, Yingkou, and Andong to inspect the Chinese passengers who took trains and ships. Soldiers along the Yalu River were sent to intercept laborers who tried to cross the frozen river to enter North Korea.[6]

The rapid deployment of epidemic governance in Russia- and Japan-controlled railway communities was achieved due to the modern systems, administrative concepts, and medical knowledge employed by the authorities. During the Japanese colonization of Taiwan between April 17, 1895, and August 14, 1945, Shinpei Goto (1857–1929) served as the chief civil affairs officer of the Taiwan Governor's Office. Goto, a professional medical doctor, established public health infrastructure in major cities in Taiwan such as isolation hospitals, crematoriums, public baths, and public toilets. These facilities significantly developed Taiwan's public health capacity. When Goto was transferred to the position of president of South Manchuria Railway Company, he used his experiences in Taiwan to face the plague outbreak in the northeast.

As it became apparent that Japan and Russia had already launched anti-epidemic operations, the Qing government began to worry about the geopolitical operations behind the plague. Russia repeatedly pressured Chinese officials in Fujiadian to take the same compulsory and modern quarantine measures and threatened to forcefully enter China's jurisdiction to initiate medical intervention. After the epidemic outbreak in Harbin, Russia positioned troops in preparation to cut off communication with Fujiadian.[7] Japan ignored the provisions of other foreign powers to cede extraterritoriality and place the anti-plague campaign under the unified administration of China, and sent the military and police to set up checkpoints along the South Manchuria Railway; Japanese authorities also deployed troops from the mainland in the name of epidemic prevention.[8] The Qing government followed a traditional approach at the beginning stage of their epidemic governance, relying on local chambers of commerce and local associations to lead the plague prevention. The state's main responsibility at that time was to provide financial supports. On a practical level, traditional Chinese medicine could not cope with the increasing spread of the plague, so on the geopolitical level, foreign powers manipulated the discourse of "modern medicine" as an excuse to expand their sphere of influence by suppressing the Chinese self-help institutions and local organizations. Japan and Russia even attempted to use compulsory anti-epidemic measures to contain the trade activities of Chinese businessmen and commercial enterprises to dominate the economy in the northeast.

In early December 1910, the Qing government, facing immense pressure, began to organize a large-scale epidemic prevention operation guided by Western medicine, with Harbin as the focus. Subsequently, the Qing government dispatched Dr. Wu Lien-teh, who had received a modern medical education at Cambridge University. Dr. Wu guided the campaign in Northeast China. On the premise of safeguarding the sovereignty of epidemic prevention, the Qing authorities made every effort to establish epidemic prevention cooperation with relevant countries. In addition, foreign doctors were employed at a high salary by the Chinese authorities, and the whole epidemic prevention process was supported by advanced Western medical means. Soon, under the command of Dr. Wu, the northeast authorities took appropriate measures to respond to the plague. Chinese authorities subsequently established epidemic prevention agencies and promulgated anti-epidemic laws. Authorities also implemented scientific medical and hygiene measures, such as the removal of corpses, cremation, disinfection, and the wearing self-made masks (Figure 7.3). Quarantine measures were carried out, especially for principal

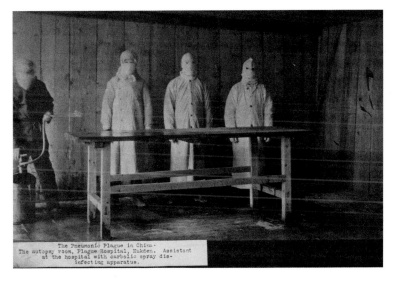

FIGURE 7.3: Doctors with modern protective clothing in the autopsy room, winter 1910–11. (Courtesy of Library of Congress/Corbis/VCG.)

cities along the railway.[9] Although China reacted slowly, with the efforts of Dr. Wu and other parties, the Qing government formed a relatively modern epidemic prevention system in a short time and gradually took initiative, particularly after facing pressure from Russia and Japan.

Epidemic governance required the cooperation and compromise of all parties to achieve the desired results. To prevent further spread of the plague, the Ministry of Foreign Affairs of the Qing government negotiated with Russia on the suspension of the Chinese Far East Railway and with Japan on the suspension of the Andong-Mukden Railway.[10] In mid-February 1911, Russia requested a joint investigation with China along the Chinese Far East Railway. Russia took charge of the railway line, while China took charge of the surroundings along the railway. At the level of domestic politics, forces from the central to the local level of the Qing government participated in the program. The Ministry of Foreign Affairs dealt with diplomatic pressure from Japan, Russia, and other foreign powers, and negotiated on specific governance issues. Local authorities were necessarily involved in disrupting urban and rural traffic, intercepting laborers and maintaining the provision of essential supplies such as vegetables, rice, oil, and salt.

The Chinese laborers were the main victims when the cross-border railway lines were blocked. When the trains stopped, the laborers were forced to continue south on foot. Moreover, to ensure the safety of Peking (Bejing) under the pressure of diplomatic missions stationed in the city, the Qing government dispatched troops to intercept laborers at Shanhaiguan, resulting in the detention of a large number of rural migrants.[11]

Conclusion

Contested governance over the prevention and control of the plague directly contributed to the formation of the modern anti-epidemic system in China, which emerged through a complex process of contradictions, compromises, and cooperation between China, Japan, and Russia. The central government, local authorities, traditional Chinese and Western medicine, officials, gentry, and doctors were involved. The control of cross-border railway lines prevented plague-infected people from spreading the disease to the principal cities along the railways on a large scale, which in turn prevented a major outbreak of the epidemic in the vicinity of the capital and its environs. Transregional traffic control became the standard method for the prevention and control of plague in the northeast. At the same time, China established a multi-level, modern epidemic prevention system based on spatial governance along the railway.

In the joint geopolitics of China, Japan, and Russia, measures to govern railways presented a complex and dynamic social-spatial process of conflict, compromise, and cooperation. Domestically, China gradually established modern anti-epidemic measures and spatial isolation policies to control the epidemic. After the end of this plague in 1911, the rule of the Qing Dynasty also came to an end. In 1917, the October Revolution, also known as the Bolshevik Coup, brought about earth-shaking changes in Russia, whose position in Northeast China was gradually replaced by Japan. The troublesome geopolitics of the northeast continued, and the frequent outbreaks of plague in the region still tested how China cooperated and compromised with foreign powers in the realm of epidemic governance.

NOTES

1. Lien-teh Wu, Yonghan Chen, Lishi Bo, and Changyao Wu, *Introduction to the Plague* (Shanghai: Harbor Quarantine Office, Department of Health, 1937), 25.
2. Lihong Du, "Qingmo Dongbei Shuyi Fangkong yu Jiaotong Zheduan" [The Prevention and Control of Plague and Shut-Down of Transportation in Northeast China in the Late Qing Dynasty], *Lishi Yanjiu* [Historical Research] 4 (2016): 74.
3. William C. Summers, *The Great Manchurian Plague of 1910–1911: The Geopolitics of an Epidemic Disease* (New Haven, CT: Yale University Press, 2012), 30–31.
4. "Manzhouli Harbin Fangyiji" [Epidemic prevention in Manchouli and Harbin], *Dongfang Zazhi* [*The Orient Magazine*] 11 (1910): 335–44.
5. Runming Jiao, "Gengxu Shuyi Yingdui yu Zhongguo Jindai Fangyi Tixi Chujian" [Responding to the Plague in Northeast China and the Beginning of a Modern Epidemic Prevention System in China], *Lishi Yanjiu* [Historical Research] 2 (2020): 15.
6. Cheng Hu, "Quarantine Sovereignty during the Pneumonic Plague in North China (November 1910–April 1911)," *Frontiers of History in China* 5, no. 2 (2010): 299, 300.
7. Shuhe Guan, "Wu Lien-teh 1910–1911 Nian zai Dongbei Fangyi zhong Renzhi 'Quanquanzongyiguan' Kao" [An Investigation of Wu Lien-teh as the Plenipotentiary General Medical Officer for Epidemic Protection in Northeast China from 1910 to 1911], *Shixue Jikan* [*Collected Papers of History Studies*] 6 (2018): 89.
8. Long Cheng, "Fangyi yu Boyi: Qingmo Shuyi Beihou de Daguo Waijiao" [Epidemic Prevention and Gaming: The Great Power Diplomacy behind the Late Qing Plague], *Dushu* 7 (2020): 6, 7.
9. Jiao, "Gengxu Shuyi Yingdui yu Zhongguo Jindai Fangyi Tixi Chujian," 16–18.
10. Fengtian Quansheng Fangyi Zongju, *Dongsansheng Yishi Baogaoshu* [Report on the Epidemic in Northeast China Volume I] (Shanghai: Harbor Quarantine Office, Department of Health, 1912), 6–7.
11. Du, "Qingmo Dongbei Shuyi Fangkong yu Jiaotong Zheduan," 78–82.

8

Print, Politics, and the Smallpox Epidemic in Terre Haute, USA, 1902–3

Allen Shotwell

The first five years of the 20th century saw a resurgence of smallpox epidemics in cities throughout the United States of America after a period of relative inactivity. Municipal responses to the disease, both from major urban centers like New York and Boston and small cities like Terre Haute on the western edge of the state of Indiana, primarily relied on the controversial approaches of quarantine and vaccination. Objections to vaccination on personal liberty grounds were voiced by a number of Americans in the early 20th century, and societies and publications were organized to oppose the practice. Quarantine was equally unpopular, although with less coordinated opposition. Implementation of both policies by city governments placed demands on municipal resources and provoked questions of legality and acceptability.[1]

The smallpox epidemic in Terre Haute began in the winter of 1902 (Figure 8.1). The Indiana State Board of Health records indicate that the disease spread during the winter and spring of 1902–3, infecting almost two hundred people. It reached its peak in March 1903, when 90 cases were recorded. The numbers followed a similar trend the next winter. Health officials from two different city administrations attempted to rein in the disease by implementing quarantines and encouraging or requiring vaccination, but perceptions of the efficacy of these policies were highly politicized. American politics in the 20th century were largely dominated by two opposing political parties: the Democrats and the Republicans. In 1902, Terre Haute's Democratic city government was criticized by the local Republican newspaper for its initial handling of the disease, but once the Democrats were voted out, the new Republican city government faced the same problems and responded in much the same way.[2]

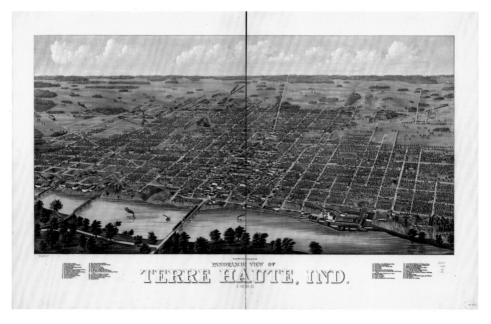

FIGURE 8.1: "Panoramic view of Terre Haute, Ind. 1880." (Courtesy of the Library of Congress, Geography and Map Division. Control No. 75693229.)

Case study: Politics and controversies of quarantine and vaccination

Major Henry Steeg led the Democratic city government of Terre Haute in 1902 at the beginning of the smallpox outbreak. Steeg appointed the city's Board of Health and Charities, which was directed by Dr. S. M. Rice and consisted of three physicians responsible for public health issues like smallpox. Funding for the Board was controlled by the City Council, also largely composed of Democrats at the time. The City's initial reaction to the outbreak was constrained by financial decisions and sensitivity to the legal ramifications of imposing strict rules on the populace. In December 1902, the Board of Health requested $2,500 from the City Council to cover costs already spent on the smallpox epidemic and to anticipate future needs. Much of the money was directed toward the local "Pest House," a building to which impoverished victims of the disease were often sent. More affluent victims were confined at home, but even this entailed the expense of hired guards, who were stationed so as to prevent infected residents from breaking quarantine.

The Board's funding request was initially shelved. In early January 1903, the City Council appropriated $25,000 for a bond to purchase land for a public park. This prompted the *Daily Tribune* to complain about the administration's reluctance to pay for combating smallpox, at just one-tenth of the cost of the park.[3]

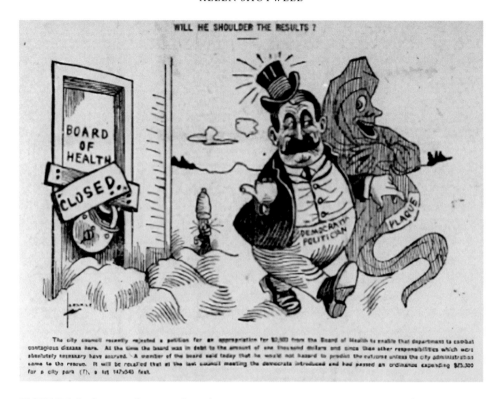

FIGURE 8.2: Cartoon from *Daily Tribune*, January 12, 1903, 1. (Courtesy of Hoosier State Chronicles.)

On January 12, 1903, political cartoonist Harry Larimer's illustration of a Democratic politician walking arm-in-arm with the specter of plague away from a closed and padlocked Board of Health was printed on the *Daily*'s front page. The next day, Mayor Steeg called for an emergency meeting of the Council to consider the smallpox funding request, which was finally approved (Figure 8.2). The city government's hesitance to fund smallpox measures continued to rankle critics. On February 4, 1903, illustrator Larimar contributed another cartoon, this time weaving together city politics and the medical crisis by depicting the city administration as a quack doctor forcing an enormous "Park Pill" down the throat of a young patient labeled "Terre Haute" (Figure 8.3).

While quarantine brought public complaints about fiscal priorities, the smallpox vaccination program brought legal challenges. Terre Haute was home to Frank Blue, secretary of the Anti-Vaccination Society of America. Other prominent opponents of vaccination, including Clerk of the Schools Walter Sharpe and several attorneys, also lived in the city. With the consent of the School Superintendent, the Board implemented a vaccination requirement for school children in

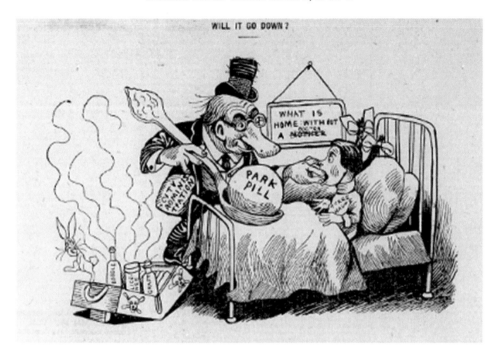

FIGURE 8.3: Cartoon from *Daily Tribune*, February 4, 1903, 1. (Courtesy of Hoosier State Chronicles.)

February 1903. In response, attorney Eli Redmon personally escorted his unvaccinated son to school and remained with him, insisting that an arrest warrant would need to be issued before he would agree to leave. The warrant was never produced. Another attorney, Ira Kisner, succeeded in getting an injunction against banning unvaccinated children from school.[4]

The school system fought back. Unvaccinated children were allowed to enter their normal classrooms only to find that their classmates and the teacher had been relocated to another room, leaving them to sit alone or return home. The Board of Health closed the schools entirely on February 28 but a judge lifted the closure and ordered the schools to reopen on March 5. The *Daily Tribune* highlighted the legal wrangling over vaccinations, printing Harry Larimer's depiction of City Attorney Peter M. Foley. As "The Modern Sphinx" who refused to reveal his thoughts on mandatory vaccination, Foley was shown failing to take an immediate and firm stand on the school vaccination requirement.[5]

In January, the Board of Health campaigned to encourage vaccination among the general population by posting photographs of smallpox victims in advanced stages of the disease in store windows around Terre Haute. In February, the secretary of the Indiana State Board of Health, J. N. Hurty, sent photographs of his

71

own to the city, which were hung in the windows of well-known downtown business Baur's Drug Store. The images warning of the consequences for the unvaccinated soon attracted the attention of hundreds of people (Figure 8.4).[6] Hurty published a letter in the *Daily Tribune* explaining that the photographs depicted "people who said they would rather have smallpox than be vaccinated" and that two of these unvaccinated individuals had already died.

People motivated by photographs of smallpox victims did not have far to go to be vaccinated. By October 1903, almost ten thousand smallpox vaccines sold by Baur's Drug Store had been administered. Another ten thousand vaccinations were provided by a rival drugstore a block east of Baur's run by D. P. Cox, and a free vaccination clinic was also set up in front of the Rose Dispensary one block north.[7] Despite these efforts, smallpox continued to spread through 1903 and the outbreak was even worse the following winter. The Terre Haute Board of Health reported 64 cases of smallpox in January 1904 and 74 cases in February. The Democrats were swept out of city government during the spring elections by the Republicans, who were led by mayoral candidate Edwin Bidaman on a ticket of reform. Bidaman selected Dr. W. E. Bell to lead the Board of Health and Public Charities, but a change in the administration did not solve Terre Haute's smallpox fiscal and political problems. In October 1904, shortly after they took over the

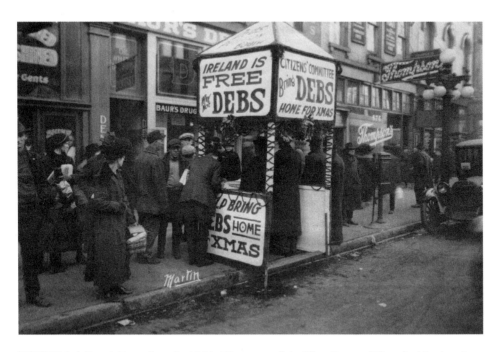

FIGURE 8.4: Baur's Drug Store in 1921. (Courtesy of the Vigo County Historical Society.)

72

government, both Bidaman and Bell were embroiled in the controversies that had plagued their predecessors.[8]

Dr. Bell made a request to the City Council for $30,000 in October to fund smallpox control. This was six times what had been spent the previous year. The Council eventually granted $3,500, but not immediately. Another smallpox case appeared in a local school, prompting the Board to order the fumigation of the home of every student attending the school where the outbreak occurred; every associated family member was to be vaccinated. When August Markle refused to comply, his daughter was not allowed to return to school and his house was placed under quarantine, prompting yet another legal battle.[9] Markle filed a case of *habeas corpus*. Under United States federal law, a writ of *habeas corpus* is essentially a claim of illegal imprisonment and generally includes a request to bring the detainee to court to determine the legality of the imprisonment. Markle broke quarantine in order to come to the courthouse where the Board of Health had him arrested and returned home. Judge Stimson ordered Markle returned to court the next day, arguing that the Constitution required the presence of a plaintiff in court for a *habeas corpus* case to proceed. Led by Dr. Bell, the members of the Board of Health left the courtroom when Markle appeared and refused to participate in breaking the quarantine. The judge proceeded without them, ruling—more or less—in Markle's favor. Frustrated by the lack of support for public health policies, Bell first threatened to inform the State Board of Health then submitted his letter of resignation, which Bidaman refused to accept.

Conclusion

The social and political frictions produced by smallpox in Terre Haute in the early 20th century were short-lived. Just eight months after their legal battle, all seemed to be forgotten and forgiven between Bell and Markle, and the doctor hired his former nemesis to work on his new home. The visual and physical effects of the epidemic on the city itself also slipped away. Baur's Drugstore and the Rose Dispensary ceased to exist, even as buildings, well before the end of the century. Only the controversial park, which received funding when smallpox measures could not, remains as a physical reminder of the smallpox epidemic in Terre Haute. Yet, even the park was long ago renamed and stripped of all associations with its origins.

The apparent disappearance of the effects of the epidemic in Terre Haute over time contextualizes the ongoing legal actions and community protests over the methods of response as artificial conflicts between the Democratic and Republican political parties. The similar experiences of two city administrations as they attempted to combat the epidemic show that the problems were financial, social, and structural rather than matters of party ideologies regarding public health. Terre Haute's urban governance did not operate in a vacuum, so its challenges did not resolve following each election. Legal challenges to vaccination requirements and the opinions about the resources devoted by the City of Terre Haute in combating the smallpox epidemic that began in 1902 came from the complex and conflicted thinking of the citizens of Terre Haute as much as from their government.[10]

NOTES

1. Smallpox is an infectious, contagious disease caused by a virus with a long history. For an overview of the disease in the early 20th century and the epidemics in American cities, see Michael Willrich, *Pox: An American History* (New York: Penguin Press, 2011), 15–40.
2. *Twenty-Second Annual Report of the State Board of Health of Indiana for the Fiscal Year Ending October 31,1903 and Statistical Year Ending December 31, 1903* (Indianapolis, IN: State Board of Health, 1904), 123–31.
3. Terre Haute Gazette Company Press, *An Index to the Journal of the Common Council, City of Terre Haute, Indiana from January 1, 1902 to January 3, 1903* (Terre Haute: Terre Haute Gazette Company Press of Star Printing,1904), 596.
4. "Trouble Occurs at City Schools," *Daily Tribune*, February 25, 1903, 1.
5. "Foley Remains Mum," *Daily Tribune*, February 21, 1903, 4.
6. "Smallpox Pictures," *Daily Tribune*, January 29, 1903. "Pictures Sent by Hurty," *Daily Tribune*, February 27, 1903.
7. "About Town," *The Spectator*, October 1, 1904, 1.
8. Gretchen Weston, "Municipal Reform and Agitation: Terre Haute 1900–1910" (MA thesis, Indiana State University Department of History, 1967), 11-13.
9. *Miscellaneous Proceedings of the Vigo County Medical Society, 1902–1954* (A. R. Markle Papers, Archives of the Vigo County Historical Society Museum, Terre Haute, Indiana).
10. Receipt, Box 1, W.E. Bell Papers, Archives of the Vigo County Historical Society Museum, Terre Haute, Indiana.

9

Colonialism, Racism, and the Government Response to Bubonic Plague in Nairobi, Kenya, 1895–1910

Catherine Odari

Nairobi, the present-day capital of Kenya, experienced frequent outbreaks of the bubonic plague at the turn of the 20th century that disproportionately impacted African natives and Indian immigrants. The outbreaks were caused by the unhealthy living conditions that the colonial forces imposed upon non-European populations. In multiracial, colonial settings where power was contested and access to resources was characterized by competition, policy decisions regarding epidemic containment were determined by the interests of the powerful colonizing group. Such policies were used to justify the entrenchment of discriminatory practices such as segregation by the minority colonizers. Consequently, disease containment efforts for the masses were often inadequate and ineffective.

Nairobi is one of Africa's largest and most populous cities today, but less than two centuries ago, it was an uninhabited swamp that the Maasai community frequented to water their cattle. The Maasai called this place *Enkare Nyorobi*, meaning the land of cool waters. The city of Nairobi originated in the late 1890s as a colonial railway settlement (Figure 9.1). Following the Berlin Conference of 1885–86, where European states deliberated on how they would partition Africa into different spheres of European influence, the British embarked on the expansion of the empire in East Africa. Part of this expansion plan involved building transport and communication infrastructure in the African interior to facilitate the extraction of raw materials for export and the integration of Africans into the global money economy. According to British colonial authorities, the Indians were best suited for facilitating this process of integration based on their centuries-long trade involvement with coastal East Africans and their experience with the Indian subcontinent's interregional railroad.[1]

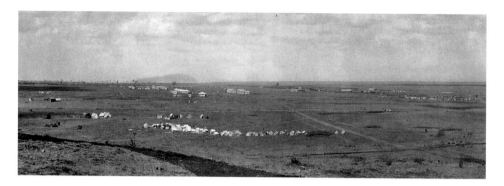

FIGURE 9.1: Early colonial Nairobi, *c.*1890. (Courtesy of the Kenya National Archives.)

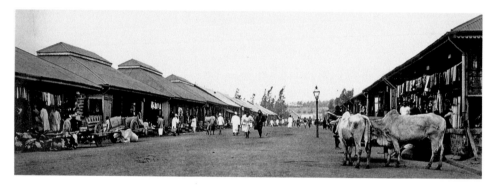

FIGURE 9.2: Indian bazaar. (Courtesy of the Kenya National Archives.)

The first group of Indian migrants arrived in Kenya, then known as the British East African Protectorate, in the late 19th century to provide indentured labor for the railroad construction. The second wave arrived in the first and second decades of the 20th century as professionals working in different sectors of the colonial economy, including administration, business, public service, and construction. The colonial government also advocated for the resettlement of British citizens in the colony. The goal was for Europeans to take advantage of the colony's agricultural potential by growing cash crops for the world market for the purposes of defraying colonial deficit.[2] The settlement of both Europeans and Indians in Kenya led to questions about racial hierarchy. Indian positionality was of especial interest in the new colony.

In many cases, European settlers saw the Indian presence as a threat to the economic prosperity the colonial state had promised them. The government had assured would-be European settlers in East Africa access to land through attractive grant schemes, cheap African labor, and the potential for huge profits.[3] The Indian presence meant competition for those profits, especially when Indian merchants set up bazaars and small shops known as *dukawallah* in Nairobi and the towns along the railway line (Figure 9.2).[4] Indians demanded rights and privileges equal to those of the British settlers since they too were British subjects. The 1921 census estimated the European population in Kenya at 9,651 people, which was far less than the native and the rapidly growing Indian populations.[5]

Despite their minority status, Europeans wielded the most political influence. Their response to Indian demands was anti-Indian discourse and portrayals of the Indians of Nairobi as duplicitous, fraudulent, unsanitary, and unworthy of equal rights with the European settlers.[6] These anti-Indian sentiments extended to the realm of public health. When an outbreak of the bubonic plague first occurred in Nairobi in 1902, European settlers blamed it on Indians because they believed Indians were inherently unsanitary.

Case study: Government intervention and bubonic plague in Nairobi, 1902–6

The plague outbreak in Nairobi in the early 20th century resulted in 69 confirmed cases; the majority of those infected died. According to Lord Cranworth, a British settler, Indians were responsible for introducing and spreading the plague (as well as venereal diseases) because they lived "in unsanitary conditions under which no English farmer would dream of keeping his pigs. He can do without what the European considers the ordinary necessities of life, such as soap and a change of clothes."[7] Contrary to this misinformed statement, understanding the spread of the bubonic plague requires the contextualization of several complex systems. Nairobi's location, poor urban planning, improper health infrastructure implementation, and inadequate sanitation facilities for the expanding population at the beginning of the 20th century together created the unsanitary conditions that led to the spread of diseases like typhoid and bubonic plague.

Nairobi sprang up along the railway line as a supply depot where the colonial administrators and railway workers would stop to replenish supplies on their way between Mombasa and the port of Kisumu on the shores of Lake Victoria. Without consulting with the colonial government, the railway administrators decided to establish the railway headquarters in Nairobi. In the years that followed, the swampy area became home to thousands of people from different racial and ethnic groups: Africans who sought jobs in the growing township, Indians who worked as laborers in the construction of the railroad and established small shops along the railway line, and European settlers attracted by Nairobi's favorable elevation and cooler temperatures.[8] Consequently, the government relocated its headquarters from Machakos to Nairobi. Despite the city's rapid growth and urbanization, health and sanitation infrastructure continued to lag, leading to frequent disease outbreaks. Additionally, the swampy ground was a source of concern for colonial administrators, who commissioned a series of reports by medical officers between 1902 and 1906 to investigate the possibility of relocating the city. In 1907, following extensive debate it was decided that relocation would be too expensive and "outside the bounds of practical politics."[9] Instead, they proposed draining the swampy areas.

Despite these obvious problems of drainage and sanitation infrastructure, colonial administrators persisted in blaming Indians for public health crises. This was demonstrated by the comments of the then commissioner of the colony, Sir Charles Elliot, who stated that "there were large numbers of 'coolies' working for the Uganda Railway, who had been allowed to congregate in crowded and ill-kept quarters, and the plague was probably introduced among them in a consignment of infected goods from India."[10] Although Elliot's suggestion is plausible, it does not explicate the colonial government's contribution to recurrent public health crises nor its responsibility for the disproportionate allocation of urban spaces in Nairobi that contributed to the city's significant sanitation problem. From the early period of colonialism, Europeans, despite their small numbers, occupied Nairobi's larger, open spaces with better drainage; Indian-owned businesses were confined to the cramped, joint commercial-residential area of the township with its limited sanitary infrastructure including inadequate sewerage and garbage disposal systems. The overcrowded, unsanitary conditions were exacerbated by Nairobi's drainage problem that made the city suitable for harboring rodents known to transmit the plague.

The result of the sanitation failure was framed as an inherently "Indian" problem and the situation was subsequently racialized by colonial policy. The government's intervention measures targeted Indians and the areas they inhabited. Goan medical doctor Rosendo Ayres Ribeiro was the first to diagnose the bubonic plague patients in 1902. Dr. Ribeiro notified the Medical Officer of Health, Dr. Alfred Spurrier, of the potential health crises, and Spurrier responded by issuing an order to burn down the Indian bazaar and relocate the Indians to the edge of the city. Having wrongly assumed that Indians and Africans were intrinsically prone to epidemics and therefore carriers and transmitters of disease, the state predicated their interventions on the separation of racial groups. The aggressive colonial pursuit to keep European settlers safe from Indians and Africans resulted in a segregation policy that divided the city into four sections. The Indian sections were established in the areas known as Nairobi South, Nairobi West, and in the north and east that covered the areas of Parklands, Pangani, and Eastleigh. The African section was established in Pumwani, Kariokor, and Donholm in the east and southeast. Finally, the European areas were set aside in the north and west in areas such as Muthaiga, Upper Parklands, Westlands, Loresho, Kileleshwa, and

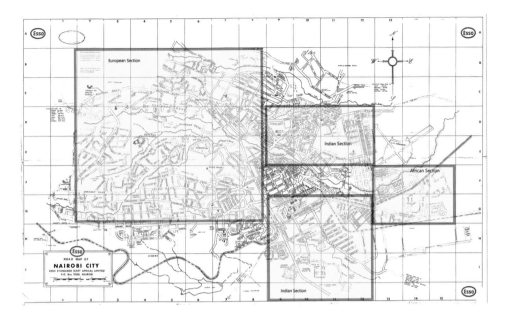

FIGURE 9.3: Map of segregated residential areas in Nairobi. (Courtesy of the Kenya National Archives.)

Kilimani (Figure 9.3).[11] The Plague Notice of 1902 built on segregationist policies to prohibit Indians and Africans from leaving Nairobi.[12] Passengers on the Uganda Railway were required to obtain a health certificate in order to travel and were quarantined in camps upon arrival at their destinations.[13] None of these actions forestalled the epidemic because the actual cause of the plague was to be found in the city's poor sanitation and drainage.[14]

In 1906, the colonial administration commissioned British engineer and sanitary advisor George Bransby Williams to investigate Nairobi's public health. His recommendations included improvements to the drainage and sewerage system and new public health legislation. Consequently, James Hayes Sadler, commissioner for the East African Protectorate, issued strict laws under the provisions of the East Africa Township Ordinance of 1903. Indian businesspeople such as the *dhobi* (laundrymen) were the obvious targets of these new laws because they operated out of the bazaar and required high volumes of water. Laundry licenses, valid for only one year, required a medical health officer inspection along with certification that the business premises had a water supply, proper ventilation, and drainage. The license applicant was also forced to submit to a medical examination. The same laws mandated contact tracing for confirmed and suspected plague cases. The *dhobi* who had been in contact with infected people were legally required to report to the medical officer and to self-quarantine, with obvious financial implications.[15]

79

Conclusion

Sadler declared the township of Nairobi free of plague on February 12, 1906.[16] However, new cases were reported until the 1990s. Stringent policies such as segregation, contact tracing, and quarantine targeted specific racial groups. While these measures may have been effective in containing the spread of the epidemic to European populations, they did not eradicate the disease, as subsequent outbreaks indicate. Total eradication required investment in public health infrastructure, for all Nairobi's populations. Proper sewerage and drainage systems, garbage disposal in all neighborhoods, urban planning in the township and residential areas, expansion of living quarters, and provision of spacious housing to accommodate the rapidly growing population were potential interventions and practical solutions to not only disease but also other social issues in the city. Instead, the colonial state and European settlers took advantage of the ongoing public health crisis to justify racially discriminatory practices such as segregation.

The colonial government both employed rhetoric that portrayed non-European groups as inherently unsanitary transmitters of disease and enacted official policies that restricted their economic and social progress. Thus, official responses to the outbreak of the plague targeted mostly Indians and Africans. However, the differential treatment extended to racial groups inevitably curtailed the colonial state's ability to forestall outbreaks of the disease in subsequent years. Colonial Nairobi's disease epidemics were framed in terms of race. This racial discourse was used to justify discriminatory public health policies and inadequate governmental infrastructural interventions, with lasting consequences for the city and its population.

NOTES

1. Frederick John Dealtry Lugard, *The Rise of Our East African Empire: Early Efforts in Nyasaland and Uganda* (London: W. Blackwood and Sons, 1893), 447. Sir Winston Churchill, in his consideration of the task of developing the East African protectorate using the labor and capital of the Indians, argued, "There are roads and railways and reservoirs which only he can make [...] The mighty continent of tropical Africa lies open to the colonizing and organizing capacities of the East." W. S. Churchill, *My African Journey* (Toronto: William Briggs, 1909), 52.
2. Caroline Elkins, *Imperial Reckoning: The Untold Story of Britain's Gulag in Kenya* (New York: Henry Holt, 2005), 2.
3. Ibid., 3.
4. Foreign Office Records 2/805, Sir Charles Eliot to Lansdowne, January 21, 1902, enclosed petition of the European settlers' committee dated January 4, 1902 (British Library, Asian and African Collection).

5. Norman Leys, *Kenya* (London: The Hogarth Press, 1924), 140.

6. Lord Cranworth, *A Colony in the Making, or, Sport and Profit in British East Africa* (London: Macmillan, 1912), 63–64.

7. Ibid., 63.

8. O. A. K'Akumu and W.H.A. Olima, "The Dynamics and Implications of Residential Segregation in Nairobi," *Habitat International* 31, no. 1 (2007): 90.

9. George Bransby Williams, *Report on the Sanitation of Nairobi* (London: Waterlow, 1907), 2–4.

10. The term "coolie" was used in the 19th and early 20th centuries to describe indentured laborers from the Indian subcontinent. Today, it is considered a derogatory term. Sir Charles Elliot, *The East Africa Protectorate* (London: Edward Arnold, 1905), 156.

11. K'Akumu and Olima, "Dynamics and Implications of Residential Segregation," 88–91.

12. The city remains segregated to date, but the segregation is along class lines rather than racial lines. Those areas that were reserved for white settlers during the colonial and postcolonial period are occupied by wealthy Africans, Indians, and the few Europeans who live in Nairobi.

13. Pheroze Nowrojee, *A Kenyan Journey* (Nairobi: Manqa Books, 2019), 30.

14. L. W. Thornton White, L. Silberman, and P. R. Anderson, *Nairobi: Master Plan for a Colonial Capital, A Report Prepared for the Municipal Council of Nairobi* (London: HMSO, 1948), 12.

15. The Official Gazette of the East Africa and Uganda Protectorates 8, No. 158 (Mombasa, June 1906).

16. The Official Gazette of the East Africa and Uganda Protectorates 8, No. 151 (Mombasa, February 1906).

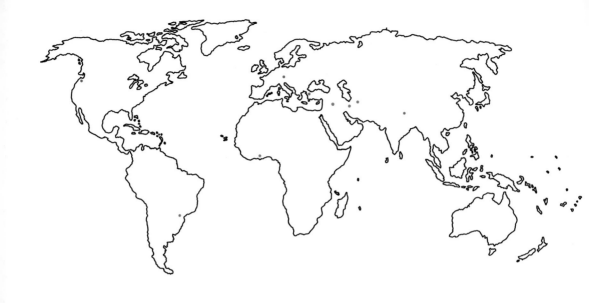

PART 2
Urban Life:
Culture and Society

Case Studies for Urban Life

Present-day cities and countries

This page: Map indicating the locations of case studies in this section of the book. (Map in the public domain, with annotations drawn by Andrew Bui)

Right page: A health officer attaching a mumps quarantine sign to the front porch of a house in Pennsylvania. Photograph, 1920/1935?. (Courtesy of the Wellcome Collection)

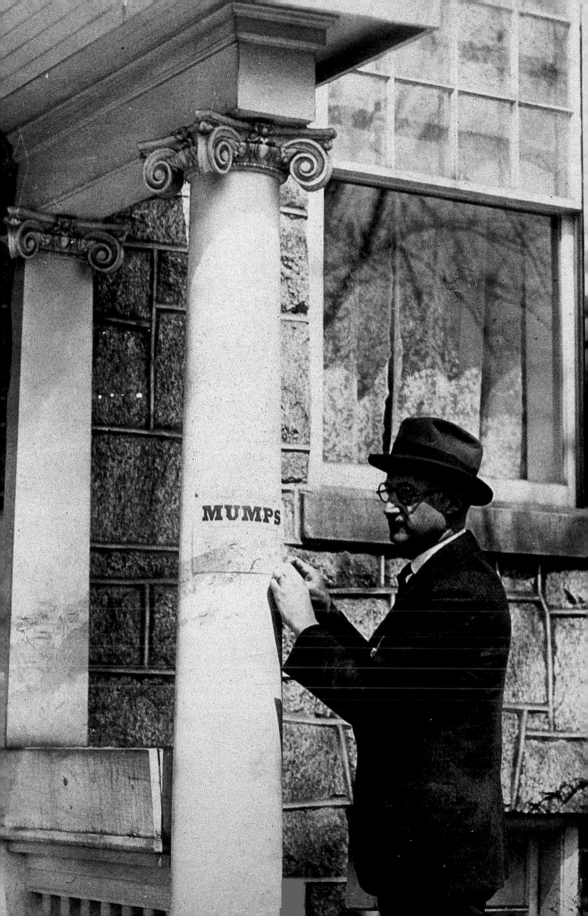

10

Women, Social Solidarities, and the Plague in 17th-Century Newcastle, England

Rachel Clamp

The threat of plague was one of the defining characteristics of the early modern era (*c*.16th–19th centuries). Primarily a disease carried by rodents, plague is transmitted to humans via infected fleas who abandon their dead or dying animal host in search of nourishment on live humans. Scholars estimate that between 60 and 80 percent of those infected with the disease ultimately succumbed to it.[1]

The social impact of this disease in England can be understood by exploring a previously overlooked urban intervention: the employment of poorer women to nurse and care for the sick in their communities. The image of the plague physician, an ominous character often depicted dressed in a long coat with gloves and a beak-like mask filled with aromatic substances, is often associated with European plague outbreaks (Figure 10.1). However, sufferers in England were more likely to be cared for by a woman hired by the parish, or by the infected household directly. In East Kent, three-quarters of all medical interventions taking place in the later 16th century took the character of nursing attendance without the assistance of what might be called a professional medical practitioner.[2]

During an outbreak of plague, the enforcement of formal plague orders received from the capital in London depended not on corporate authorities or professional medical practitioners but on the efforts of lay individuals. Patients needed to be cared for, bodies needed to be counted, the cause of death identified, and the houses of the deceased fumigated and cleansed. Most of these responsibilities fell upon the shoulders of early modern women. Evidence taken from contemporary wills and inventories, probated either during or shortly after major outbreaks of plague in the city of Newcastle between the years 1570 and 1637, suggests that these women were responsible for a significant portion of medical provision during the early modern period. They were part of relatively organized systems of health care that proved essential to the well-being of their neighbors.

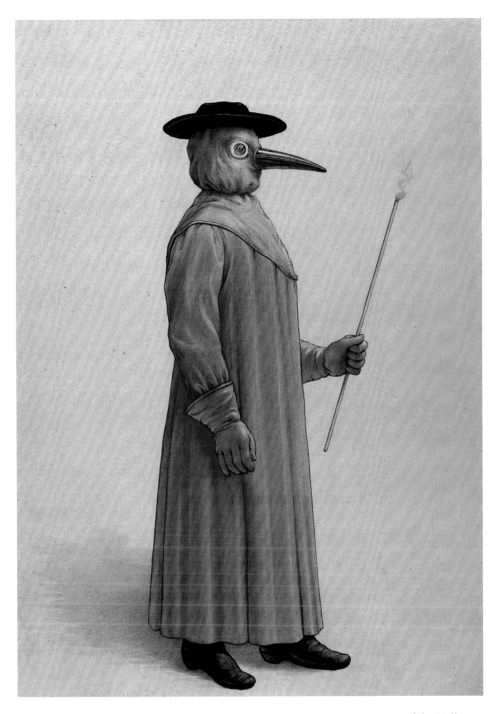

FIGURE 10.1: Physician wearing a 17th-century plague preventive. (Courtesy of the Wellcome Collection.)

Case study: Women health care workers in Newcastle, 1570–1637

Newcastle was one of the largest provincial towns in England with an estimated population of ten thousand people by 1600.[3] Its vibrant, medieval port made it the regional center for trade in wool, corn, and coal, and its position on the east coast provided close links across to the North Sea to the Baltic and the Netherlands, down the coast to London and the intermediate ports, and up to Scotland's east coast (Figure 10.2).[4] Driven by the requirements of London's insatiable fuel

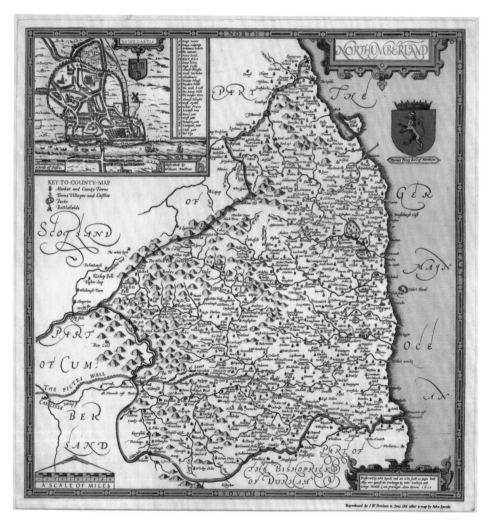

FIGURE 10.2: Map of Northumberland with inset map of Newcastle taken from John Speed, *The Theatre of the Empire of Greate Britaine*, 1610. Ref D.NCP/1/9. (Courtesy of Tyne and Wear Archives and Museums.)

demands, the town's coal industry grew exponentially after 1550.[5] By the mid-17th century, Newcastle and coal had become almost synonymous. This is demonstrated by the phrase "to carry coals to Newcastle," meaning to do something plainly superfluous.[6]

Although outbreaks of plague in Newcastle tended to follow upon those in London, the town had its own epidemic history. Through close trading links with the capital, plague found its way into Newcastle in 1570–71, 1576, 1579, 1604, and 1625.[7] International trade links also made the town susceptible to additional sources of infection. In the outbreak of 1588–89, Newcastle was afflicted a year ahead of other major English cities.[8] Plague was also identified in Newcastle in 1593, 1597–98, 1620, and, most severely, in 1636.[9]

There has often been an unspoken assumption that women's healing was limited to the domestic sphere. Part of the untold story of women's engagement in the commercial realm of healing concerns their involvement in emergency responses to outbreaks of epidemic disease. This story is particularly relevant to early modern urban environments, which struggled to cope with growing population density and increasing demands on sanitation services.[10] Traditional resources and procedures for medical relief were inadequate to cope with outbreaks of plague, and it was in these distinctive, crisis-filled conditions that women's "unofficial" healing skills were put to "official" use in several innovative and gainful ways.[11] Within this "plague industry," the occupation that appeared most frequently in the wills and inventories of plague victims was the cleanser.[12] Cleansers, although sometimes charged with caring for the sick, were largely responsible for disinfecting the house and goods after the recovery, or death, of infected individuals.

Of the 38 surviving Newcastle plague inventories consulted for this study, 67 percent list payments to a cleanser alongside debts owed by the deceased. The probate records registered at Durham Cathedral are unusually detailed, making it possible to reconstruct the regime and economy of care as well as the community's methods for trying to contain the disease. The yeoman Thomas Creake, for example, paid fourteen shillings for the "clenssinge & dightinge" of his home. He also accounted for the daily maintenance of the cleansers, for he owed 44 shillings for "meat & drincke to Iszabell creake and the clenssers that was in the house frome sainct luke days unto christenmes daye," nine weeks in total. We are even told what materials were used, as he paid nine shillings for "colles to the clensinge of the house."[13]

The keeper is the second most frequently listed plague occupation in the Newcastle probate records.[14] These women were appointed to infected households to nurse and care for the sick in their homes, often being shut up for weeks at a time (Figure 10.3).[15] In return, many were the recipients of generous testamentary bequests in addition to their wages. Ann Milborne, a survivor of the 1636 outbreak

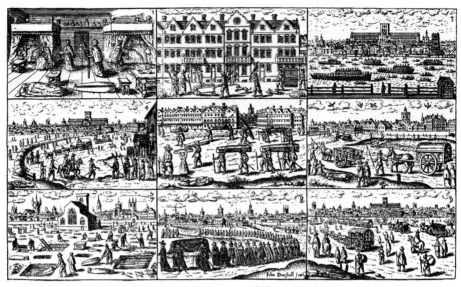

FIGURE 10.3: Scenes of the plague in London, 1665. The image in the top left corner depicts women performing various healing duties in a sick chamber. (Courtesy of the Wellcome Collection.)

of plague in Newcastle, thanked her keeper, Jane Forster, with twenty shillings and some linen. John Laverrock, another survivor of the 1636 outbreak, gave five shillings to Anne Bell "for her paynes' in nursing him."[16]

In addition to their medical duties, keepers were also responsible for maintaining contact between the infected and the outside world. Robert Greenwell, a contemporary merchant, told his keeper Elizabeth Browne "how he would dispose of his estate", information that she related out of the window to John Netherwood, who prepared a will on Greenwell's behalf.[17] Similarly, we know from testimony that same year of chapman (itinerant dealer or peddler) William Robson's former keeper that he "declared his mind" to her "by worde of mouth" since "noe Clarke could be gott to write the same."[18] It appears that, although appointed for a short period of time in severe circumstances, a great deal of trust existed between the sufferer and his or her keeper.

Keepers and cleansers were taken from the lowest levels of the social strata. Many were poor, old, and widowed, but this does not appear to have had an impact upon their employability by those above them in social standing. The majority of those who employed these women were listed as "yeomen" in their wills. This term was often used to describe status, rather than occupation.[19] The remaining occupations included millers, slaters, cordwainers, tailors, musicians/

minstrels, skippers, merchants, coopers, weavers, bakers, and beer brewers.[20] The homes of such individuals in the city would likely have been clustered around the main thoroughfare that lay from the central market down to the populous Sand-hill area and on toward the quayside. Poor, female healers would regularly have traversed the boundaries between the crowded, poorer areas of the city and into the larger, wealthy homes and premises of the middling sort.

In paying recipients of poor relief to assist plague sufferers, London parishes drew upon a circle or cycle of obligation in which tasks performed by women, previously performed as a result of private arrangements, slowly became institutionalized during the late 16th and early 17th centuries. This gradual shift may be why poor women were eventually appointed to be the hands and eyes of the state in the domestic spaces of the parish, because they were already there.[21] In Newcastle, however, it appears that this phenomenon of labor had not yet risen to the level of requiring parish compensation and relied almost entirely on existing structures of obligation within the community. The evidence of this labor exists in payments to keepers and cleansers listed in the inventories of the deceased and in testamentary gifts and bequests, rather than institutional arrangements. The plague thus provided the impetus for the creation of organized networks of care, but these networks relied upon the strong bonds of mutual assistance already present in the community.

Conclusion

The wills and inventories of Newcastle plague victims demonstrate that the city's inhabitants were cared for by a relatively informal sisterhood of women who continued to serve the needs of their community at great risk to their own well-being. The keepers and cleansers of Newcastle were an essential part of the city's attempts to control and monitor the spread of disease. But that is not all. Their existence also challenges assumptions concerning the divisive nature of this disease. Writing in 1636, the Newcastle cleric Robert Jenison asserted that the plague was a force that "scatters us from one another" and "deprives a man of comforters in his greatest agonie and need."[22] Historian James Amelang has since argued that the disease caused "the breakdown of the normal relations of friendship, neighborhood, and family and kin obligations, which had previously united and bound the urban community."[23]

However, a historical micro-study of the 1636 outbreak of plague in Newcastle challenged this interpretation of the socially divisive nature of plague by demonstrating the strength of individuals' relationships with neighbors, fraternities, guilds, and kin.[24] The actions of the cleansers and keepers of Newcastle provide further evidence of these significant social relationships as an essential part of plague response. Through their commitment to their communities, these women reveal that the bonds of mutual trust and obligation held strong even during times of crisis. The distinctive conditions created by the plague facilitated the creation of informal networks of care, which traversed both social and geographical boundaries and ultimately strengthened social solidarities within urban communities.

NOTES

1. Jean-Noël Biraben, "Plague in Britain," in *The Plague Reconsidered: A New Look at Its Origins and Effects in Sixteenth- and Seventeenth-Century England* (Derbyshire: Local Population Studies, 1977), 27; Paul Slack, *The Impact of Plague in Tudor and Stuart England*, (Oxford: Oxford University Press, 1991), 8; A. Appleby, "Disease or Famine? Mortality in Cumberland and Westmorland 1580–1640," *The Economic History Review* 26, no. 3 (1973): 404.

2. Ian Mortimer, *The Dying and the Doctors: The Medical Revolution in Seventeenth-Century England* (Woodbridge: Royal Historical Society, 2004), 206.

3. Andrew Burn, "Work before Play: The Occupational Structure of Newcastle upon Tyne, 1600-1700," in *Economy and Culture in North-East England 1500–1800*, ed. Adrian Green and Barbara Crosbie (Suffolk: Boydell and Brewer, 2019), 118.

4. Andrew Burn, "Work and Society in Newcastle upon Tyne, c. 1600–1710" (Ph.D. diss., Durham University, 2014), 17.

5. John Hatcher, *The History of the British Coal Industry: Vol I: Before 1700: Towards the Age of Coal* (Oxford: Oxford University Press, 1993), 45.

6. Burn, "Work and Society," 39.

7. Keith Wrightson, " 'That Lamentable Time': Catastrophe and Community in the Great Newcastle Plague of 1636," in *Newcastle and Gateshead before 1700*, ed. Diana Newton and A. J. Pollard (Chichester: Phillimore, 2009), 241–64.

8. Ibid.

9. Richard Welford, *History of Newcastle and Gateshead Vol III: Sixteenth & Seventeenth Centuries* (London: Walter Scott, 1887), 56, 116, 117, 123, 230, 263, 337. For the 1636 plague outbreak, see Keith Wrightson, *Ralph Tailor's Summer: A Scrivener, his city and the plague* (New Haven, CT: Yale University Press, 2011).

10. Leona Skelton, *Sanitation in Urban Britain, 1560-1700* (London: Routledge, 2016), 36–40.

11. See Diane Willen, "Women in the Public Sphere in Early Modern England: The Case of the Urban Working Poor," *The Sixteenth Century Journal* 19 (1988): 559–75.

12. See Neil Murphy, "Plague Ordinances and the Management of Infectious Disease in Northern French Towns c. 1450–c.1560," in *The Fifteenth Century XII: Society in an Age of Plague*, ed. Linda Clark and Carole Rawcliffe (Suffolk: Boydell and Brewer, 2013), 23.

13. Durham University Library Archives and Special Collections (DUL), DPRI/1/1570/C5/2–3. *Colles* (coal) was often used for cleansing as a cheaper alternative to frankincense, pitch, and resin.

14. Twenty-six percent of the surviving plague inventories consulted in this study refer to the services of a keeper.

15. Richelle Munkhoff, "Poor Women and Parish Public Health in Sixteenth-Century London," *Renaissance Studies* 28, no. 4 (2014): 579–96.

16. DUL, DPRI/1/1636/M6/1; DPRI/1/1637/L4/1.

17. DUL, DPRI/1/1636/G12/1–2.

18. DUL, DDR/EJ/CCD/2, fo. 2v.

19. Keith Wrightson, *English Society 1580-1680* (London: Routledge, 2002), 28.

20. DUL, DPRI/1/1585/G1; DPRI/1/1610/K1; DPRI/1/1625/C8; DPRI/1/1636/C5; DPRI/1/1636/R10; DPRI/1/1636/G8; DPRI/1/1636/G12; DPRI/1/1636/E2; DPRI/1/1636/H6; DPRI/1/1637/W1; DPRI/1/1637/R12; DPRI/1/1637/H10.

21. Munkhoff, "Poor Women and Parish Public Health," 581.

22. Robert Jenison, *Newcastle's Call to Her Neighbour and Sister Townes and Cities throughout the Land, to Take Warning by her Sins and Sorrows Lest This Overflowing Scourge of Pestilence Reach Even to Them Also* (London: Printed for Iohn Coleby at the signe of the Vnicorne neere to Fleet Bridge, 1637), 35.

23. James Amelang. "Introduction: Popular Narrative and the Plague," in *A Journal of the Plague Year: The Diary of Barcelona Tanner Miquel Parets 1651*, ed. James S. Amelang (Oxford: Oxford University Press, 1991), 4–5.

24. See Wrightson, " 'That Lamentable Time'."

11

The Jewish Ghetto as a Space of Quarantine in Prague, 1713

Joshua Teplitsky

In the cities and towns of what was once Habsburg Bohemia and Moravia, now part of the Czech Republic, the memory of plague is often built into the public spaces of urban life. Looming over many a town square stands a memorial pillar at the top of which rises a statue of the Virgin Mary, glorious in her triumph over two contagions: the heresy of Protestantism and epidemic disease (Figure 11.1). These columns mingle civic commemoration with imperial pomp in defining the dominant culture of urban space in the centuries following the Catholic Counter-Reformation of the 16th and 17th centuries.[1] Like much of the rest of Europe, which experienced an outbreak of pestilence at least once a generation during this period, the cities of the Habsburg Monarchy lived under the regular threat of disease. Epidemic disease ravaged Prague in 1649 and again in 1679–80; 30 years after that, plague reared its head one final time in the late summer of 1713. While Prague's Marian column represents the collective civic piety of its Catholic majority, it obscures the epidemic experiences of a sizeable population that was not part of the Catholic fold but was nonetheless part of the fabric of urban life: the large Jewish community. The collective, seemingly uniform, grace commemorated by the pillars stands in stark relief to the ways in which political, social, and medical responses to plague were differentiated by religion and legal standing. These circumstances affected minorities who, at the same time that they became victims of epidemic trauma, were subjected to discriminatory, human-made policies.

Spatial differentiation was a significant component of Habsburg plague policy. In the early 18th century, Habsburg authorities labored to distinguish between healthy and unhealthy regions, even going so far as to establish a

92

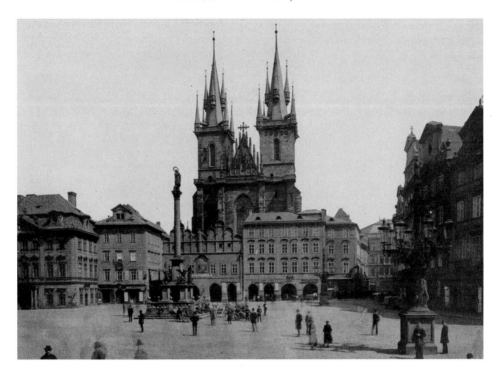

FIGURE 11.1: Marian column, Prague, December 1894. The column was erected in the mid-17th century and demolished with the fall of the Austro-Hungarian monarchy in 1918. (Courtesy of Wikimedia Commons.)

lengthy sanitary cordon on its frontier with the Balkan region of the Ottoman Empire.[2] That approach to differentiated space found a parallel within the topography of the city of Prague, as the physical walls of the Jewish ghetto distinguished between neighborhoods and their inhabitants, even as those areas were sequestered according to the identity of their residents. The urban space of the Prague Jewish ghetto, with its instruments of enclosure, doubled as a site for containment of both the disease and the people accused of its hastening its spread. This already-differentiated space within the Prague cityscape was further accentuated during the outbreak of an epidemic, as the ghetto walls came to serve as a site of collective quarantine. At the same time, however, that space maintained a degree of porousness. The concerted efforts on the part of civil authorities to enclose the city's Jews within the ghetto could not fully diminish the points of contact that crossed religious lines and urban spaces before the outbreak and were part of the rhythms of neighborly exchange between Christians and Jews in the city.

Case study: Quarantine and cultural responses
to the plague in Prague, 1713

Jews had lived in Prague since the early medieval period, and by the start of the 18th century their numbers had risen to over eleven thousand, making them nearly a quarter of the city's population.[3] A tolerated minority in the city, in many ways more tolerated than Protestants, Jews enjoyed the formal protection of the Habsburg monarchs on account of their economic utility; yet this economic role was often the basis of local challenges to their presence.[4] Prague's Jewish Ghetto, called the "Jewish Town" by contemporary authorities, held a semiautonomous status (Figure 11.2). The Jewish Town was distinct politically as well as spatially and was separated from the rest of the city by walls with entrance gates.[5] The neighborhood had its own town hall, in which sat a Jewish elected leadership, its

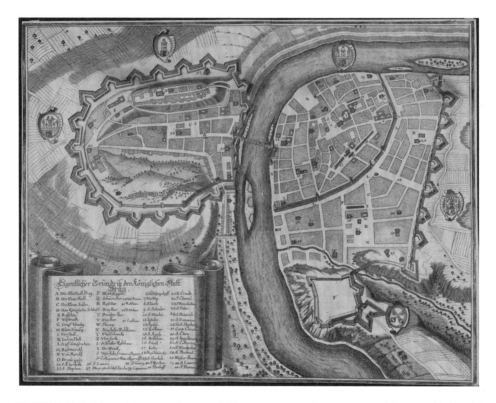

FIGURE 11.2: Map of Prague. The Jewish Town was spatially a portion of the so-called "Old Town" of the city, on the northern portion of the right bank of the Moldau. In this map, from ca. 1650, the ghetto walls are not presented. ("Eigentlicher Grundtriss der königlichen Statt Prag," in Merian Matthäus and Martin Zeiler, *Topographia Bohemiae, Moraviae et Silesiae*, Frankfurt am Main, 1650.)

own places of worship, and a separate welfare sector of schools, charitable institutions, midwives, apothecaries, and surgeons.[6] It was also an overcrowded site,
with thousands of residents distributed throughout only a few hundred buildings.

When the plague struck Prague in July 1713, the Habsburg offices paid particular attention to this crowded urban neighborhood. Edicts issued from the capital in Vienna often distinguished between the instructions for the city as a whole
and for the Jewish Town, ostensibly to protect the non-Jewish residents of the city
from contact with Jews, who were thought to be the vector for contagion.[7] On
August 7, 1713, imperial authorities called for the total sealing of the ghetto and
the prohibition of all transit in and out, as well as the closure of the Jewish market,
which stood outside of the ghetto walls and was a site of commerce and exchange
between Christians and Jews. This policy marked the differentiation between the
Jewish Town and the rest of Prague: while the prescribed course of action for the
city called for the sealing of individual houses, the mandated action for the Jewish
quarter sought a wholesale enclosure of the entire neighborhood.

The enclosure policy for Prague's Jewish neighborhood reflects a tension
between containment of Jews within the city and their complete exclusion from
it. During an earlier outbreak in 1680, civil authorities considered expelling the
entire population of the Jewish Town and relocating the Jews to a nearby village.[8] In 1713, rather than seeking the expulsion of Jews and the attendant risk of
spreading the disease further afield in the process, the empire prioritized the Jews'
concentration and isolation to a particular quarter of the city, tightly regulating
their movement through urban and regional space.

The wholesale sealing of the ghetto sowed chaos and bred confusion and
trauma. Repeated edicts sent from Vienna to Prague in the later weeks of August
and the start of September 1713 reveal that although the order to seal the ghetto
was issued in early August the execution of that order was only implemented
slowly. The Habsburg imperial offices vented their frustration on August 18,
finding it "not a little strange" that their instructions to temporarily seal the
Jewish ghetto and shut down its market were not fulfilled.[9] The failure to follow
these orders would certainly, they believed, result in "the wider lingering of the
infection" and its spread to other locations.[10] Compounded with the eviction of
all foreign Jews from the city and the refusal of the rural nobles to grant Jews permission to stay on their lands, the state's initial efforts to halt the rapid spread of
the disease had been undermined by local interests.

Still, the grip of the authorities on the ghetto continued to tighten, prompting
the flight of Jews who possessed the resources and contacts to escape and seek
refuge elsewhere. This process of flight bred further chaos and fear as the departure
of the Jewish economic and cultural elite undermined solidarity and upset the
social order. A Yiddish narrative written after the plague's end mourned the way

that "this departure created great turmoil in the community, enough to break one's heart and spirit."[11] The ghetto's complete enclosure by late August had calamitous effects. On September 11, 1713, some four weeks after the decision was issued to seal the ghetto and shut the marketplace down, the Prague Elders wrote to the authorities expressing the dire straits of the Jewish community, which had been left "helpless and wretched and desperate."[12] Sealing the ghetto had made food scarce, cut off medical supplies and personnel, had made even the removal of the dead extremely difficult, and had consigned the healthy to inevitable infection and death.

Yet the very orders that conveyed the efforts of the state to turn the ghetto into a site of quarantine also offer evidence of the regular urban contacts across religious lines that the authorities sought to diminish. The enclosure of the space of the ghetto and the curtailment of Jewish-Christian encounters reveal the preexisting norms of neighborliness that preceded the crisis. For example, the state's early plague instructions, from July 31, aimed to end the interactions that resulted from the domestic labor practice of Christian and Jewish washerwomen who regularly conducted their tasks side by side.[13] On the opposite end of the social spectrum, the potential for mutual trust across religious lines was expressed in the language of an edict that condemned healthy Jews who, fleeing from the city and fearing for the belongings they would necessarily leave behind, deposited their goods with Christian householders in the healthier areas outside the Jewish Town rather than with other Jews.[14] In other instances, Jews who were trapped inside of the sealed ghetto who sought exemptions from the harsh measures of the ghetto's closure relied upon the familiarity of Christian neighbors to attest to their responsible behavior (Figure 11.3). Such was the case for a Prague Jew named Anschel Güntzburger, who marshalled the support of Christian neighbors in mid-September to demonstrate to his vigilance in isolating his home from social contact. Güntzburger's neighbors signed an affidavit, indicating that such familiarity and reliance were not severed by the epidemic's arrival nor by the state's fiat.[15]

The Prague plague of 1713 claimed between a quarter and a third of the lives of the city's residents. For the Jews, a combination of long-standing urban neglect and direct discrimination resulted in a horrific number of deaths, experiences of chaos, disorder and emotional and psychological trauma, and the lasting guilt and pain resulting from the indignities suffered by the dead. Jewish life resumed some of its rhythms in the months and years that followed, but the plague left its impact in the loss of life and on memorial and commemorative activities within the Jewish community. Plague may even have facilitated fresh efforts at reducing the Jewish population of the city: a month after the worst of the plague subsided, the authorities began to devise a strategy to further reduce the Jewish population.

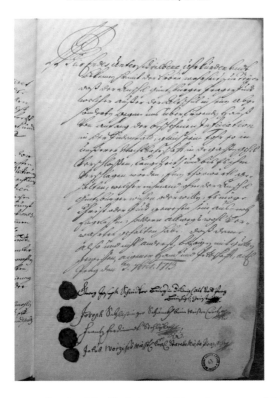

FIGURE 11.3: Signatures and seals of the Christian neighbors in support of Anschel Güntzburger (September 11, 1713). Three of the signatories give their names in German, the fourth in Czech. (Courtesy of Národní Archiv, Prague, Ms. SM 842/E2/16: fol. 63v.)

Conclusion

The surviving sources from the Prague plague of 1713 highlight the dynamics and dynamism of plague response in this urban center. As a minority in the city, the Jewish population experienced both the impact of disease as well as discrimination at the hands of policy-makers. Yet the language of edicts and affidavits reveals that social contacts with Christian neighbors of all social classes continued even under duress. Minorities are often vulnerable to neglect in public health initiatives and can disproportionately feel the impact of an epidemic. Anti-Jewish plague policy caused great hardship, even as the contribution to overall public health remains in question.

The impact of the epidemic response in the urban space of the Prague ghetto was built upon the indifference of the state, preexisting policies, political arrangements, and social exchanges. On the one hand, the ghetto was a space ready for wholescale enclosure, and on the other, it maintained points of contact and support. The encounter between ordinary Jews and Christians in plague-ridden Prague was based on the rhythms of engagement and the domains within which neighbors shared urban spaces and the structures of daily and civic life across social divides. In spite of Habsburg desires, plague did not respect walls, boundaries, or borders, meaning Prague in 1713 was only as healthy as its least healthy neighborhood.

NOTES

1. R. J. W. Evans, *The Making of the Habsburg Monarchy, 1550–1700: An Interpretation* (Oxford: Clarendon Press, 1979), 444–46; Howard Louthan, *Converting Bohemia: Force and Persuasion in the Catholic Reformation* (Cambridge: Cambridge University Press, 2009), 273–74.

2. Gunther E. Rothenberg, "The Austrian Sanitary Cordon and the Control of the Bubonic Plague: 1710–1871," *Journal of the History of Medicine and Allied Sciences* 28, no. 1 (1973).

3. On the built environment of Prague and Jewish life, see Rachel L. Greenblatt, *To Tell Their Children: Jewish Communal Memory in Early Modern Prague* (Stanford, CA: Stanford University Press, 2014), 11–46.

4. Jaroslav Prokeš and Anton Blaschka, "Der Antisemitismus der Behörden und das Prager Ghetto in nachweißenbergischer Zeit" [The Anti-Semitism of the Authorities and the Prague Ghetto in the Post-White Mountain Era], *Jahrbuch der Gesellschaft für Geschichte der Juden in der Čechoslovakischen Republik* 1 (1929): 41–262.

5. Milada Vilímková, *The Prague Ghetto* (Prague: Aventinum, 1993), 33–34.

6. On the terminology of Jewish quarters and ghettos, see Benjamin Ravid, "All Ghettos Were Jewish Quarters but Not All Jewish Quarters Were Ghettos," *Jewish Culture and History* 10, nos. 2–3 (2008): 5–24.

7. Národní Archiv, Prague, Ms. Stará manipulace (hereafter SM) 842/E2/16, box no 663: fol. 16v.

8. Michael Rachmuth, "Der Plan einer Verlegung des Prager Ghettos nach Lieben 1680" [The Plan to Move the Prague Ghetto to Lieben in 1680], *Jahrbuch der Gesellschaft für Geschichte der Juden in der Čechoslovakischen Republik* 6 (1934): 145–56.

9. Národní Archiv, Prague, Ms. SM 842/E2/16, box no 663: fol. 10v.

10. Ibid.

11. Moses ben Hayyim Eisenstadt, *Eyn Nay Kloglid* (Amsterdam, n.d.), 2r. For a variant translation of this text into English, see Sylvie Anne Goldberg, *Crossing the Jabbok: Illness and Death in Ashkenazi Judaism in Sixteenth- through Nineteenth-Century Prague*

(Berkeley: University of California Press, 1996), 163. See also Chava Turniansky, "Yiddish Song as Historical Source Material: Plague in the Judenstadt of Prague in 1713," in *Jewish History: Essays in Honour of Chimen Abramsky*, ed. Chimen Abramsky, Ada Rapoport-Albert and Steven J. Zipperstein (London: Peter Halban, 1988), 189–98.

12. Národní Archiv, Prague, Ms. SM 842/E2/16: fol. 67r.

13. Ibid., fol. 3v.

14. Jewish Museum of Prague Ms. 120064 "Kopialbuch of David Oppenheim," §145, 462.

15. Národní Archiv, Prague, Ms. SM 842/E2/16, box no 663: fols. 62–64.

12

Hygiene and Urban Life in the "District of Death" in 19th-Century Istanbul

Fezanur Karaağaçlıoğlu

The arrival of the Black Death in Istanbul during the mid-14th century heralded a nasty cycle of plague epidemics that would continue to ravage the city periodically until the final outbreaks occurred in the mid-19th century (Figure 12.1). During this time, plague appeared in the city regularly, although differing in severity and duration. The last two most severe epidemics—in 1812–13 and 1836–37—caused the combined death of more than two hundred thousand people and shaped how the city was perceived by both Europeans and Ottomans.[1] Although plague outbreaks in Europe had largely subsided by the 18th century, their stubborn persistence in the Eastern Mediterranean led to the perception that the incidence of plague was "spatially anchored" to the "diseased" lands of the Levant.[2] Western European visitors who came to Istanbul in the early 19th century and wrote about their visits could contrast the Ottoman city with the plague-free conditions of their cities. The scourge of plague epidemics thus became one of the many exotic features of Istanbul and the subject of accounts by mainly French, German, Austrian, and English travel writers.

Western European visitors would typically stay in the neighborhoods of Galata and Pera, also known as the Frankish district. Located north of the city center and across the Golden Horn, Galata was established in the late 13th century as a Genoese trading colony and grew into a walled town beside Byzantine Constantinople. Pera was an *extra muros* northern extension of Galata, which flourished in the early 18th century. The densely populated district of Galata-Pera was home to a bustling port that saw a constant exchange of people and goods from across the Mediterranean (Figure 12.2). Until 1822, five plague hospitals were administered by Pera's Armenian, Greek, French, Austrian, and Italian communities, each one attached to a cemetery originally reserved for the victims of various epidemics. European sources commonly referred to this stretch of burial grounds as

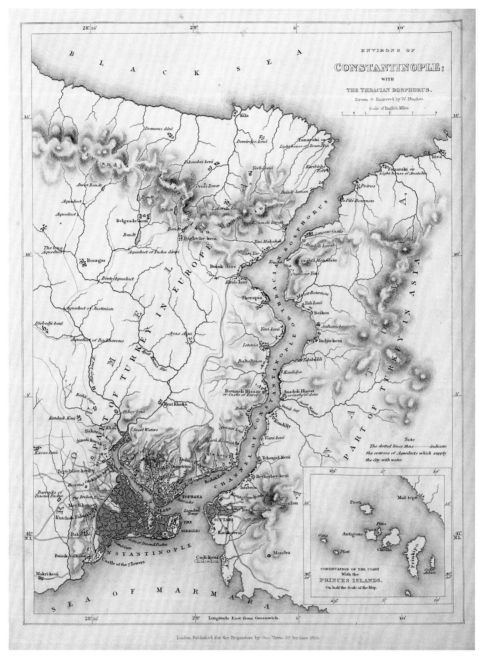

FIGURE 12.1: Map of Istanbul and the Bosporus, 1838, Julia Pardoe, *The Beauties of the Bosphorus* (London, 1838). (Courtesy of Aikaterini Laskaridis Foundation.)

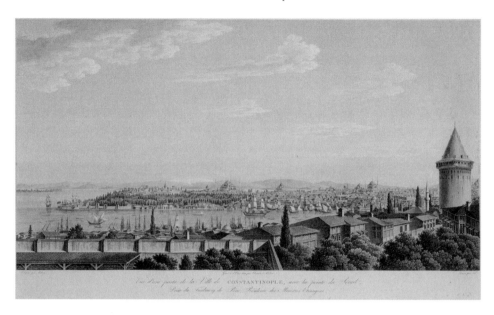

FIGURE 12.2: View of Istanbul from Pera, 1819, Antoine Ignace Melling, *Voyage pittoresque de Constantinople et des rives du Bosphore* [Scenic Journey through Constantinople and the Shores of the Bosporus] (Paris, 1819). (Courtesy of Aikaterini Laskaridis Foundation.)

the *Grands-Champs-des-Morts* (or the Great Burial Ground). European physicians took an interest in Istanbul's plague hospitals, where they had the opportunity to study the disease, test their hypotheses about contagion, and publish their observations.

Case study: Plague visibility in Galata-Pera

In its uncomplicated form, plague is a vector-borne infectious disease that is not directly transmitted through physical contact or close proximity between humans. The bacillus may be carried from person to person via ectoparasites such as fleas or body lice. However, if bubonic plague advances to the lungs and becomes pneumonic, it can turn contagious. This must have contributed to the misconception that it was a "contagious" illness. Still, the theory of "contagion" offered a seemingly convincing explanation for the spread of plague: that immediate contact with the patient or their belongings caused infection. In particular, it was thought that the disease spread via invisible, poisonous "seeds," which were not always differentiated from miasmatic emanations but believed to reproduce within the sick body and stick onto anything it touched. This theory remained popular—but not unchallenged—in European medicine throughout the early 19th century. Europeans in Istanbul became known for their "Frankish measures," including quarantine, which, while long in use in Europe, was not officially established and broadly implemented in the Ottoman Empire until 1838–39. That same year, the Ottomans collaborated with the European community on political, educational, commercial, and sanitary issues to establish the Quarantine Council in Galata.

Galata-Pera was inhabited by both non-Muslim and Muslim Ottomans as well as Western Europeans. Daily life presented manifold possibilities to come into contact with the different communities living in the city. European accounts record the potential for shock and inspiration in encounters between different ethno-religious groups. These impressions were, of course, based on outsiders' perceptions of the Ottoman people filtered through the prism of confessional identities as well as influenced by the orientalizing images found in travel literature.[3] Muslims were always described as essentially different in their response to the plague—such that being physically near them during outbreaks could be a frightening experience.[4] Western European visitors portrayed non-Muslims as followers of the principles of quarantine and sanitary measures such as fumigation. European accounts also reveal the extent to which the plague affected and infected the spaces of Galata-Pera. Hospitals, cemeteries, churches, and altars dedicated to intercessory figures such as St. Roch, St. Anthony, St. Charalambos, and Panagia (the Virgin Mary) filled the neighborhood while "plague priests"[5] and physicians sporting waxed taffeta cloaks perambulated. The northern end of Pera was viewed eerily as the somber grounds for hospitals and cemeteries (Figure 12.3).[6]

During plague seasons, wealthy Perote (the non-Muslim Ottoman dwellers of Pera) and European merchants and embassy staff would retreat to their country estates or summer embassies in the villages along the Bosporus Strait or on the Princes' Islands off the Istanbul coast. This practice of seasonal relocation reflected an awareness of the need to flee Pera to avoid contact with infectious individuals, as well as their clothes and belongings, on crowded streets. The wealthy could afford to arrange for separate living spaces for the sick if necessary, as well as to delegate the conduct of their business affairs in Galata-Pera to non-Muslim intermediaries. With matters settled so, they could avail themselves of the fresh air and sea breeze of the coast—a beautiful and freeing environment that was widely thought to be effective in beating the plague.

In certain neighborhoods—especially those that were known for other menaces—disease outbreaks were sometimes understood as a natural and inevitable occurrence. More broadly, European authors would describe the climatic and topographical conditions or the habits of "nations" (religio-cultural groups) as factors in the spread of diseases. Specifically, they would ascribe the persistence of epidemic diseases in some districts, but not others, to differences in living

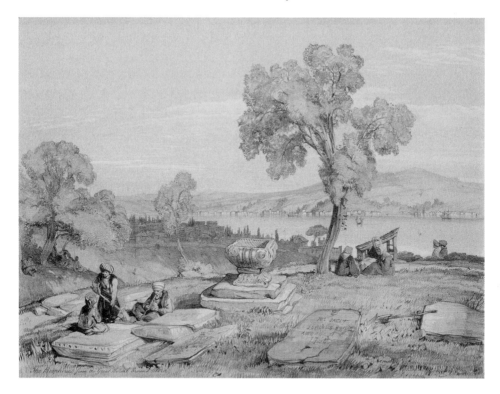

FIGURE 12.3: The Great Burial Ground, 1838, John F. Lewis, *Lewis's Illustrations of Constantinople Made during a Residence in That City in the Years 1835–6* (London, 1838). (Courtesy of Aikaterini Laskaridis Foundation.)

conditions, poverty levels, and urban planning and public health and hygiene policies. European authors' observations concerning Galata-Pera's neighboring districts, largely inhabited by Greeks and Jews, address the links between poverty and the socio-economic backgrounds of the victims of epidemics.[7]

Western European visitors to Istanbul vividly described their fears of the near-constant exposure to supposed contagion while walking in the streets of Galata-Pera. First and foremost, the "Turks" (Ottoman Muslims) embodied this danger, as they seemingly would not take any precautions or care for securing distance between themselves and others.[8] Regular commuters between Galata-Pera and other parts of the city, including dragoman guides and Armenians who visited Pera for religious services and family gatherings, were also feared as groups whose actions could not be controlled or checked. The Europeans and the Perote would try to protect themselves by using intermediaries to engage with the outside world. They would also avoid the restaurants and cafés where merchants, chefs, bachelors, voyagers, seamen, and other potentially infected people spent time, as well as customs such as handshaking or card games. Plague was often the concluding theme of conversations; one would never—despite one's good manners—pick up a lady's handkerchief from the floor, and no social gatherings could take place at theaters, balls, clubs, and salons.[9] However, churches remained open and, indeed, crowded with Perote, Catholic Armenians, and Greeks.[10]

Plague hospitals were associated with impoverished patients, servants, and migrants to Pera. The visiting European and Perote tended to be suspicious of servants, who they feared would not reveal their illness unless absolutely necessary. Plague hospitals were possibly dreaded as much as the plague itself. Indeed, "fear" was a common theme throughout contemporary European accounts, both in reference to others and as a personal feeling.

The European physicians who worked in or visited the local hospitals in Istanbul were highly critical of the operations of these facilities. For example, they identified the practice in the hospitals of keeping or selling the personal belongings of patients who died of plague as problematic and as evidence of failure to adhere to protective measures. Already in the 18th century, European scholars had begun to expect other professionals to contribute to the development of scientific knowledge for the good of humanity. Accordingly, Western European physicians in Istanbul sought equivalent scholarly motivations and endeavors in the Ottoman Empire but were met with disappointment, which became a recurrent theme in their writings.[11] They attributed the Ottoman doctors' lack of interest in researching the severe and continuous presence of the plague to a kind of "Islamic fatalism." Some Europeans even speculated that the Ottomans may have had ulterior motives for not researching diseases. For instance, the French physician Albert Brayer (1775–1848), who resided in Istanbul between 1815 and 1827 to do research on plague, supposed that it was possibly a deliberate choice to leave the incidence of plague largely unexamined, because, wickedly, one could more easily blame a murder on the plague if there was no one to call for a thorough inspection.[12]

Conclusion

How and in what terms people define diseases, not only medically but also culturally, influence how they are approached and dealt with. In cases of epidemics, these definitions influence perceptions of all the actors involved in urban life by underscoring certain aspects of city topographies and common practices. In accordance with these influences, cities may be classified as either salubrious or insalubrious, safe or dangerous. In Istanbul, plague had a definite and immediate impact on urban life. Since the nature of this disease had remained misunderstood for centuries, outbreaks brought about different responses.

In contrast to the majority of the Ottomans, many Western European and Perote contemporaries were in search of safety from disease in the openness of fresh air and wide spaces. Galata-Pera appeared to them as damp, dark, and dirty—a poisonous landscape. European visitors, including physicians, saw in Galata-Pera a kind of medical topography, both in terms of contagion and miasma. This topographical view provided visitors with guidelines for safely navigating the city. The writings of Western European visitors suggest that they believed this view was indecipherable for both Muslim and non-Muslim Ottomans. Consequently, visitors to Istanbul would often say that the movements and actions of the local population were dangerous and arbitrary with regard to mitigating the spread of diseases. The accounts reveal an experience of Galata-Pera that was based on knowledge and awareness for which writers could find no cognate in the district. Due to the different responses and epidemiological experiences, the plague was easily instrumentalized in Orientalist discourses.

Acknowledgement: This article is produced from the author's MA thesis: "Epidemics, Urban Life, and Sanitation: Pera and the End of the Plague" (Boğaziçi University, 2019). A version of this article with the title "Exotic and Toxic? Plague in Early Nineteenth-Century Galata-Pera" is published in *YILLIK: Annual of Istanbul Studies* 2 (2020): 7–34.

NOTES

1. Nükhet Varlık, "İstanbul'da Veba Salgınları," trans. Ahmet Aydoğan, in *Antik Çağ'dan XXI. Yüzyıla Büyük İstanbul Tarihi Cilt IV (Toplum)*, ed. Coşkun Yılmaz [Plague Epidemics in Istanbul] (Istanbul: İstanbul Büyükşehir Belediyesi Kültür Yayınları, 2015), 146–51.

2. Nükhet Varlık, " 'Oriental Plague' or Epidemiological Orientalism? Revisiting the Plague Episteme of the Early Modern Mediterranean," in *Plague and Contagion in the Islamic Mediterranean*, ed. Nükhet Varlık (Kalamazoo, MI: Arc Humanities Press, 2017), 66.

3. Sonja Brentjes, "Introduction," in *Travellers from Europe in the Ottoman and Safavid Empires, 16th–17th Centuries: Seeking, Transforming, Discarding Knowledge*, ed. Sonja Brentjes (London: Routledge, 2016), ix–xxix.

4. See and cf., e.g., Helmuth von Moltke, *Briefe über Zustände und Begebenheiten in der Türkei aus den Jahren 1835 bis 1839* [Letters about the Conditions and Occurrences in Turkey from the Years 1835 to 1839] (Berlin: Ernst Siegfried Mittler, 1841), 116; Albert Brayer, *Neuf années à Constantinople: observations sur la topographie de cette capitale, l'hygiene et les moeurs de ses habitants, l'Islamisme et son influence, la peste ses causes, ses variétés, sa marche et son traitement; la non-contagion de cette maladie; les quarantaines et ses lazarets avec une carte de Constantinople et du Bosphore de Thrace* [Nine Years in Constantinople: Observations on the Topography of This Capital, the Hygiene and Customs of Its Inhabitants, Islamism and Its Influence, the Plague Its Causes, Its Varieties, Its

Progress and Its Treatment; the Non-Contagion of This Disease; the Quarantines and Its Lazarets with a Map of Constantinople and the Bosporus of Thrace] (Paris: Belizard, 1836), vol. 2, 102–4.

5. The priests who administered the plague hospitals and for whom Christians would send for when suspecting having caught the disease. See ibid., 470–72.

6. See, e.g., Anton Prokesch von Osten, *Denkwürdigkeiten und Erinnerungen aus dem Orient, vol. I* [Memorabilia and Memories from the Orient] (Stuttgart: Hallberger'sche Verlagshandlung, 1836), 483; François-Alphonse Belin, *La Latinité de Constantinople: champs du repos, rites funéraires d'après les Comptes-rendus du Cimetière latin* [Constantinople of the Latins: Cemeteries, and Funerary Rites according to the Records of the Latin Cemetery], ed. Rinaldo Marmara (Montpellier: Université Paul Valéry, Université Montpellier III, 2004).

7. See Brayer, *Neuf années à Constantinople*, vol. 1: 25, 399; Francis Hervé, *A Residence in Greece and Turkey with Notes on the Journey through Bulgaria, Servia, Hungary and the Balkan*, vol. 2 (London: Whittaker, 1837), 122–23; Antonio Baratta, *Bellezze del Bosforo ossia panorama del maraviglioso canale di Costantinopoli preceduto da un' accurata descrizione dello stretto dei dardanelli e del Mar di Marmara...* [Beauties of the Bosporus or Panorama of the Marvelous Channel of Constantinople Preceded by an Accurate Description of the Dardanelles Strait and the Sea of Marmara...] (Torino: Stabilimento Tipografico Fontana, 1841), 416; Charles Maclean, *Results of an Investigation Regarding Epidemic and Pestilential Diseases Including Researches in the Levant Concerning the Plague*, vol. 1 (London: Thomas and George Underwood, 1817), 259–65.

8. Nükhet Varlık, *Plague and Empire in the Early Modern Mediterranean World: The Ottoman Experience 1347–1600* (New York: Cambridge University Press, 2015), 72–88.

9. Hervé, *A Residence in Greece and Turkey*, vol. 2: 179; Prokesch von Osten, *Denkwürdigkeiten und Erinnerungen*, vol. 1: 482–488; Moltke, *Briefe über Zustände*, 119.

10. French contagionists were known for avoiding mass.

11. See Brayer, *Neuf années à Constantinople*, vol. 2: 471–72; Dr. Burghardt, "Nachricht über die Behandlungsweise der Pestkranken in den Pestspitälern zu Konstantinopel" [Information on How the Plague-Infected are Treated in the Plague Hospitals of Constantinople], *Medizinische Jahrbücher des kaiserlichen königlichen österreichischen Staates* 4, no. 1 (1817): 109–14.

12. Brayer, *Neuf années à Constantinople*, vol. 2: 122. It is possible to detect the trope of the "Oriental intriguer" in the European accounts. However, there are Ottoman documents which give a similar impression that it was not unlikely that some people would try to conceal a murder as a natural death from plague. Varlık, *Plague and Empire*, 264, 288, 289.

13

Religious Rituals and Cholera in the Shrine Cities of 19th-Century Iran

Fuchsia Hart

The Iranian cities of Mashhad and Qom are associated with the highly venerated shrines around which they have developed. Mashhad (with the literal meaning of "martyrium") in the far east of today's Iran is home to the shrine that, according to Twelver Shi'i traditions, houses the remains of 'Ali b. Musa (*d. c.*818), who is commonly referred to as Imam Reza (Figure 13.1).[1] Imam Reza is recognized as the eighth of the Twelve Imams, the religious and political leaders revered by Twelver Shi'i Muslims. His sister, Fatima (*d. c.*817), commonly referred to by the epithet *Ma'sumeh* (the Infallible One), is buried in the central Iranian city of Qom (Figure 13.2). These two sites have long been among the most significant holy complexes within Iran, canonized as pilgrimage destinations since the 10th-century crystallization of Twelver Shi'i practice.

These shrines and the cities in which they are situated have long suffered from epidemic disease, such as plague. A record of one such outbreak is given by the Qajar court poet Fath 'Ali Khan Saba in a poem lamenting an outbreak of plague in Qom in the early 19th century.[2] However, throughout the rest of the 19th century, the shrine cities of Mashhad and Qom became the victims of a new disease, experiencing numerous outbreaks of cholera, as did Iran more widely. Cholera is an acute diarrheal infection of the intestine, spread through food and water carrying *Vibrio cholerae* bacteria. The disease can be described as a "fecal-oral" infection, as food and water may be contaminated by traces of the feces of victims.[3] The bacteria are incubated by the warmth of the stomach, but it is only when the body begins to destroy the bacteria that its harmful poison is released. The main symptoms are vomiting and acute diarrhea, which causes a severe loss of body fluid that can lead to death.

Cholera bacteria first entered Iran from India, where the earliest recorded epidemic of the infection broke out in 1817. James Baillie Fraser (1783–1856), the Scottish artist and writer, arrived in Iran shortly after the first wave of cholera and

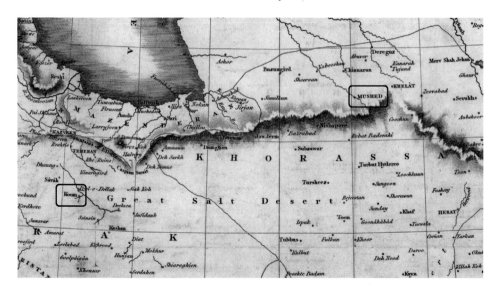

FIGURE 13.1: Detail from Aaron Arrowsmith's "Map of Persia and adjacent countries, for Sir John Malcolm's History of Persia" (London: I. Murray, 1815), showing Qom ("Koom") to the south of Tehran and Mashhad ("Mushed") in the east of the country. (Courtesy of Library of Congress, Geography and Map Division.)

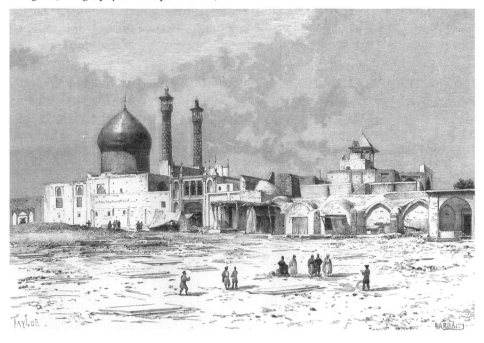

FIGURE 13.2: Mausoleum of Fatima in Qom with cemetery in the foreground. Jane Dieulafoy, "Tombeau de Fatma a Koum," *La Perse, La Chaldée et La Susiane* (Paris: Librarie Hachette et Cie, 1887), 187.

lamented the lack of understanding of the dreadful infection at the time: "[L]ittle on the whole could be gathered, either here or at Muscat, calculated to throw much additional light either on the nature of epidemic cholera, or on the means by which the disease is propagated or conveyed."[4] Largely due to this lack of knowledge, cholera went on to plague Iran and its inhabitants for much of the century, and became the most common epidemic throughout the period.[5]

Importantly, religious shrines and a number of practices associated with them—namely pilgrimage, communal use of water, and burial—were simultaneously affected by and contributed to the spread of cholera in the 19th century. Accounts, largely written by Europeans in Iran, describe the sacred urban landscape of Shi'i shrines and their role within religious life in the context of cholera epidemics. Medical reports and official rulings convey a range of responses to these outbreaks and likewise illuminate the ways in which those responses affected shrines and religious rituals.

Case study: Cholera in 19th-century Qom and Mashhad

Within the context of urban life, shrines facilitated divine intercession, blessings, and salvation, and served as places where people gathered, accessed water, and were buried. These uses may have contributed to the urban spread of cholera. Mashhad, home to the only burial place of an Imam outside of Iraq and the Arabian Peninsula, attracted pilgrims from the east of Iran, as well as from many neighboring countries. During the 19th century, cholera was largely spread by those infected with the bacteria who moved from place to place, including during pilgrimage.

Devotees would be encouraged to touch and even kiss the fabric of the shrines of these great religious institutions, moving from the thresholds and doors to the structures covering the graves themselves. Ritual praxis within these spaces from their foundation until the 19th century likely changed very little, and the small, dim, enclosed central shrine chambers would often be densely packed with a throng of pilgrims, all jostling for contact with the holy tomb. When East India Company (EIC) officer Arthur Conolly (1807–1842) traveled through Iran on his way to India in the Islamic month of Muharram in 1829, he entered the mosque within the Mashhad shrine complex, finding it "crowded to the extremity."[6] The shrines were frequented all year round for myriad reasons, so several factors could compound the potential efficiency of these spaces as vectors for infection.

A pilgrim would commonly resort to a shrine on the occasion of prayers made for relief from illness. An example is given in the memoirs of the Qajar prince 'Ayn al-Saltana (1872–1945), who recorded that he visited the shrine of Fatima in Qom when afflicted with malaria. He sought to treat himself with a list of remedies, among them a drink of water that had been poured over the locks of the tomb (*ab-i qufl*) and a pill made of dust from the tombcover (*zarih*).[7] Another example by Edward Stirling (1797–1873), working in the service of the EIC, recounted the story of a member of the clergy staying in the neighboring chamber while on pilgrimage in Mashhad. The cleric had fallen ill and while he would not take earthly medicine, he claimed to have been offered a drink by Imam Reza during the night, which cured him of his ailments.[8]

Streams and canals associated with the shrines acted as a conduit for waterborne bacteria, such as those that cause cholera. In 19th-century Mashhad, there was "a canal [... which] appears to unite the uses of a drinking fountain, a place of bodily ablution and washing of clothes, a depository for dead animals, and a sewer."[9] This canal ran down the center of the city's principal thoroughfare and through the main courtyard of the shrine, where it would be used for drinking and ablutions (Figure 13.3). At Qom, the British traveler Isabella Bishop (*d.* 1904) described the main waterway as equally noxious: "[T]he Ab-i-Khonsar, which supplies the drinking water, percolates through 'dead men's bones and all

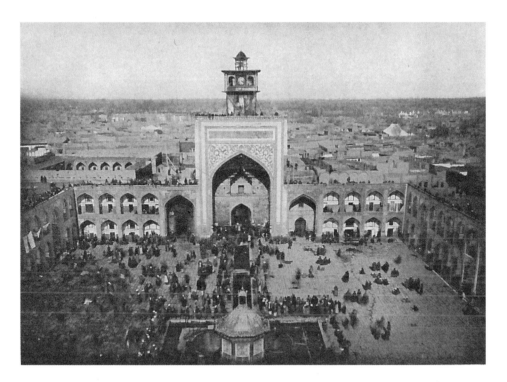

FIGURE 13.3: Canal running through the main court of the shrine of Imam Reza. Major P. M. Sykes, "The 'Old Court,' Showing Nadir's Fountain in the Foreground," in *The Glory of the Shia World: The Tale of a Pilgrimage* (London: Macmillan, 1910), 241.

uncleanness'."[10] The living would wash both themselves and their dead in this water, as well as drinking from it. At the time of a cholera outbreak, such a combination of uses of the water would certainly have accelerated the spread of the disease. To make matters worse, it was believed that submerging a cholera victim in cold water could provide a cure.[11] This certainly did not help the patients and would have had the unfortunate side effect of polluting water systems. This risk was compounded by the religio-legal understanding of running water as pure (*tahir*); stagnant water exceeding one *kurr* (350 liters), regardless of possible pollutants, was also acceptable.[12]

Not unconnected from the matter of water was the practice of burial at these shrines. The presence of so many corpses could compromise the cleanliness of any nearby water sources. Devotees desired burial alongside Imam Reza or his sister to benefit from the blessings brought by proximity, even in death. The dead would be brought from all over the country to their final resting places at Qom and Mashhad, potentially bringing illness with them. At Qom, "the famous *imamzada* [shrine] is preceded by an immense cemetery of tombstones so close together that they cover the ground like paving," and Mashhad was no different, with vast burial grounds radiating from the shrine outwards.[13] The dead were largely transferred to these holy sites in boxes lashed to camels or donkeys. Stirling reported that the corpses underwent "proper cleansing and purifying of the entrails"; the process continued by "somehow drying up the flesh and adding proper spices for the preservation of the flesh, and afterwards wrapping the whole up well in new clothes and putting the corpse in a long box [...] made airtight by wax and other means" (Figure 13.4).[14]

Far from the report of cleansed and spiced burials, others wrote of the noxious smells emanating from the coffins. Lady Sheil (1825–1869), wife of the British Ambassador, explained that "the boxes [were] nailed in the most imperfect manner, admitting of the free exit of the most dangerous exhalations."[15] This final journey of the deceased would often be delayed by practical matters such as inclement weather conditions or the need to accumulate the funds to pay for the burial. Therefore, the dead would be buried immediately, often in shallow graves close to their place of death, to be exhumed and taken to their final, holy resting place at a later date. Sometimes nothing more than a pile of bones remained, but other temporary burials would be in varying states of decomposition and "were generally announced by the most offensive smell."[16] In this way the relocation of burials may have been "sowing not improbably the seed of a fresh outbreak."[17]

Measures to halt the spread of cholera were enacted throughout the 1800s in response to the numerous outbreaks, with scientific sophistication developing as the century proceeded. The most common response to an outbreak, or an impending one, was to leave an urban area for a rural setting. When news reached

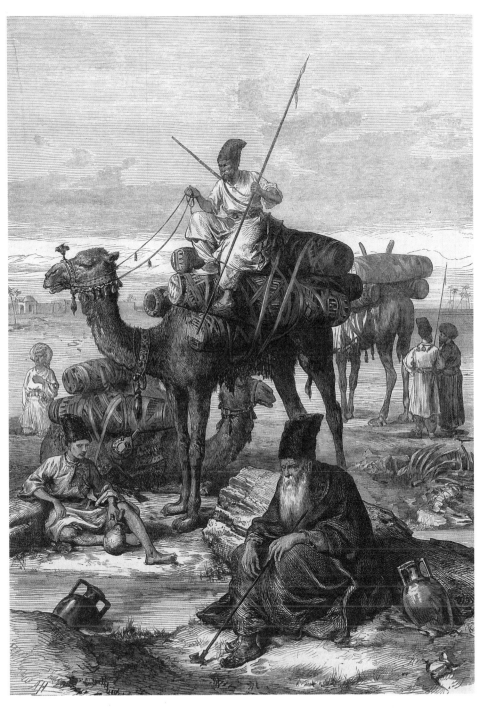

FIGURE 13.4: "Pilgrims with Their Dead Going to the Shrines of Kerbala and Meshid Ali," *London Illustrated News*, June 14, 1873.

Mashhad of the epidemic spreading from the Afghan border early in 1892, those who could do so left the city and "fled to the mountains."[18] Some groups isolated themselves, as seen during the 1892 outbreak in Khorasan, during which tribes from Bujnurd and Ghuskan successfully "interrupted all intercourse between their camps."[19] There were, however, a number of more official and institutionalized responses to the many cholera outbreaks of the 19th century.

The International Sanitary Conference held in Istanbul in 1866 tackled the problem of pilgrims carrying disease directly. Iran was advised to close its borders to devotees making pilgrimages during outbreaks. The problem of transporting the dead was also addressed, with suggestions that the deceased should only be moved in the cooler months and that the coffins should be well sealed.[20] In 1882, following a meeting of the Sanitary Council of Khorasan, a ruling was issued consisting of ten orders that were created "in the interest of the public health of the people of this province" to address public sanitation and use of water.[21] Number three forbade the washing of "clothes and old things" in the city's streams and reservoirs; number eight outlawed latrine pits; number ten emphasized that latrines and wells for drinking water must be dug far apart. In spite of these measures, one out of every nineteen residents of Mashhad died during the 1892 outbreak.[22] In 1897, following the closure of the Herat-Mashhad road by Russian forces in an attempt to stem the flow of disease-carrying pilgrims from Afghanistan, Muzaffar al-Din Shah (r. 1896–1907) issued a decree instituting a program of disinfection and quarantine (unfortunately generally ineffectual) on Iran's eastern border.[23] The Russians, dissatisfied with these measures, maintained the closure of the route until mounting pressure from religious authorities forced them to relent.[24]

Conclusion

The pressure from religious leaders to maintain access to the shrine in Mashhad, along with their ultimate success in doing so, is indicative of the desire to preserve religious life in and around these sacred sites, even during outbreaks of deadly infections such as cholera. The pilgrims who would have continued to flow toward these sites interacted both with the shrines and with wider urban spaces as well. Both of the sites discussed here were, as they still are, embedded within highly urban geographies. Moreover, the shrines and the key aspects of religious life that they supported were in many ways the defining features of the urban life of their respective cities at this time. The crowds that flocked to both urban spaces were drawn by the blessing-bestowing shrines, a pull that did not abate even during times of the most severe epidemics—devotees may have actually been more likely to fill these spaces in times of greatest need, such as during illness. While other cities may have emptied during outbreaks as their inhabitants fled to rural areas, Mashhad and Qom would have continued to see people coming into the city through pilgrimage and burial traffic.

While it was certainly recognized that the practices discussed above—pilgrimage, communal water usage, and burial—may have contributed to outbreaks of disease, access to shrines and the ongoing ability to perform religious rites remained priorities and would have remained a distinctive feature of the urban life of Qom and Mashhad. There is no evidence that access to the shrines was ever restricted in the 19th century with a view to halting the spread of disease. Shrines in urban contexts affected their surroundings during an epidemic, but measures enacted for the prevention of disease never outweighed the seemingly vital continuation of urban, social, and religious life.

NOTES

1. This chapter is based on an article written for the Ajam Media Collective, published in May 2020.

2. Fatḥ ʿAlī Khān Kāshānī Ṣabā and Muḥammad ʿAlī Najātī. *Dīvān-i Ashʿār-i Malik Al-Shuʿarā' Fatḥ ʿAlī Khān Ṣabā* (Tehran: Iqbāl, 1962), 33.

3. Amir Afkhami, "Disease and Water Supply: The Case of Cholera in Nineteenth-Century Iran," in *Transformations of Middle Eastern Natural Environments*, ed. Jeff Albert, Magnus Bernhardsson, and Roger Kenna (New Haven, CT: Yale University Press, 1998), 207.

4. James Baillie Fraser, *Narrative of a Journey into Khorasan in the years 1821 and 1822* (London: Longman, Hurst, Rees, Orme, Brown and Green, 1825), 36.

5. Ahmad Seyf, "Iran and Cholera in the Nineteenth Century," *Middle Eastern Studies* 38, no. 1 (January 2002): 169.

6. Arthur Conolly, *Journey to the North of India, Overland from England, through Russia, Persia, and Affghaunistaun* (London: Richard Bentley, 1834), 273.

7. Willem Floor, *Public Health in Qajar Iran* (Washington, DC: Mage, 2004), 83.

8. Jonathan Lee, ed., *The Journals of Edward Stirling in Persia and Afghanistan, 1828–29, from Manuscripts in the Archives of the Royal Geographical Society* (Naples: Istituto Universitario Orientale, 1991), 129; Floor, *Public Health in Qajar Iran*, 80.

9. Curzon, *Persia and the Persian Question* (London: Longmans, Green, 1892), 152.

10. Isabella Bishop, *Journeys in Persia and Kurdistan Including a Summer in the Upper Karun Region and a Visit to the Nestorian Rayahs* (London: John Murray, 1891), 168.

11. Fraser, *Narrative of a Journey into Khorasan*, 62.

12. Afkhami, "Disease and Water Supply," 215.

13. Jane Dieulafoy, *La Perse, La Chaldée et La Susiane* (Paris: Librarie Hachette et Cie, 1887), 186 ("ce célèbre imamzaddè est précédé d'une immense nécropole aux pierres tombales si rapprochées qu'elles recouvrent la terre comme le ferait un dallage").

14. Lee, *Journals of Edward Stirling*, 66.

15. Mary Sheil, *Glimpses of Life and Manners in Persia* (London: John Murray, 1856), 197.

16. George Fowler, *Three Years in Persia, with Travelling Adventures in Koordistan* (London: Henry Colburn, 1841), 28.

17. Gertrude Bell, *Persian Pictures* (London: Ernest Benn Limited, 1928), 68; Afkhami, *A Modern Contagion*, 11.

18. Bell, *Persian Pictures*, 59.

19. Camposampiero, "On the Recent Outbreak of cholera in Persia. Report by Dr Camposampiero, Ottoman Sanitary Delegate at Tehran, to the Constantinople Board of Health. Summarised and Reported to the Epidemiological Society by Dr. E. D. Dickson, Physician to the British Embassy at Constantinople," *Transactions of the Epidemiological Society of London* 13 (1893–94): 156.

20. Afkhami, *A Modern Contagion*, 31.

21. Floor, *Public Health in Qajar Iran*, 244–45; Niẓām al-Salṭana Māfī, Husayn Qulī Khān, and Maʻṣūma Niẓām Māfī, *Khāṭirāt va Asnād-i Ḥusayn Qulī Khān Niẓām al-Salṭana Māfī* (Tehran: Nashr-i Tārīkh-i Īrān, 1361/1982), vol. 2, 27–28.

22. Afkhami, *A Modern Contagion*, 72, table 2.2.

23. Ibid., 85 and 181 (Appendix B).

24. Ibid., 86.

14

Social Life, Illness, and the Marketplace in Kumasi, Ghana, from the 20th Century to the Present

George Osei and Shobana Shankar

Kumasi, capital city of the Ashanti Region of Ghana, has a rich history as a cross-roads of long-distance trade in Western Africa. It is known in the modern world economy for commodities like cocoa and gold. Kumasi was the seat of power of the Asante Empire, founded in the 18th century. The city is iconic for the Asante people as the spiritual and political center of their traditional ruler the Asantehene and as a symbol of their collective ability to adapt to major changes while retaining their historic cohesion. The British invaded Asante many times between 1800 and 1900 before finally conquering and incorporating it into the Gold Coast Colony. Even these violent foreign intrusions did not erase essential features of the city, such as its palace and market.

Kumasi and other West African cities with early and lasting commercial networks have effectively maintained public well-being and health through their markets and market institutions. African informal markets (including traditional markets and unregulated trade) are used by all strata of society. The market community combines commonsense approaches to the preparation and storage of foods and indigenous knowledge to prevent both foodborne and communicable disease in urban and rural Africa.[1]

During the Spanish influenza pandemic of 1918–19, public activity in the markets in Kumasi was a measure of disease and devastation;[2] yet the importance of the connection between public markets and disease prevention goes beyond any single epidemic or health concern. The markets in Kumasi play an important role in social communication and therefore provide a useful lens through which to understand how diseases have been combatted and health maintained and restored. Organized public spaces may be sites for possible infections, but the marketplace can also be envisioned as a crucial institution for social collaboration and cohesion to combat

117

disease and preserve well-being. Kumasi Central Market, one of the largest in West Africa, operates as a commercial and noncommercial system with actors including merchants, producers, political authorities, and consumers jockeying for power.[3]

Women make up well over half of the merchants in Kumasi market's web of power relations.[4] Many of the insights into the social, economic, and public health dynamics in the Kumasi Central Market presented here come from fieldwork interviews with four women who have an intimate understanding of the functions of the market. Their experiences show the gender dynamics of the market, where women are central actors, just as in the domestic realm. As intermediaries between Kumasi market and households, women's experiences also suggest how information and practices related to health and disease flow between the market and residential neighborhoods.[5]

Case study: Kumasi's markets in public life and public health since 1900

British colonial authorities in Kumasi confronted a bubonic plague outbreak in 1924–25, just a few years after the influenza pandemic of 1918. A number of public health measures were enacted in the central market as well as the trading area of the *zongo*, the multiethnic enclave of immigrants from the northern savanna and sahelian regions. The colonial authorities used a public health rationale to blame disease transmission on so-called African behaviors and to destroy Kumasi residents' houses in and around the markets. These authorities did not see how their own policies, which expanded Gold Coast cocoa production, had contributed to the rapid and haphazard growth of these commercial areas. Roads connecting regional networks for the transportation of market commodities to the coast facilitated the transmission of disease. According to earlier European travelers' accounts, Kumasi and its markets had been orderly, and a major reason for those earlier public welfare management efforts had been the presence and activism of political leaders in the market. The British relied on such leaders to mitigate the plague outbreak in the 1920s: it was the chief of the *zongo* who marshaled volunteers to clean up city streets and conduct other sanitation efforts.[6]

In the 21st century, the Ghanaian government has relied on social mobilization in and around the crowded market areas to combat a series of outbreaks of cholera, a bacterial infection caused by contaminated food and water. The disease can spread rapidly because of urban crowding and poor hygiene, but the Ghanaian Disease Control Unit has been able to cover these areas with public messages to bring down transmission rates.[7] Public health information can travel quickly in a city like Kumasi through public institutions with established leaders and experts, like traditional political authorities and respected market traders. The physical location of the Kumasi Central Market, at the locus of prominent neighborhoods in the city, helps explain its centrality in relationships across different segments of society.

The market's use as a space for the commemoration of death shows its intricate role in public life. Funerals, which the Akan peoples conduct to maintain good relations between the dead and living, are held in the market to allow public mourning and healing.[8] Given the specificity of washing and other funerary rites in the market, it is clear that Kumasi dwellers appreciate order and can accept regulation in emergencies like epidemics. Additionally, most members of Kumasi society have an attachment to the market, which makes it a useful point of social communication. This is an indispensable aspect of voluntary, noncoercive public health measures. Many wealthy traders built homes near the market, suggesting that the wealthy and powerful have an investment in maintaining commercial areas of the city. Such an attachment can be compared to the wealthy of other cities who flee to suburbs or reside in enclaves outside the city center, often on private grounds that are heavily fenced and guarded.

The Asante royal family has a crucial role in the market. The various sections of the market have different leaders who report to the Asantehemaa (Queen mother of Asante), and these market patrons oftentimes offer gifts to the Queen Mother in the form of foodstuff and other products. The traders believe that the land where they live and trade is maintained at the benevolence of the Asantehene (King of Asante). His role in public health campaigns, for example in the COVID-19 pandemic, reveals his watchful protection (Figure 14.1). The investment endures in the hereditary sections of the market that are given to Adehye (Royals) who are the descendants of the Asantehene. In these ways, the traditional authority of the King and Queen Mother is maintained in the market and plays a role in the health and well-being of those who work there.

The gendered nature of Asante royal power in the market is mirrored by the significant social, political, and economic authority of the women market traders. Market associations strengthen relationships between market women and provide assistance in times of sickness, need, and misfortune. These associations also show how social relationships exist outside of family and kinship. Market women form commodity groups and market associations, and the commodity group leaders and market queens are instrumental in decision-making processes that concern the market. Some market groups are engaged in political activism and openly support political reforms. Some of these market women are very wealthy due to their trade in large volumes of goods. There are market leaders who regulate the prices of goods to prevent exorbitant rates, as determined by market forces. Decisions about pricing and distribution are sometimes reflected in the planning of family meals based on availability of particular produce, the passage of information related to

119

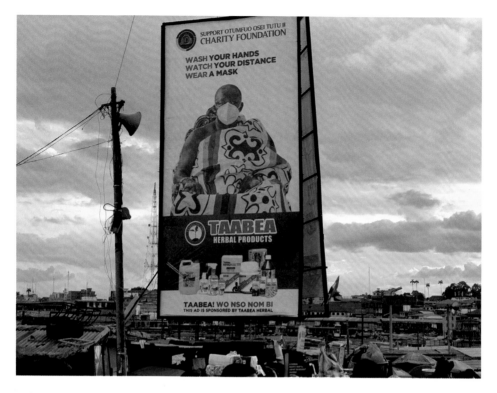

FIGURE 14.1: Asantehene on Covid-19 billboard, 2020. (Photograph by George Osei.)

food availability and scarcity, and other kinds of social communication related to the economy of health. Elderly market women are also skilled at assessing and predicting market changes after many years of plying their trade.[9] Such knowledge helps guide them and their families in making investments, for example, in property and houses, and in saving resources for emergencies. Such women can be very important in chains of public health communication and prevention.

Women's involvement in the market shapes health, well-being, and disease prevention through ethnopharmacology and the sales of herbal medicines in Kumasi and in the rest of the country. In Ghana, women control much of the trade in medicinal herbs and are the primary customers for such plant-based treatments (Figure 14.2).[10]

The internal regulation of the market in the 21st century includes safety measures regarding livestock and abattoirs in order to prevent the zoonotic transmission of disease and the contamination of soil, water, and other public resources by animal products. The sale of livestock was not prevalent inside the central market in the precolonial period as the indigenous Akan of the Kumasi area reared their own livestock in their home compounds; the sale of livestock brought to the

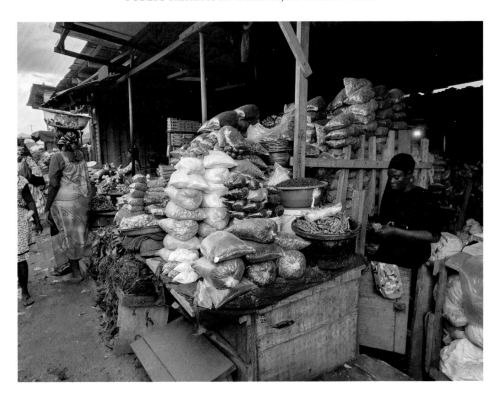

FIGURE 14.2: Herbal medicine trader, 2020. (Photograph by George Osei.)

central market by Dagomba traders from the northern part of the country only began sometime around the mid-20th century. Although the numbers of animals brought into the central market were regulated, the animals were not subjected to any health checks. Livestock brought from outside Ghana today continue to be sold in separate markets such as the *zongo*, where immigrant and itinerant traders have more of a presence. The Ghanaian Department of Game and Wildlife attempts to regulate bush meat from wild animals, but this is largely to ensure that hunters do not capture animals during periods of gestation to allow continuity of game species.[11] This animal control system may need to be adapted to future needs for disease-prevention.

The regulatory system of the market has encountered other challenges, notably in the area of freshwater preservation. In the past, as late as the 1960s, Kumasi authorities issued town ordinances to protect rivers and streams by establishing green belt zones on their banks. The Subin River, which serves as the main source of water for the central market traders and the nearby community, has been polluted due to population growth and unregulated building construction (Figure 14.3).[12] In recent times, city authorities have constructed a storm drain over the river to

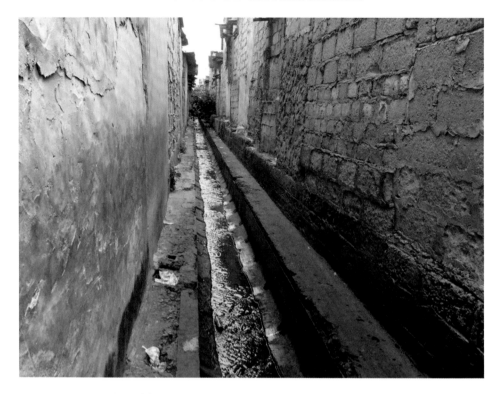

FIGURE 14.3: Section of the Subin River, 2020. (Photograph by George Osei.)

prevent flooding, which has enabled the extension of the market with the new stalls placed over the drains. Market encroachment is an example of the "unplanned, runaway urbanism" that has resulted in competition for water resources in Kumasi (Figure 14.4).[13] The social regulatory mechanisms in the market have been compromised with the growth of the population in and around the market. Older structures of authority and organization might be revisited to better use the social resources of the market in Kumasi.

Conclusion

Markets mean more than economic exchange in cities like Kumasi. They have fostered social, political, and cultural relationships over centuries and across institutions including the traditional monarchy, mercantile classes, kin groups, and producers. They also function significantly in both health and disease. While markets have sustained livelihoods, the sale of medicines, and the bestowal of the blessings of esteemed personages as protectors of the community, in modern times, they have

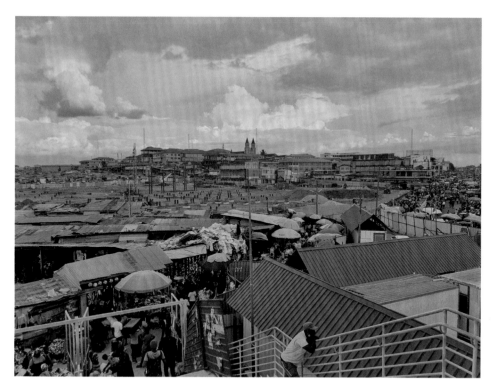

FIGURE 14.4: Kumasi Central Market reconstruction, 2020. (Photograph by George Osei.)

represented dangerous spaces where contagions may spread easily from person to person or from animals to people and where modern sanitation has been difficult to construct and maintain. Government authorities, particularly the British colonial authorities in the 20th century and postcolonial public health experts, have approached the market through the prism of epidemics and their prevention. But the people who work in and live near markets reveal its other sides, particularly its social communication functions and its mutual aid networks that can influence collective action and communal responses to disease outbreaks.

Kumasi's public health history, like that of other African cities, reveals how, even with centralized political authority, "health services have never been provided exclusively by the state."[14] Indeed, the public health duties of the modern state—"the protection and care of the health of its citizens"—were performed by the Asante monarchy and public institutions that had an independent role in public life. Economic and health interests have long been intertwined in a West African conceptualization of the public good. This perspective has been vitally important as Ghanaians have managed epidemics and developed an important body of indigenous knowledge with which to meet future threats.

NOTES

1. Kristina Roesel and Delia Grace, eds., *Food Safety and Informal Markets: Animal Products in Sub-Saharan Africa* (New York: Routledge, 2015), xxiii, 3, 4.

2. David K. Patterson, "The Influenza Epidemic of 1918-1919 in the Gold Coast," *The Journal of African History* 24, no. 4 (1983): 485–502.

3. Gracia Clark, *Onions Are My Husband: Survival and Accumulation by West African Market Women* (Chicago: University of Chicago Press, 1994). See Chapter 1.

4. Ibid.

5. Informant 1, interview with authors, Kumasi, Ghana, July 22, 2020 (age 70. Occupation: currently on retirement from a lifetime of trading in the market); Informant 2, interview with authors, Kumasi, Ghana, July 23, 2020 (age 58. Occupation: used to sell cosmetic products in the market and is now a poultry farmer); Informant 3, interview with authors, Kumasi, Ghana, July 23, 2020 (age 62. Occupation: currently a retired teacher, whose mother used to sell in the market and who accompanied her to work as a child); Informant 4, interview with authors, Kumasi, Ghana, October 3, 2020 (age 59. Occupation: Currently sells clothes in the market and has been selling in the market for about 30 years).

6. Benjamin Talton, " 'Kill Rats and Stop Plague': Race, Space, and Public Health in Postconquest Kumasi," *Ghana Studies* 22, no. 1 (2019): 95–113.

7. Frank Badu Osei and Alfred Stein, "Temporal Trend and Spatial Clustering of Cholera Epidemic in Kumasi-Ghana," *Scientific Reports* 8, no. 1 (2018): 1–11.

8. Kwame Arhin, "The Economic Implications of Transformations in Akan Funeral Rites," *Africa* 64, no. 3 (1994): 312.

9. Gracia Clark, "Consulting Elderly Kumasi Market Women about Modernization," *Ghana Studies* 12, no. 1 (2009): 97–119.

10. Tinde Van Andel, Britt Myren, and Sabine Van Onselen, "Ghana's Herbal Market," *Journal of Ethnopharmacology* 140, no. 2 (2012): 368–78.

11. Bush meat was checked by British colonial authorities before it was brought to market. Public Records and Archives Administration, Accra, Ghana. CSO 20/1/ 19 Cape Coast Town Council Annual Report, 1929–1930. File No. 1478/30.

12. Abubakari Ahmed and Romanus D. Dinye, "Impact of Land Use Activities on Subin and Aboabo Rivers in Kumasi Metropolis," *International Journal of Water Resources and Environmental Engineering* 4, no. 7 (2012): 241–51.

13. Tom C. McCaskie, " 'Water Wars' in Kumasi, Ghana," in *African Cities: Competing Claims in Urban Spaces*, ed. Francesca Locatelli and Paul Nugent (Leiden: Brill, 2009), 135–55.

14. Ruth J. Prince and Rebecca Marsland, eds., *Making and Unmaking Public Health in Africa: Ethnographic and Historical Perspectives* (Athens: Ohio University Press, 2014), 5.

15

The City as Field Hospital and the Influenza Epidemic in Seattle, USA, 1918–19

Louisa Iarocci

The Saturday meeting of the City Council of Seattle, Washington, on September 21, 1918, included an unscheduled visit from the city's health commissioner, Dr. J. S. McBride. According to newspaper reports, McBride informed the assembled civic officials that not a single case of so-called Spanish influenza, the mysterious disease that was sweeping across Europe, had appeared in the city. He declared "that a fall of rain would make its presence in Seattle almost impossible."[1] Two weeks later, McBride announced that new cases were being reported to his office every few minutes and that the death toll included both civilians and military personnel.[2] On his advice, the Mayor of the city, Ole Hanson, ordered immediate, drastic steps to control the movement of people and the spread of the disease. In Seattle, as in other cities across the United States, the influenza epidemic would alter the character of public space and of urban life for at least the next year.

The highly virulent respiratory illness known as the "Spanish flu" made its way across the United States in a series of waves between the spring of 1918 and the spring of 1919, coinciding with the final months of World War I. Estimated to have infected around a quarter of the country's population, the epidemic would result in the deaths of over half a million people.[3] While commonly known as the "Spanish" flu, the origins of this virulent strain of influenza, now known as H1N1 1918, continue to be debated to the present day.[4] But the factors that contributed to its lethality are more certain, foremost among them the rapid spread and progression of the illness to pneumonia and potential death.[5] With the lack of effective treatment, influenza had a high fatality rate, especially among young and otherwise healthy adults.[6] The spread of this "disease of crowds" in the United States and Europe has been linked to the congregation and movement of military personnel and wartime workers during World War I.[7] The epidemic reached the United States at a time when the expansion of mass transportation and commerce had increased the scale and density of major cities, providing the optimal environment for it to spread.[8]

For most of the summer of 1918, newspaper headlines in Seattle, and in other US cities, were dominated by news of the war overseas, with occasional reports of the spread of the "mysterious plague" relegated to the back pages. But the arrival of the second most deadly wave of influenza in late August made headlines as the death toll began to rise in east coast cities.[9] The epidemic officially reached Seattle by the last week of September, with hundreds of cases reported at military bases in Washington State.[10] Having doubled its population in the first two decades of the 20th century, the youthful "big city" of the Pacific Northwest provided a ready place of entry for the disease.[11] As the busiest port on the west coast, the Seattle area was home to several large military and naval training stations, in addition to the shipbuilding industry that was critical to the wartime effort (Figure 15.1). The city became a battleground in the war against one of the deadliest infectious outbreaks of all time, taking on the role of a "great field hospital" that acted as both a target and a weapon for civic officials and local residents.

Case study: Prevention, isolation and treatment of disease in Seattle, 1918

The local press in Seattle served as the primary communication conduit between local government and the public with three major dailies and countless other newspapers.[12] Despite the grim news that the flu had taken its first civilian victims in the first week of October, health commissioner McBride and Mayor Hanson presented a united front as newspaper headlines declared "Seattle Is Ready to Fight."[13] On October 5, 1918, the mayor announced an immediate citywide ban on all public gatherings and the immediate closure of all theaters, moving picture halls, poolrooms, saloons, churches, schools, and public libraries.[14] Police officers were dispatched to enforce the order, placing locks on the doors and arresting owners who refused to comply with restricted store hours.[15] A special "influenza squad" was assigned to "break up all street meetings or gatherings [...] whether of the open-air kind or not," including assemblies for religious services and funerals.[16] Those who had to come downtown for essential work in wartime-related industries or in food and drug stores were instructed to avoid crowding in the streets and streetcars and to "keep moving" at all times.[17]

As the usual crowds of theatergoers and shoppers downtown were replaced by empty storefronts and darkened signs, the city's public buildings became visible barricades, preventing public gatherings and disease transmission. The transition within the urban space was so quick that on the evening of the ban announcement

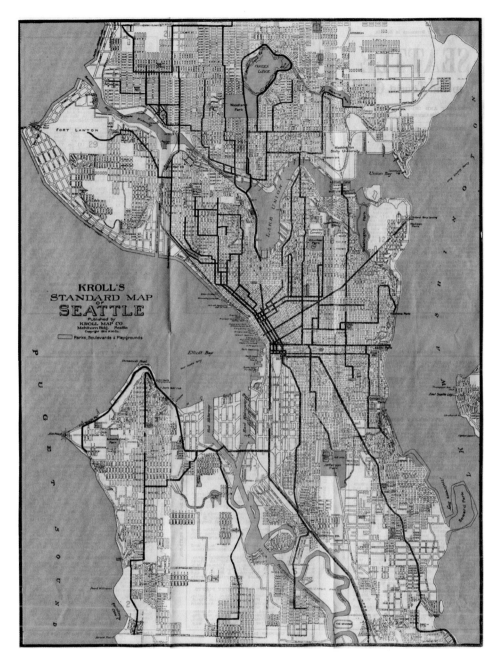

FIGURE 15.1: Kroll's standard map of Seattle (Kroll Map Co. Seattle, 1914). The black lines represent street cars, cable cars, and interurban railway lines. (Reprinted with the Permission of Kroll Map Company and courtesy of Rob Ketcherside.)

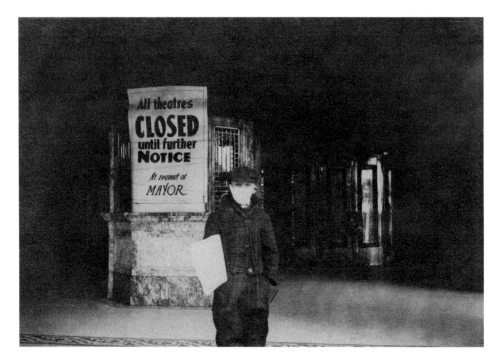

FIGURE 15.2: Newspaper boy wearing flu mask outside closed theater, Seattle, 1918. (Courtesy of the Museum of History & Industry, Seattle, shs6338B.)

the press reported that "the streets were a mass of humanity, moving aimlessly back and forth with no place to go."[18] The blank, shuttered storefronts of the city's once lively places of entertainment displayed official notices of closing orders, with only essential workers remaining in this barricaded city "gone dark" (Figure 15.2).[19]

As the number of infections and related deaths rose through the month of October, Seattle and Washington State authorities waged a campaign to inform and motivate the public.[20] Citizens were encouraged to consider fighting the disease as their patriotic duty in order to protect themselves and their community, as well as the city's essential wartime industries.[21] "Respiratory etiquette" was emphasized by health officials, who cautioned against unsanitary behaviors like spitting, coughing, and sneezing in public along with sharing drinking and eating utensils.[22] But by far the most visible preventative strategy was wearing a mask in public—first required for workers in direct contact with the public and then made mandatory for all citizens on October 29, 1918.[23]

The local chapter of the Red Cross, mostly made up of women, produced thousands of the regulation six-ply gauze masks for free distribution to the public.[24] Storeowners and streetcar conductors were tasked with the responsibility of denying entry to anyone not wearing a mask. Local newspapers aided with enforcement by publishing the names of those who had received fines or been arrested for noncompliance.[25] *The Seattle Star* reported that most citizens were wearing masks but scolded those "bare faced individuals" who were conspicuous for the "openness of [their] countenances which were generally defiant or contrite."[26] The "face-apron" was the subject of frequent news reports discussing its impact on fashion, crime, and social life.[27] Despite the often light-hearted tone, the *Post-Intelligencer* complained that the "ghastly masks" were intensifying the collective sense of fear and panic in the city and were thus detrimental to the aim of defeating the epidemic.[28]

The coordination between the mayor's office and public health officials at the city and state levels was reported to be as well organized as a military campaign. City officials did not impose a general quarantine on residents, but army and navy camps were locked down in mid-October.[29] Those with access to a private physician were instructed to stay in their homes if they became sick; the less privileged were told to voluntarily isolate themselves in a city hospital.[30] Police drove physicians to make house calls and to forcibly escort sick patients to local facilities. When local hospitals reached capacity, officials announced that shuttered city buildings like halls and churches would be repurposed to serve as temporary emergency hospitals.[31] For example, the former courtrooms on the third floor of the old courthouse building were renovated to provide approximately 240 beds in separate wards for men and women. Civic officials were often quoted in newspaper reports that assured the public of the cleanliness and efficiency at the "old courthouse" hospital (Figure 15.3).[32] However, the lack of a full understanding of the disease and of effective treatments meant that only palliative care was offered to patients.

Daily newspaper reports of the deaths of workers from the shipyards and other industrial sites suggest that the hospital was seen as the destination for the "destitute sick" to go to die.[33] Health commissioner McBride even directly accused those who "lived in congested rooming houses and hotels" of driving up infection rates by waiting too long to admit themselves for treatment.[34] The news that two patients, delirious with fever, had "escaped" from the Old Court House Hospital reinforced the impression that the facility was less an institution of healing and more a place of incarceration for flu sufferers with no other options.[35]

The image of the city as a place of contagion caused by the uncontrolled mingling of working bodies and airborne germs was reinforced in influenza reports from the rest of the country. Dire updates from hard-hit cities like San Francisco and Philadelphia described coffin and grave shortages as well as morgues overflowing with flu victims.[36] On October 18, 1918, the Seattle Union Record painted a grim picture with a headline claiming that Seattle's morgue was "jammed with dead bodies."[37] Public officials cautioned residents to avoid downtown, where the air was "full

OLD COURTHOUSE CONVERTED INTO EMERGENCY HOSPITAL

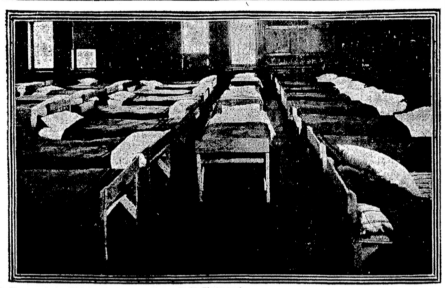

—Photograph by Webster & Stevens, Times Staff Photographers.
This photograph shows some of the cots in the old courthouse that were formerly used by the Soldiers and Sailors' Club to accommodate men visiting Seattle, which have been taken over by the City Health Department.

City Health Commissioner McBride this morning, with permission of the Board of County Commissioners, took over the entire third floor of the old courthouse to convert it into an emergency hospital. The Soldiers and Sailors' Club had been using the ten rooms, formerly occupied by the Superior Courts and the county clerk, as dormitories for men who could not obtain sleeping accommodations elsewhere in the city.

Dr. McBride and City Building Superintendent J. A. Johnson inspected the rooms this morning and left them in charge of John P. Dixon, district sanitary inspector, for fumigation. The health department was also given the use of 241 cots with bedding, which are being fumigated today.

Inspector Dixon said this morning that while the ten rooms will be put in readiness for occupancy that at present the city will only use the large courtrooms that were formerly Judges Kenneth Mackintosh and Boyd J. Tallman's departments. Each cot will be given sixty-four square feet of floor and 512 cubic feet of air space. This will permit the placing of forty-one cots in the southern courtroom and twenty-four in that in the north side of the building.

OPEN-AIR SERVICES HELD BY CHURCHES

Congregations Gather in Rain Because of Ban Put on All Indoor Meetings.

DIVIDED AS TO EFFECT OF RAIN ON INFLUENZA

Diversity of opinion was found today among physicians in Seattle that the rainfall that was general throughout Western Washington yesterday will have a beneficial effect against the influenza epidemic. Rainfall at this period of the year is customary and many physicians hold it not only lays the dust and clears the atmosphere, preventing to some extent the spread of germs, but also has a general beneficial effect to the health of residents.

HOSPITALS UNABLE TO ADMIT ALL GRIP CASES

Accommodations Inadequate to Handle Patients Afflicted With Influenza.

FIGURE 15.3: Old courthouse converted into emergency hospital, *Seattle Daily Times*, October 7, 1918, 7. (Public domain.)

of influenza germs" and the very act of breathing was "likely to draw them into your nose and throat."[38] At the same time, residents were told to get outdoors to breathe as much "fresh pure air as possible" as a way to not simply prevent the flu but allegedly cure it.[39] Street cars, the primary means of transportation for workers, were ordered to be fully ventilated at all times, with a third of windows kept open.

Citizens were told to keep their bodies and property clean and municipal crews washed city streets and removed refuse.[40] Touting the healing effects of cleanliness and fresh air, health commissioner McBride continued to promote his theory that the abundant rain in Seattle would serve as a "foe of influenza [...] by checking the germ-laden dust of the streets."[41] The notion that the built fabric of the city itself, along with its citizens, could assist in the prevention of the spread of disease would gather strength with the opening of public inoculation stations for the administration of an "anti-influenza" serum (Figure 15.4). Familiar urban locations like police stations, libraries, and department stores were adapted to serve as temporary medical stations that prioritized inoculating industrial workers with the aim of ensuring that the war effort could continue.[42] Although the "vaccine"

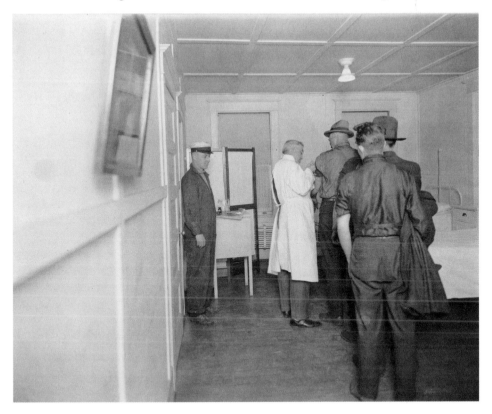

FIGURE 15.4: Flu serum injection: Influenza in Seattle, December 1918. (Courtesy of the National Archives, photo no. 165-WW-269B-9.)

was likely ineffective, the provision of this free service gave authorities a way to promote their competence and allay people's fears with the illusion of protection.

Conclusion

The announcement of Armistice on November 11, 1918, brought the masses downtown to pack the streets for an impromptu parade. Reports claimed that many of the jubilant attendees had "burn(ed) their detested cheesecloth and tape" masks.[43] Despite continued warnings from civic officials, the return of crowds to public spaces seemed to signal that the epidemic had ended along with the war. The following day, the city and state announced the reopening of public gathering places but maintained the masking order. This cautious approach proved prescient as "dangerously high" totals of influenza cases returned in the first week of December.[44] This time, officials responded by fanning throughout the city to quarantine the sick by placing yellow "flu cards" on hundreds of homes.[45] Despite anxieties about holiday crowds, the flu lost its grip on the city by the end of the year.[46]

Almost 1,500 people died from influenza in Seattle in 1918, although this excessive death rate remained one of the lowest among US cities of a similar size.[47] In early 1919, Mayor Hanson proposed that a memorial to the war's military victims from Washington State take the form of a "highly ornamental and useful hospital" to be built in Seattle.[48] While not realized, this effort to leave a permanent trace of the role the city played as an improvised medical unit reflected how closely the distant war and the local fight for the health of Washington's citizens were intertwined. The story of urban life of Seattle during the influenza epidemic reveals how the city acted as both a transmitter of contagion and as the nucleus of healing. In its official response to disease, the city defended against a viral enemy from the outside that exposed the social inequities within.

NOTES

1. "'Investigation' is Mild Affair," *Seattle Star*, September 21, 1918, 2.
2. "Spanish Flu Takes First Victims Here," *Seattle Star*, October 4, 1918, 1.
3. David Patterson and Gerald F. Pyle, "The Geography and Mortality of the 1918 Influenza Mortality," *Bulletin of the History of Medicine* 65, no. 1 (Spring 1991): 4–21.
4. Sandra Opdycke, *The Flu Epidemic of 1918: America's Experience in the Global Health Crisis* (New York: Routledge, 2014), 4.
5. Fred R. Van Hartesveldt, "Influenza Pandemic, 1918–1919," in *Encyclopedia of Pestilence, Pandemics, and Plagues Vol. 1*, ed. Joseph P. Byrne (Westport, CT: Greenwood Press, 2008), 313–17.

6. Sarah Boslaugh, "Influenza," In *Encyclopedia of Epidemiology*, ed. Sarah Boslaugh and Louise-Anne McNutt (Thousand Oaks, CA: Sage, 2008), 534–36.

7. Howard Phillips, "Influenza Pandemic," *1914–1918 online: International Encyclopedia of the First World War*, https://encyclopedia.1914-1918-online.net/article/influenza_pandemic (accessed July 10, 2020).

8. Nancy Tomes, "'Destroyer and Teacher': Managing the Masses during the 1918–1919 Influenza Pandemic," *Public Health Reports* 125, no. 3 (2010): 48, 52–53.

9. Howard Markel, Harvey B. Lipman, J. Alexander Navarro, Alexandra Sloan, Joseph R. Michalsen, Alexandra Minna Stern, and Martin S. Cetron, "Nonpharmaceutical Interventions Implemented by US Cities during the 1918–1919 Influenza Pandemic," *Journal of the American Medical Association* 298, no. 6 (2007): 644–54.

10. "Navy Camp at 'UW' Has 650 Influenza Cases," *Seattle Times*, September 30, 1918, 19; "Bremerton Hit by Spanish Influenza," *Seattle Times*, October 4, 1918, 16.

11. Between 1900 and 1920, the population of the city almost quadrupled, reaching over three hundred thousand in 1918. "Decennial Population: City of Seattle 1900-2000," City of Seattle Strategic Planning Office (April 12, 2001), https://www.seattle.gov/Documents/Departments/OPCD/Demographics/DecennialCensus/1900to2000DecennialPopulationOverview.pdf (accessed July 10, 2020).

12. Nancy Tomes observes that the 1918 influenza epidemic was the first "mass-mediated pandemic" in the United States, taking place during the height of the popularity of newspaper reading. Tomes, "'Destroyer and Teacher'," 51.

13. "Seattle Is Ready to Fight Spread of Influenza," *Seattle Post-Intelligencer*, October 5, 1918, 1.

14. "Mayor Closes Theaters, Schools and Churches," *Seattle Star*, October 5, 1918, 1; "Ban Gatherings in an Effort to Halt Influenza," *Seattle Post-Intelligencer*, October 6, 1918, 1.

15. "All Stores are Closed by Hanson," *Seattle Star*, October 31, 1918, 1.

16. "Churches Meet Quarantine Order," *Catholic Northwest Progress*, October 11, 1918, 1. "Total of 1,921 Cases in Seattle Now," *Seattle Star*, October 12, 1918, 2.

17. "Five Die of Flu Last 24 Hours," *Seattle Star*, October 8, 1918, 1.

18. "Ban Gatherings," 10.

19. "Epidemic Shows No Signs of Immediate Abatement," *Variety*, October 11, 1918, 1.

20. "Calls 'Flu' Fight Individual's Job," *Seattle Post-Intelligencer*, December 11, 1918, 2.

21. "Preventive Measures against Spanish Influenza in Force," *Labor Journal* 27, no. 24 (October 11, 1918): 1. Opdyke, *The Flu Epidemic of 1918*, 101.

22. The US Surgeon General even issued recommendations asking members of the public to learn to breathe through their noses. "How to Fight Spanish Influenza," *Cayton's Weekly* 3, no. 18 (October 12, 1918): 4.

23. "Influenza Mask Order Extended," *Seattle Daily Times*, October 26, 1918, 12. "Seattle Ordered to Wear Masks Beginning Today," *Seattle Post-Intelligencer*, October 28, 1918, 1.

24. Nancy Rockafellar, "'In Gauze We Trust': Public Health and Spanish Influenza on the Home Front, Seattle, 1918–1919," *Pacific Northwest Quarterly* 77, no. 3 (July 1986): 104–5.

25. "Failure to Wear Masks Causes Arrest of Ten," *Seattle Daily Times*, October 31, 1918, 8; "Four Arrested for Ignoring Mask Edict," *Seattle Star*, October 31, 1918, 4.

26. "Put on that Gauze Mask and Smile," *Seattle Daily Times*, October 30, 1918, 1.

27. Newspapers reported that masks were used as fashion accessories, advertising banners, and criminal disguises. A local attorney was reported to have cut a hole in his mask in order to smoke cigars. "Flu Fashions," *Seattle Star*, October 31, 1918, 6; "Is It On Straight?: Flu Masks Are Not Chest Protectors!," *Seattle Star*, October 29, 1918, 4; "Flees Bandits Who Utilize Flu Masks," *Seattle Star*, October 30, 1918, 10.

28. "Pandemic and Panic," *Seattle Post Intelligencer*, October 29, 1918, 6.

29. The decision not to impose a general quarantine on residents appears to have come from the federal government, at least in part due to concerns about the impact on the economy. Tomes, "Destroyer and Teacher," 52.

30. "City Hastens to Curb Influenza," *Seattle Post-Intelligencer*, October 8, 1918, 1.

31. "Halls and Churches to be Flu Hospitals," *Seattle Star*, October 7, 1918, 9.

32. "Three Deaths from Influenza," *Seattle Post-Intelligencer*, October 9, 1918, 1; "Hospitals Unable to Admit All Grip Cases," *Seattle Daily Times*, October 7, 1918, 7.

33. "Close Hospital in Court House," *Seattle Post-Intelligencer*, November 21, 1918, 18.

34. "Influenza Mask Order Extended," 12.

35. "Epidemic Losing Hold on Seattle," *Seattle Daily Times*, October 23, 1918, 9.

36. "Hundreds Are Dead of Spanish Disease," *Seattle Star*, October 12, 1918, 3; "Use Steam Shovel to Dig Influenza Victims Graves," *Seattle Daily Times*, October 28, 1918, 5.

37. Influenza Mask Order Extended," 12.

38. "Spanish Influenza Is Epidemic Here," *Seattle Star*, October 18, 1918, 4.

39. E. C. Rodgers, "Nation's Capital Battling for Life against the Flu," *Seattle* Star, October 19, 1918, 2.

40. "City Expected to be Free of Epidemic Soon," *Seattle Daily Times*, November 3, 1918, 12.

41. "Heavy Rain Aids Influenza Fight," *Seattle Daily Times*, December 2, 1918, 10.

42. "To Open Public Serum Stations," *Seattle Post Intelligencer*, November 3, 1918, 9.

43. "Seattle, Now Unmuzzled, Puts the Day Resting Tired Feet at Movies," *Seattle Post Intelligencer*, November 13, 1918, 10.

44. "500 Flu Cases Daily Average," *Seattle Star*, December 10, 1918, 1.

45. "Flu Cards Nailed on Seattle Homes," *Seattle Star*, December 6, 1918, 1; "Influenza Cases All Quarantined," *Seattle Daily Times*, December 11, 1918, 15.

46. "Influenza Is Again Showing a Decline," *Seattle Star*, December 18, 1918, 1; "Flu Loses Its Grip on City," *Seattle Star*, December 26, 1918, 4.

47. "Seattle, Washington," *American Influenza Epidemic of 1918–1919: A Digital Encyclopedia*, https://www.influenzaarchive.org/cities/city-seattle.html (accessed August 11, 2020).

48. "How About a Hospital for a Memorial," *Seattle Star*, December 9, 1918, 4.

16

Rural Migrants, Smallpox, and Civic Surgery in 20th-Century Baghdad, Iraq

Huma Gupta

In 1978, the Republic of Iraq issued a postage stamp in support of the World Health Organization and its attempts to eradicate smallpox or the variola virus (Figure 16.1). In addition to celebrating this international campaign, the stamp also highlighted the central role that nurses played within this effort. The 25 Fils stamp featured a heroic figure of a nurse, whose upper torso was suspended before a large institutional structure. On top of the structure, the illustrator placed a white flag bearing a red crescent to indicate that it was a hospital. The building's modernist, concrete column-slab construction equipped with ribbon windows was a nod to the Iraqi state's expansive mid-century hospital-building project. From 1973 onward, the state began building a complex of medical teaching hospitals in Baghdad, collectively known as *Madinat al-Tabb* or Medical City. Therefore, the stamp's iconography was intended to reify two major accomplishments of the Iraqi state: expansion of the state's medical infrastructure on the one hand and eradication of smallpox—a disease that had plagued the state with repeated outbreaks since the British-installed Hashemite monarchic regime took power in 1921—on the other.[1]

While the worldwide campaign to eradicate smallpox would not be completed until 1980, Iraqi authorities had made considerable progress toward smallpox eradication since the 1940s when they began mass vaccination and public awareness campaigns.[2] In fact, the last major smallpox appearance occurred in Iraq between 1971 and 1972, when an outbreak in nearby Mashhad, Iran, spread into Iraq along pilgrimage routes. An international pilgrim visiting religious shrines in Basra and Baghdad contracted smallpox in February 1972 and brought it back with him to Yugoslavia, subsequently causing a large outbreak of the disease and tens of deaths. While Iraq was able to quickly contain the smallpox outbreak of 1971–72, this had not the case in previous decades when the country's beleaguered

135

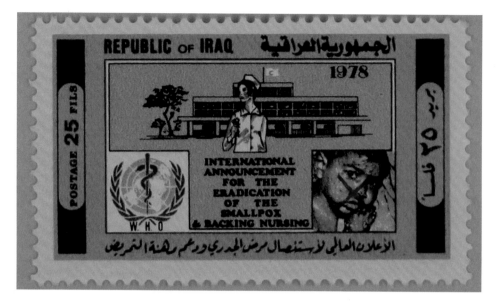

FIGURE 16.1: Republic of Iraq. 1978 postage stamp for the International Announcement for the Eradication of the Smallpox & Backing Nursing. (Personal Collection of Huma Gupta.)

medical personnel battled smallpox outbreaks in 1921, 1926, 1929, 1932, 1941, 1948, 1951, and 1956–57.

In response to these recurrent outbreaks, the government launched nationwide vaccination campaigns in 1949 and most notably in 1956 under the supervision of the newly established Ministry of Health. While the 1978 stamp described above put forth a triumphal national narrative of smallpox eradication, it also obscured the lesser-known story of how the specter of smallpox also enabled a campaign of mass displacement in the rural migrant settlements of Baghdad.

Case study: Civic surgery and the campaign to eradicate smallpox

The 1956 Iraqi Housing Census enumerated 16,413 *sarifa* (reed mat) and 27,491 *kukh* (mud) dwellings for a total of 43,904 transient or semi-transient structures in the capital city of Baghdad. These fragile constructions comprised nearly half (44.8 percent) of the 98,019 houses recorded in greater Baghdad (Figure 16.2).[3] These mud and reed dwellings coexisted with large villas and equally defined the urban landscape of the capital (Figure 16.3). In cities, migrants (formerly dispossessed cultivators or *fellahin*) were employed as low-ranking members of the army, police, civil service, construction, dairy industries, and the domestic servant class.

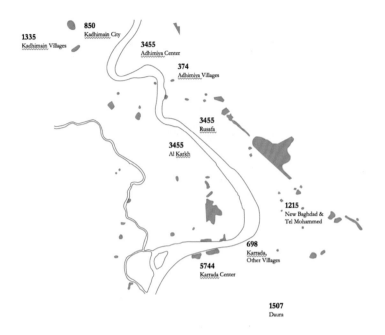

FIGURE 16.2: Spread of migrant settlements in 1950s Baghdad. (Map by Huma Gupta.)

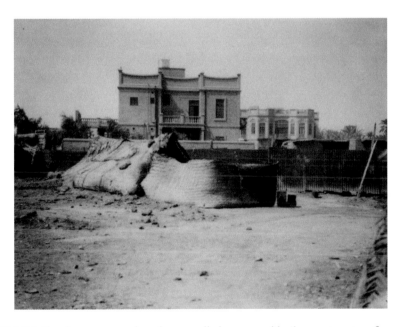

FIGURE 16.3: Reed structure and reed-mat walled courtyard built next to a two-floor villa in Baghdad. Taken by Kamil Chadirji. Kamil and Rifat Chadirji Photographic Archive Binder B10, Photo 10/110. (Courtesy of Aga Khan Documentation Center, MIT Libraries.)

Despite the fact that migrants formed the backbone of the human infrastructure that sustained the building of a modern Iraqi state, descriptions of them as vectors of disease commonly circulated in the Iraqi press. What press circulars often failed to mention, however, was that Baghdad's more affluent residents were dumping their waste and sewage in migrant neighborhoods, causing water and soil contamination, along with outbreaks of disease.[4] In 1957, Iranian social worker Sattareh Farman described a typical migrant dwelling in Baghdad:

> [A] single room must provide for all the household functions, which include living, sleeping, eating, cooking, washing and the occasional accommodation of animals and fowl. Arising from this congested and highly unsanitary form of living are conditions which create an ideal environment for the development and spread of disease, squalor and general ill-health. Such diseases as smallpox, TB, and typhus are known to be prevalent, and the inhabitants in the areas under study unfortunately represent a continual danger to the health of the entire urban population.[5]

Contrary to public perceptions, migrants were often well informed about the gravity of smallpox and eager to receive the vaccine. For example, the Greek architect Maria Zagorissiou reported how, when walking through the migrant settlement of Shakriya in 1957, residents repeatedly mistook her for a doctor and asked her to inoculate their children.[6] The Iraqi novelist Abdullah Sakhy also recounted how, when he was five years old in 1956, a group of female nurses clad in white skirt suits descended upon Asima, his neighborhood of reed and mud dwellings that was located beyond the eastern flood dyke in Baghdad.[7] The nurses went from dwelling to dwelling in an effort to gather children like him for inoculation. While these frontline health workers were represented by the nurse displayed on the 1978 stamp, the face of the smallpox-infected child on the stamp was meant to represent the heretofore-unvaccinated children like Sakhy, who lived in Iraq's rural peripheries or Baghdad's migrant settlements.

Vaccination campaigns were conducted alongside other projects that served the Iraqi state's developmental agenda. The nurses administering the vaccine were frequently accompanied by civil servants: police officers who feared resistance from migrants who opposed the monarchic regime, officials collecting census information, and municipal officials marking migrant dwellings for demolition. Therefore, in this historic moment, the migrant body in Baghdad was perceived as a vector of disease that threatened the governing economic and political classes both through a resurgence of the smallpox epidemic in 1956 and, eventually, an anti-monarchic revolution that would bring down the Hashemite regime in 1958.[8]

From 1956 onward, the language and logic of city planning in Iraq was medicalized in order to justify dispossessing migrant communities for speculative land development, and the migrant worker's settlement was diagnosed as an infectious pox itself, calling to be excised from the purportedly healthy growing body of the Iraqi state through "civic surgery." Sanitation, water supply, space, and fresh air had already become central design principles in modernist architecture and urban planning following World War I as discourses of hygiene and the germ theory of transmission gradually gained acceptance among medical practitioners between the 18th and 20th centuries.[9] The understanding of the city as a biological organism was perhaps best exemplified by Le Corbusier's 1925 text *Urbanisme*—translated into English in 1929 as *The City of To-morrow and its Planning*—which decreed a causal relationship between health and design: "Hygiene and moral health depend on the lay-out of cities. Without hygiene and moral health, the social cell becomes atrophied."[10]

However, ideas of town planning as a form of "conservative surgery" were already in use during the late 19th century in the work of Scottish proto-town planner Patrick Geddes. These ideas traveled from the British Isles and reappeared in a more drastic form as calls for "civic surgery" in programs drafted by the British town planner Max Lock for the development of Basra (1956) or in the National Housing Program designed by the Greek town planner Constantinos A. Doxiadis of Doxiadis Associates (D.A.) for Baghdad (1957).[11] Both these programs were meant to eradicate reed and mud dwellings, first in large cities, later to be followed by the rest of the country. Therefore, during the year following the 1956 Housing Census and alongside the smallpox vaccination campaign, the Baghdad Health Directorate began enacting programs of forceful disinfection and fumigation of migrant dwellings. These took place a few weeks before D.A. unveiled plans at the 1957 National Housing Exhibition of conducting a massive program of slum clearance that would displace the first batch of 28,500 migrant families in Baghdad over the next five years.[12] The simultaneous deployment of sanitation, vaccination, and urban planning interventions in migrant settlements was intended to be mutually reinforcing and helped to generate broad consensus around the displacement of tens of thousands of families that was to take place over the next decade.

Migrant residents understood that sanitation and vaccination campaigns were a double-edged sword that could lead to displacement, and they were often put in the impossible position of either attempting to hide from vaccination teams or rejecting necessary health interventions. A D.A. report recounted such an encounter in 1956:

> As a result to the action taken by the Asimah [Capital] Health Directorate of moving the Sarifas from the neighborhood of dirty water, some of the inhabitants refused, and about 300 of them stood in the way of the official clerks and prevented them from doing their jobs, which obliged *Amanat Al Asimah* to ask for Police help, to investigate and punish the people responsible for that.[13]

A further complication was created by the fact that a significant portion of the inhabitants in many migrant neighborhoods were employed as low-ranking members of the army and police. In these interactions, police officers were put in a position where they were required not only to enforce vaccination campaigns but also to arrest, discipline, and even raze the dwellings of their neighbors.

Hashim Barakat, the Director of Health in Baghdad, claimed that migrants would be resettled to new housing schemes, where they would be provided with clean water, roads, electricity, and access to schools and health clinics. What Dr. Barakat failed to mention that the land that these migrants were occupying had become more valuable due to growing investment in public infrastructure and the completion of the Wadi Tharthar Flood Control project (1956). The flood control project meant that former flood zones where migrants had built their neighborhoods had now become prime real estate for suburban development. Despite attempts at resistance, by the early 1960s migrant settlements like Asima and Shakriya were completely destroyed. Dr. Barakat's promises, however, were never realized.[14] And new peripheral migrant settlements faced the same challenges regarding access to water and sanitation as before. While the smallpox vaccination campaign would eventually reduce the incidence of the virus among migrant communities, the campaign itself provided health and municipal officials an opportunity to collect statistical and household information from unsuspecting rural migrants that would later enable the destruction of their homes.

Conclusion

Epidemics and epidemic responses amplify existing patterns of social inequality, in turn shaping urban life and social practices. Public discourse on smallpox eradication in 1950s Iraq demonstrates the ways marginalized populations like rural migrants are perceived as vectors of disease; by association, their settlements are seen as epicenters of outbreaks, regardless of the actual source of disease. Following smallpox outbreaks in 1948 and 1956, the Iraqi state made rural migrants and their settlements the central subject of medical and urban planning interventions. State-wide inoculation campaigns took place as Iraq experienced an exponential growth in the oil revenues that fueled the rapid expansion of its financial, medical, statistical, and urban planning institutions.

Iraqi institutions did work in concert to eradicate smallpox. Yet, they also utilized the broad mandate to improve the health of Iraqi citizens in order to execute a covert expansion of the state's surveillance activities in the capital city of Baghdad through household studies, censuses, and the accelerated displacement of poorer residents from valuable urban land.[15] It is therefore important to interrogate triumphal state narratives of disease eradication and examine how the specter of disease also enables campaigns of mass displacement and eviction. Moreover, broad public health campaigns can provide cover for the ruling government to deploy police officers in targeted campaigns of intimidation, directed at groups who engage in any form of resistance to the displacement that accompanies vaccination and sanitation campaigns. Finally, epidemics often give rise to the medicalization of city planning programs and vocabulary, such as "civic surgery," which can permit the reconfiguration of political dissidents and the urban poor as cancerous growths or an infectious pox that needs to be excised from the healthy growing body of the city or state.

NOTES

1. For an overview of the medical apparatus of the 20th-century Iraqi state, see Sara Farhan, "The Making of Iraqi Doctors: Reproduction in Medical Education" (Ph.D. diss., York University, 2019).

2. For an overview of mid-century smallpox eradication efforts in Iraq, see Sara Farhan and Huma Gupta, "The Campaign to Eradicate Smallpox in Monarchic Iraq," Jadaliyya.com, April 23, 2020, https://www.jadaliyya.com/Details/41002.

3. Ministry of Economics, *Report on the Housing Census for Iraq* (Baghdad: Government Press, 1956), 15.

4. Maria Zagorissiou, "The Slums of Buffalo Holders," March 20, 1958, Iraq Reports v. 126, Archive Files / 24000, Constantinos A. Doxiadis Archives, 1.

5. Sattareh Farman, "The Social Problems of Urbanization in Iraq, Prepared for the Government of Iraq." New York: United Nations Technical Assistance Programme, TAA/IRQ/4, 1958, 16, 17, 20.

6. Maria Zagorissiou, "The Slums of Sarifa Holders," July 13, 1958, Iraq Reports v. 127, Archive Files / 24001, Constantinos A. Doxiadis Archives, 15.

7. Abdullah Sakhy, phone interview with Huma Gupta, April 10, 2020.

8. "The inability of the medical authorities to bring the recent smallpox epidemic rapidly under control emphasized to wealthy Iraqis the necessity of supplying sanitation and medical care to the urban slums, if for selfish reasons alone." Doris G. Phillips, "Rural-to-Urban Migration in Iraq," *Economic Development and Cultural Change* 7, no. 4 (1959): 420.

9. UK Ministry of Health, *Manual of Unfit Housing* (London: UK Ministry of Health, 1919); American Public Health Association, *Principles of Healthful Housing* (Washington, DC: American Public Health Association, 1939); Margaret Campbell, "What Tuberculosis Did for Modernism: The Influence of a Curative Environment on Modernist Design and Architecture," *Medical History* 49, no. 4 (2005): 463–88.

10. Le Corbusier, *The City of To-Morrow and its Planning* (New York: Dover, 1987), 84.

11. "Town Planning is the science of 'civic surgery'. Before derelict and blighted areas can be removed, new communities grafted on, traffic congestion eased, a thorough 'medical examination' or penetrating 'civic diagnosis' is needed." Max Lock & Partners, *The New Basrah: A Survey and Planning Report for the Basrah Municipality* (London: The Millbrook Press, 1956), 13.

12. *Iraq Times*, January 26, 1957; *Housing Program of Iraq (1st Roll-Negative), Motion Pictures and Videorecordings / 29200*, Constantinos A. Doxiadis Archives, 9.

13. B. Kachachi, "Sarifa Dwellers Baghdad/Re: CQA 172/ 12.6/1956," July 10, 1956, *Archive Files / QB 197*, Constantinos A. Doxiadis Archives.

14. For the national housing program and slum clearance efforts in Iraq, see Huma Gupta, "Migrant Sarifa Settlements and State-Building in Iraq" (Ph.D. diss., Massachusetts Institute of Technology, 2020).

15. Farhan and Gupta, "Campaign to Eradicate Smallpox."

17

House, Social Life, and Smallpox in Kathmandu, Nepal, 1963

Susan Heydon

In the early 1960s, many parts of the world were free of smallpox but in the small Himalayan kingdom of Nepal, the disease remained widespread and much feared. The 1961 census recorded that almost 97 percent of a population of nearly 9.5 million lived in rural areas at the time. Nepal was one of the least developed countries in the world, with the majority of rural residents living at a subsistence level. The daily grind of life for most Nepalis had changed little since Prithvi Narayan Shah (1723–1775) conquered the Kathmandu Valley kingdoms in 1768.[1] The British colonized much of the wider South Asian region, but the rugged landscape and supply of Gurkha soldiers to fight British causes helped Nepal remain independent. Education and health had little place in government philosophy.[2]

Sandwiched between the large regional powers of India and China, Nepal is rectangular in shape, approximately 800 kilometers long and 200 kilometers wide, and divided into three broadly horizontal areas: the flat Tarai to the south, the central hills, and the mountains to the north. In the early 1960s, the population of 450,000 living in the Kathmandu Valley in the central hill region included the residents of three ancient cities and multiple townships and villages. The largest city, the capital Kathmandu, was the center of government, which in 1963 was firmly in the hands of the king. Kathmandu was also the most densely populated region of Nepal (Figure 17.1).[3]

Smallpox was an acute and contagious viral disease that entered through the respiratory tract and was primarily spread by contact with an infected person.[4] Despite smallpox's long presence in Nepal, no accurate data exist from before the 1960s and little has been written about the disease's impact on the country. The first figures appear in international statistics in 1961, when five cases and two deaths were recorded in West Nepal among Tibetan refugees.[5] Everyone was at risk, particularly in crowded, urban areas such as Kathmandu. In 1816, even the young king died from the disease.

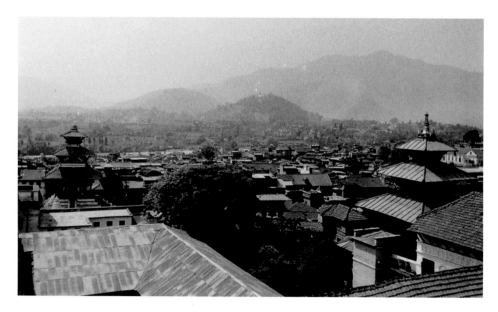

FIGURE 17.1: Kathmandu rooftops. (Courtesy of Tod Ragsdale, Nepal Peace Corps Photo Project.)

The severe variola major form of the virus with a case fatality rate of over 20 percent was endemic among the population. Every four or five years the disease became epidemic, as occurred in 1963; the virus was also endemic to India, Nepal's southern neighbor. Nepalis understood that smallpox was infectious, without a known cure, and disfiguring but that survivors acquired long-lasting immunity. It was also understood that the disease could be prevented through vaccination or variolation (inoculation with live smallpox matter). However, Nepal had an extremely limited health infrastructure and even in the capital most Nepalis were unable to access vaccination.[6] The country operated a single infectious disease unit at Bir Hospital in Kathmandu; there were few trained health workers. Without quarantine procedures or facilities, smallpox cases throughout Nepal were looked after and managed in the domestic environment.[7]

Case study: Smallpox in Kathmandu, 1963

The epidemic in Kathmandu and the surrounding area in 1963 was part of Nepal's last major smallpox epidemic, but it is largely missing from the historical record. In late February, cases in the remote Mt. Everest region were traced to a porter, who was infected in Kathmandu while looking for work with an overseas climbing expedition.[8] The first cases in Nepal were only recorded in the World Health Organization's (WHO) official *Weekly Epidemiological Record* at the end of April.[9] The infected area was listed as Kathmandu, and although the disease was widespread in many parts of the country no notifications were given for cases elsewhere. Weekly totals began to rise steeply at the end of September, peaking with 319 cases and 112 deaths in the week ending on December 14. Numbers subsequently dropped and no further cases were recorded after January 25, 1964. With the absence of a formal reporting system, these figures likely underrepresented the situation.

Smallpox management in 1960s Nepal is also largely missing from the historical record. Smallpox was common, particularly in childhood; its lesions were highly visible. Smallpox spread from contact with an infected person and many people thought that they could be infected through the practice of spitting out of windows. An infected person typically exhibited a fever as an early symptom, but as this was common for many illnesses, the virus could be present before people realized. The disease was most infectious during the first week. Many elderly people today remember having the disease or caring for their children; their stories relate their anguish from the time but also bring to light the social practices that surrounded looking after someone with smallpox. These family-centered practices were mostly learned from other family members and oral tradition. Beliefs and practices about smallpox varied among Nepal's many ethnic groups, but the Newar, the main inhabitants of the urban environment of old Kathmandu city and the valley, addressed three common threads while talking with me about smallpox: isolation of the person with smallpox, care of the ill, and the importance of religious rituals.[10]

Newar society was structured around caste and occupation; over centuries, this determined the allocation of space in the city, with elites living nearest to the center. Kathmandu's streets were narrow and daylight hardly penetrated the tightest alleyways. Such crowded conditions allowed disease to spread easily. Multi-storeyed individual houses, typically home to an extended family, were crowded together, opening on to the street with a shop or built around small common courtyards. Most private dwellings were small, dark, and cold, with low ceilings and without indoor running water and sanitation. Sometimes residents needed to pass through another house to get to their own, and much of the activities of daily life took place in the semi-public space of the courtyard, or the public areas of the street and neighborhood squares (Figure 17.2).[11]

Word spread quickly when a case of smallpox appeared in the community. People recall that there were many cases and many deaths in 1963. Children were kept inside and visitors did not enter homes. Those who contracted the disease were isolated in a part of the house away from other members of the household

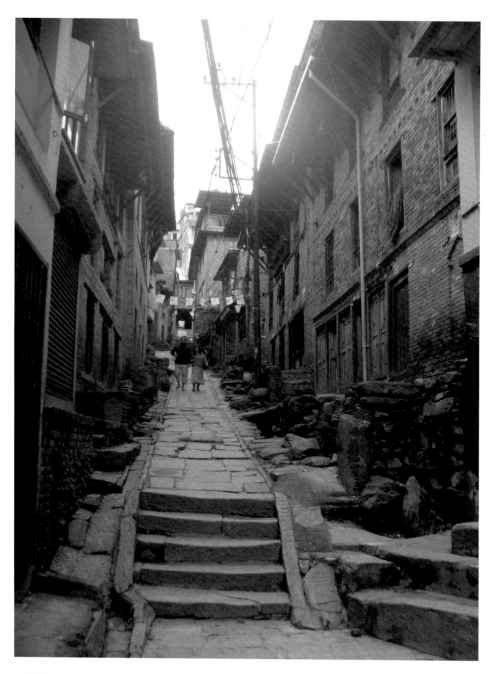

FIGURE 17.2: Narrow city streets. (Courtesy of Susan Heydon.)

and family activities. Although a Newari house becomes ritually purer in the higher storeys, the decision about where to isolate diseased family members was more pragmatic. Where possible, the person was put in a separate room, had their own bed and sheets, and did not share family food and utensils. Severe cases of smallpox required considerable care, and once confined to a bed, an infected person often did not leave until they recovered or died. A single carer, usually a senior female member of the household, was designated. Mothers recalled the demands of the role as they attended to every need and want of their severely ill children: smallpox was painful. Some had more than one child with the disease to look after and struggled with the exhaustion. An outside healer was rarely called upon as people knew there was no treatment and little that could be done. Children often found the time lonely and boring. Much later they still remembered the intense itchiness of the scabs as the pustules healed, at which time they might be sent out to the outside courtyard so that people passing by could tell them not to scratch.

Spiritual offerings were an integral part of people's responses to smallpox. Rituals were first carried out in the home in a special area or room, mostly by women. The obligation to carry out rituals also took carers into public spaces, both locally and further afield. The main Newar site was the Buddhist temple complex at Swayambunath to the west of Kathmandu city, which had a small double-storeyed temple dedicated to a goddess known by various names—Hariti or Ajima to local Newar, or Sitala to Hindu believers (Figure 17.3). Kathmandu's roads were poor and access to transport was limited, so the carer usually went on foot on a trip that could often take all day.

During the peak of the epidemic, the government increased its vaccination activities by focusing in and around the Thimi area of the valley where the number of cases was highest. The township was not yet part of the Smallpox Control Pilot Project begun in 1962 as a joint effort of the Government of Nepal and the WHO. Extra health workers, students, police, and government workers were brought in to help. Most Nepalis supported vaccination, although some Newar groups voiced opposition. The head of the government response, Dr. Ram Bhadra Adiga, considered this to be due more to a lack of education than religious prohibitions.[12] Vaccinators targeted people on the move, such as pilgrims and holy men traveling from India for the annual Shivaratri festival. In February 1964, the government passed legislation making vaccination compulsory for children under the age of twelve years, although in practice this policy made little difference to the number of recorded cases. The epidemic was over, births were not registered, and health services were limited. Vaccination against smallpox only reached the whole country in 1973.

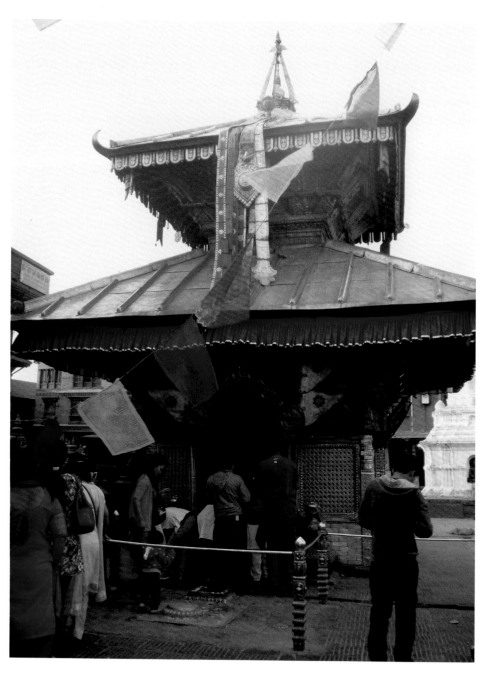

FIGURE 17.3: The temple at Swayambunath. (Courtesy of Susan Heydon.)

Conclusion

Infectious disease spreads most easily where people congregate and live together in crowded conditions. Social practices during the smallpox epidemic in Kathmandu in 1963 were an aspect of the complex relationship between people and their environment and influenced what was done to address the disease and how domestic and public spaces were used. Such practices were also shaped by the unique features of smallpox as a highly visible disease transmitted only through human to human contact. Knowledge of these features meant that people were aware when smallpox was present and that authorities could eliminate the involvement of other vectors.

The spread of the disease could be controlled with a viable vaccine and other measures, but health infrastructure in Nepal was extremely limited. From a public health perspective, the government response to the epidemic focused on increasing vaccination activities rather than management of the Kathmandu urban environment. Mass vaccination was the generally accepted international strategy; the World Health Assembly adopted a proposal in 1959 to eradicate the disease globally. Progress in Nepal was initially slow because of the country's enormous physical and human challenges, but eventual success came by adapting the eradication program to Nepali conditions. The last case of smallpox in Nepal was recorded in 1975. Until eradication was achieved, people coped with cases of the disease as best as they could within the context of their daily lives. Newari social practices relied upon smallpox management in the home through isolation, although carers often traveled across the city to carry out ritual obligations. A family's multi-storeyed house made isolation possible in a crowded urban environment, as did the love and nursing care mothers gave to their sick children. In places such as Nepal in the 1960s, smallpox outcomes at home were better than in an institution.

NOTES

1. See John Whelpton, *A History of Nepal* (Cambridge: Cambridge University Press, 2005).
2. Hem Narayan Agrayal, *The Administrative System of Nepal: From Tradition to Modernity* (New Delhi: Vikas, 1976), 132.
3. 1900 per square mile/4920 per square kilometer.
4. For the standard English-language international textbook of the time, see C. W. Dixon, *Smallpox* (London: J. & A. Churchill, 1962).
5. World Health Organization, *Weekly Epidemiological Record* (WER) 36, no. 15 (April 14, 1961), 158. This publication listed notifications reported under the International Sanitary Regulations.

6. For the development of Nepal's health services, see Hemang Dixit, *Nepal's Quest for Health* (Kathmandu: Educational Publishing House, 2014).

7. For a survey of smallpox cases admitted to Bir Hospital, see M. R. Pandey, I. L. Acharya, and A. Moyeed, "Clinical Survey of Small Pox," *Journal of Nepal Medical Association* 2, no. 1 (1964): 8–11.

8. Sir Edmund Hillary, *Schoolhouse in the Clouds* (London: Hodder and Stoughton, 1964); James Ramsey Ullman, *Americans on Everest* (Philadelphia: J. B. Lippincott, 1964).

9. *WER* 38, no. 21 (May 24, 1963): 262.

10. Interviews took place in April 2015 in Kathmandu and May 2017 in Kathmandu and Kirtipur. I would like to thank my colleague Kiran Bajracharya for his assistance in organizing and with interpreting.

11. Ulrike Müller, *Thimi: Social and Economic Studies on a Newar Settlement in the Kathmandu Valley* (Giessen: Geographical Institute, Justus Liebig University, 1981), 22–23.

12. Ram Bhadra Adiga, "Smallpox Epidemic in Nepal (1963–1964)." I am very grateful to the family of Dr. Edward Crippen (USAID) for providing a copy of this unpublished paper.

18

Meningitis, Shared Environments, and Inequality in São Paulo, Brazil, 1971–75

Daniela Sandler

In 1971, a meningitis outbreak slowly entered the outskirts of the city of São Paulo, in the southeast of Brazil, by then the country's largest and richest urban center. São Paulo was a fast-growing metropolis of eight million people, and the uptick in cases was mostly limited to a low-income neighborhood far from the denser areas of the city. Since 1964, Brazil had been under a right-wing military dictatorship. The regime systematically neglected issues of poverty and inequality and failed to prioritize the plight of those first affected by the illness. Early attempts by doctors and journalists to sound the alarm were censored; the military dictatorship, which controlled the government at the city, state, and federal levels, did not want bad news to mar the official narrative of Brazil's growth and its "economic miracle."[1]

Meningitis, an inflammation of the fluid and membranes, or meninges, that surround the brain and spinal cord, can be caused by bacteria, viruses, or fungi. The prognosis and treatment of meningitis varies depending on the pathogen.[2] The São Paulo outbreak was initially caused by the "C" strain of the *Neisseria meningitidis* bacterium, but it was compounded later by illness caused by the "A" strain, which was more aggressive and affected populations in slightly different age categories. In São Paulo, meningitis was allowed to spread unchecked, transmitted through close personal contact by exposure to respiratory and throat secretions. The disease thrived in low-income neighborhoods where residents lived in overcrowded dwellings without adequate ventilation and sanitation, and far away from health clinics and hospitals. The epidemic traced concentric circles in the city's territory, first in peripheral areas, then inching closer to the wealthier neighborhoods in the center, until the entire city was engulfed in 1974.[3] By then, the epidemic was augmented by a parallel outbreak of the aforementioned aggressive "A" strain of the bacterium. The outbreak peaked in the second half of 1974.[4] An estimated

151

900–2,500 people died from the epidemic in São Paulo alone, and cases later spread from São Paulo to other cities and states in Brazil.[5]

Residents of São Paulo's peripheral neighborhoods commuted to the wealthier districts to work in service and commerce, allowing the pathogen to reach the entire city with time. The meningitis epidemic was finally contained by a massive vaccination campaign in 1975, with numbers tapering down and only returning to endemic levels in 1977.[6] With the introduction of a vaccination program, the city was saved by herd immunity, through which a threshold of vaccinated residents protected the wider population. The vaccination campaign brought an end to a period of suffering and anxiety and prevented the epidemic from engulfing the whole nation. However, the relatively swift and sweeping effect of the vaccine pushed aside any discussion about improving the environmental and socioeconomic factors that had allowed the epidemic to fester in the first place. Overcrowded dwellings in far-flung neighborhoods lacked infrastructure, sanitation, clean water, access to local health care facilities, and efficient transit connections to the hospitals in the center of the city. São Paulo's chronic social ills were left untreated.

Case study: Meningitis in São Paulo, 1971–75

The São Paulo meningitis outbreak and the reasons why it lasted so long must be understood in relation to the sociopolitical context of São Paulo and Brazil in the mid-1970s. São Paulo had been experiencing intense urban growth since the 1950s as the new center of industrial and financial activity in the country, which was accompanied by migration from rural areas, especially from the northeast of Brazil.[7] These migrants found low-income jobs in factories and on construction sites in São Paulo, but little adequate housing. Some laborers found affordable housing in tenement houses in the center, but most went to live in undeveloped areas on the outskirts of the city.

These peripheral neighborhoods were the districts with the fastest demographic growth between the 1950s and 1980s. New residents in so-called self-built settlements lacked basic infrastructure such as paving, water, electricity, education, health, parks, public safety, and public transportation. Initially the density of these areas was low, but the dwellings themselves were overcrowded, as families built what they could afford and lived in close quarters. The severe inequalities that still define São Paulo were ingrained in the urban fabric at a metropolitan scale for the city and its metro region.[8]

Attempts to address inequalities faced political difficulties. The right-wing military coup in 1964 was motivated by fears of communism, and demands to address spatial and economic inequities through land or income reform were viewed with suspicion.[9] Residents of peripheral areas of São Paulo and other large cities were mostly left to their own devices.[10] Public housing programs were insufficient to meet the demand and compounded the problem through standardized and massified designs and cut-rate construction.[11] In spite of these political failings, academics, urbanists, and economists began to turn their attention to the disparities between the center and the margins of the city, and periphery residents began to organize themselves, but they did not wield sufficient power to change conditions.[12]

This was the climate in which, in 1971, meningitis cases increased in the Santo Amaro neighborhood in the southern periphery of the city (Figure 18.1). A few months later, cases went up in neighborhoods in the far eastern periphery, not contiguous to the southern districts. The illness jumped across the city, skipping over wealthier neighborhoods in a pattern, going from south to east to north to

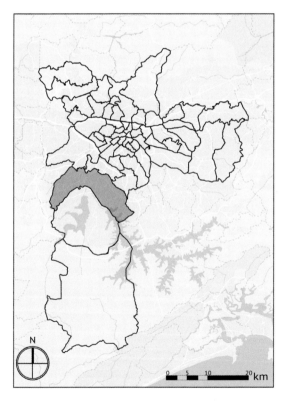

FIGURE 18.1: Map of district with epidemic levels of meningitis in São Paulo, 1971: Santo Amaro district highlighted. (Map drawn by Mary Dahlman Begley, based on the work of Rita de Cássia Barradas Barata, 1988.)

west, and then finally closing in on the center. Epidemiologists and infectious disease doctors explained this as a function of the living conditions in the peripheries where residents were "living in overcrowded dwellings, malnourished, performing strenuous labor, ill-adjusted to the climate, physically and emotionally stressed by the metropolitan way of life." Doctors believed "their immune systems were possibly more vulnerable to the meningococcus."[13] In the first three years of the epidemic, higher-income neighborhoods in the central core with adequate living conditions were spared. Decades later, public health experts would recognize "social conditions as fundamental causes of disease."[14]

The relationship between poverty and the epidemic is clear. Residents of the peripheries commuted via public transit from home to work and shared these spaces, so the bacterium must have traveled with them to be passed around in crowded buses and tight workspaces. But by the second semester of 1974, every single neighborhood, including the wealthy areas, registered cases at the epidemic level (Figure 18.2). The disease eventually affected the entire city, not merely the crowded periphery.

Other types of shared spaces may explain the urban spread. While many residents of the peripheries worked in factories or construction, somewhat separately from other socio-economic classes, others worked in service and commerce jobs in middle- and upper-class neighborhoods, commuting to work as shop clerks, cab drivers, janitors, nannies, and maids. Domestic workers have been pervasive in Brazil since the end of slavery in 1888 and often shared living spaces daily with higher-income residents.[15] Maids cleaned, cooked, and often looked after children, feeding, bathing, and comforting them. The meningitis pathogen, spread through saliva and respiratory secretions, thrives in situations of such close contact. Many asymptomatic carriers could still transmit the disease. Although central neighborhoods offered a significantly higher quality of life including adequate living space

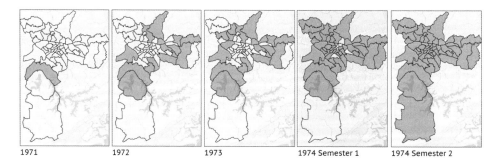

| 1971 | 1972 | 1973 | 1974 Semester 1 | 1974 Semester 2 |

FIGURE 18.2: Progression of districts with epidemic levels of meningitis (highlighted) in São Paulo, 1971–74. (Map drawn by Mary Dahlman Begley, based on the work of Rita de Cássia Barradas Barata, 1988.)

for most families and urban and health infrastructure and sanitation, they were not beyond the reach of the disease.

Bacterial meningitis progresses rapidly and is sometimes overlooked during initial diagnosis. Patients with a fever were often sent home, only to deteriorate in a few hours. Mothers would beg for doctors to run spinal taps on their children to test for the disease, a scary-sounding exam that most people normally wanted to avoid.[16] Patient recovery depended on quick diagnosis and immediate treatment with antibiotics. This was much more of a problem for residents of the peripheries, who had to commute over long distances to centrally located hospitals. The journey, often via public transportation, could take two hours or more given the congested traffic of São Paulo.

The intimacy of inequality in São Paulo spread the disease to all socio-economic groups. This was also the turning point for the epidemic. Once groups with more political and economic clout were affected and demanded action, the government changed its stance. News outlets were able to publish more openly on the epidemic, which helped raise public awareness and put pressure on the government.[17] News stories reported on the rising number of cases, overcrowded hospitals, and the overwhelmed public health system. Most patients were sent to the Emílio Ribas Hospital, the official hospital for infectious diseases. Located in a central neighborhood, it had 450 beds, but at the peak of the disease it held 1,046 patients, many of them lying on the floor in hallways. Maria Aparecida Basile, a doctor who worked at Emílio Ribas at the time, recounted that sinks were converted into makeshift beds for babies and toddlers.[18] Lines formed outside of the hospital, which, as a public institution, could not turn down patients (Figure 18.3). The lines made the epidemic terrifyingly visible—not only did newspapers publish photos, but the hospital was located on a busy thoroughfare, and people in cars and buses could see the overcrowding from the street.

The federal government swooped in with a monumental vaccination campaign, a heroic gesture that appeared to save the day, quenching the epidemic. The government imported 80 million doses of a vaccine from the Meriéux Institute in France, the only laboratory capable of manufacturing it.[19] The vaccine had never been administered at this scale, and the Meriéux Institute had to build new facilities in order to produce the doses in a relatively short period of time. The vaccination campaign began in March 1975; ten million people were vaccinated in the first five days and the entire national campaign took ten months (Figure 18.4).[20] But the vaccine obviated the need for environmental measures such as adequate housing, sewage and trash collection, street paving, green spaces, potable water, public transportation, and access to local health care, which could have reduced the impact of the epidemic in the city's peripheries. The precarious conditions in these areas were allowed to grow unchecked, just as the pathogen had been, and

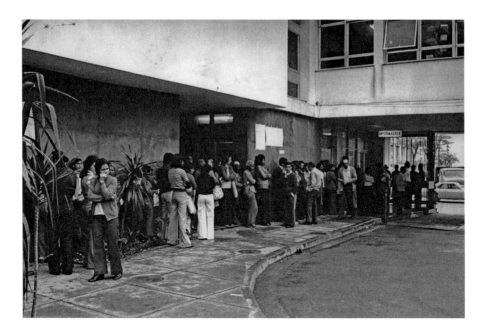

FIGURE 18.3: Parents and relatives line up waiting to visit meningitis patients in the Emílio Ribas Hospital, São Paulo, 1974. (Courtesy of Folhapress.)

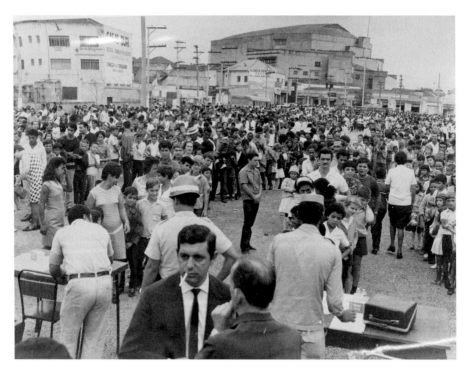

FIGURE 18.4: Vaccination campaign, metropolitan region of São Paulo, 1976. (Courtesy of the Archives of the Emílio Ribas Museum of Public Health – Butantan Institute/Acervo Museu de Saúde Pública Emílio Ribas – Instituto Butantan.)

today the urban challenges of the peripheries, home to almost nine million people, two-thirds of the entire population of São Paulo, are more daunting than ever.

Doctors who focus on clinical medicine and pharmaceutical interventions such as antibiotics and vaccines reiterate the critical need to improve living conditions, noting that they are as important as the toolkit of medicine.[21] Such improvement, of course, is much more costly, time-consuming, and politically demanding than a ten-month vaccination campaign, particularly in the context of a right-wing military dictatorship uninterested in social equality.

Conclusion

The conditions of inequality in the periphery of São Paulo allowed meningitis to rise above endemic levels and to spread to the entire city. Peripheral areas suffered due to overcrowded living conditions and to their distance from health care, which meant worse outcomes. The epidemic revealed the need to see decentralized health care as integral to urban infrastructure in a metropolis as vast as São Paulo and made clear the distinction between population density and housing overcrowding. The most affected areas, both in terms of case numbers and deaths, were not the densest areas at the time. The older neighborhoods where the middle- and upper classes lived in high-rise apartments in the center of the city were dense and verticalized, but living conditions were adequate and there was no overcrowding: residents had access to ventilation, fresh air, direct sunlight, playgrounds, and parks. In addition, these populations had prompt medical care, better nutrition, support systems, and access to information about the disease and its progression. It was not urban density that allowed the disease to propagate: it was overcrowding, coupled with lack of sanitation and urban infrastructure.

The success of the meningitis vaccine might suggest that herd immunity was a form of urban infrastructure, residing not in the physical spaces of the city but in the bodies of its residents. If so, vaccines could be seen as a public urban improvement. But, as with comparable public improvements such as water treatment to prevent cholera or fumigation to curb mosquitoes, vaccination is a narrow-spectrum measure. Although the 1970s meningitis outbreak in São Paulo was contained, several other epidemics have since plagued the city: dengue fever, zika, and chikungunya. In all cases, the peripheries have fared much worse than the urban center. The interconnectedness of the city means, however, that when the peripheries fall ill, the entire city ails in more ways than one.

NOTES

1. Carlos Giannazi, *A Doutrina de Segurança Nacional e o "Milagre Econômico" (1969/ 1973)* [The National Security Doctrine and the "Economic Miracle" (1969–1973)] (São Paulo: Cortez Editora, 2014).

2. If the *Neisseria meningitidis* bacterium is the source, the illness is referred to as meningococcal disease, which can include meningitis and other illnesses like septicemia. There are six subtypes, or serogroups, of *Neisseria meningitidis*, so a vaccine that works for some subtypes might not work for others.

3. Rita de Cássia Barradas Barata, "Epidemia de Doença Meningocócica, 1970/1977" [Meningococcal Disease Epidemic, 1970–1977], *Revista de Saúde Pública* 22, no. 1 (1988): 19–23.

4. At that time, cases rose to 179.71 per 100,000 people, far above the endemic level of 2.16 per 100,000. José Cássio de Moraes and Rita de Cássia Barradas Barata, "A Doença Meningocócica em São Paulo, Brasil, no século XX: Características Epidemiológicas" [Meningococcal Disease in São Paulo, Brazil, in the 20th Century: Epidemiological Features], *Cadernos de Saúde Pública* 21, no. 5 (September–October 2005): 1462.

5. "A Epidemia de Meningite que a Ditadura Militar no Brasil Tentou Esconder da População" [The Meningitis Epidemic That the Military Dictatorship in Brazil Tried to Hide from the Population], *Faculdade de Ciências Médicas da Santa Casa de São Paulo*, June 9, 2020, https://fcmsantacasasp.edu.br/a-epidemia-de-meningite-que-a-ditadura-militar-no-brasil-tentou-esconder-da-populacao/; Conceição Lemes, "Meningite: Um Crime da Ditadura Brasileira" [Meningitis: A Crime of the Brazilian Dictatorship], *A Voz Dissonante*, March 22, 2009, https://vozdissonante.livejournal.com/56761.html; Rita de Cássia Barradas Barata, *Meningite: Uma Doença Sob Censura?* [Meningitis: A Disease under Censorship?] (São Paulo: Cortez, 1988).

6. "De Olhos Bem Fechados: Meningite, a Epidemia que a Ditadura Não Conseguiu Esconder" [Eyes Wide Shut: Meningitis, the Epidemic the Dictatorship Couldn't Hide], *Revista Ser Médico*, no. 33 (October/November/December 2005), https://www.cremesp.org.br/?siteAcao=Revista&id=216.

7. See Paulo Fontes, *Migration and the Making of Industrial São Paulo* (Durham, NC: Duke University Press, 2008).

8. United Nations Habitat and Fundação Sistema Estadual de Análise de Dados, *São Paulo: A Tale of Two Cities* (Nairobi: United Nations Settlements Program, 2010), 13–25.

9. Vera da Silva Telles, "Anos 70: Experiências, Práticas e Espaços Políticos" [The 1970s: Experiences, Practices and Political Spaces], in *As Lutas Sociais e a Cidade: São Paulo Passado e Presente*, ed. Lúcio Kowarick (São Paulo: Paz e Terra; Centro de Estudos de Cultura Contemporânea; Instituto de Pesquisas das Nações Unidas para o Desenvolvimento Social, 1988), 247–86.

10. Erminia Maricato, ed., *A Produção Capitalista da Casa (e da Cidade) no Brasil Industrial* [Capitalist Production of the House (and the City) in Industrial Brazil] (São Paulo: Editora Alfa Omega, 1982).

11. Erminia Maricato, *Política Habitacional no Regime Militar: Do Milagre Brasileiro à Crise Econômica* [Housing Policy in the Military Regime: From the Brazilian Miracle to the Economic Crisis] (Petrópolis: Vozes, 1987).

12. Ana Claudia Castilho Barone, "A Periferia como Questão: São Paulo na Década de 1970" [The Periphery as an Issue: São Paulo in the 1970s], *Revista da Pós* 20, no. 33 (2013): 64–85.

13. Lygia Busch Iversson, "Aspectos Epidemiológicos da Meningite Meningocócica no Município de São Paulo (Brasil), no Período de 1968 a 1974" [Epidemiological Aspects of Meningococcal Meningitis in the Municipality of São Paulo (Brazil), from 1968 to 1974], *Revista de Saúde Pública*, no. 10 (1976): 12.

14. Bruce Link and Jo Phelan, "Social Conditions as Fundamental Causes of Disease," *Journal of Health and Social Behavior*, Extra Issue (1985): 80–94.

15. Priscila de Souza Silva and Silvana Nunes de Queiroz, "O Emprego Doméstico no Brasil: Um Olhar para o 'Trabalho da Mulher' na Perspectiva Histórica e Contemporânea," *Revista de Ciências Sociais*, no. 49 (July/December 2018): 188–204.

16. Maria Aparecida Basile, interview with author via videoconferencing, July 2020.

17. Catarina Schneider and Michele Tavares, "O Retrato da Epidemia de Meningite em 1971 e 1974 nos Jornais *O Globo* e *Folha de São Paulo*" [The Portrait of the Meningitis Epidemic in 1971 and 1974 in the Newspapers *O Globo* and *Folha de São Paulo*], Paper presented at Alcar 2015: 10º Encontro Nacional de História da Mídia, Universidade Federal do Rio Grande do Sul, Porto Alegre, June 3–5 2015.

18. Basile, interview.

19. Baptiste Baylac-Paouly, "Confronting an Emergency: The Vaccination Campaign against Meningitis in Brazil (1974–75)," *Social History of Medicine*, hkz120 (December 2019), https://doi.org/10.1093/shm/hkz120.

20. Denis Delbecq, "Charles Mérieux, le roi des vaccines, s'est éteint" [Charles Mérieux, the King of Vaccines, Has Passed Away], *Le Libération*, January 20, 2001, https://www.liberation.fr/societe/2001/01/20/charles-merieux-le-roi-des-vaccins-s-est-eteint_351771.

21. Basile, interview.

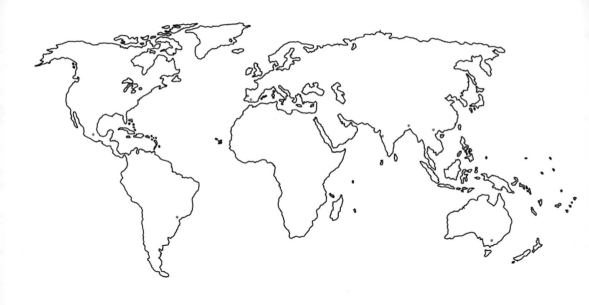

PART 3
Urban Infrastructure:
Permanence and Change

Case Studies for Urban Infrastructure

Present-day cities and countries

19. Lisbon, Portugal (Plague, 1480–95)
20. Seville, Spain (Plague, 16th Century)
21. Puebla, México (Plague, 1737)
22. Dhaka, Bangladesh (Cholera, 1858–1947)
23. Ilha Grande, Brazil (Cholera, 1886)
24. Mumbai, India (Plague, 1896)
25. Hanoi, Vietnam (Plague, 1885–1910)
26. Culion Island, The Philippines (Leprosy, 1898–1941)
27. Melbourne, Australia (Influenza, 20th Century)

This page: Map indicating the locations of case studies in this section of the book. (Map in the public domain, with annotations drawn by Andrew Bui.)

Right page: Bombay plague epidemic, 1896–97: interior of a plague hospital. Photograph attributed to Clifton & Co. (Courtesy of the Wellcome Collection.)

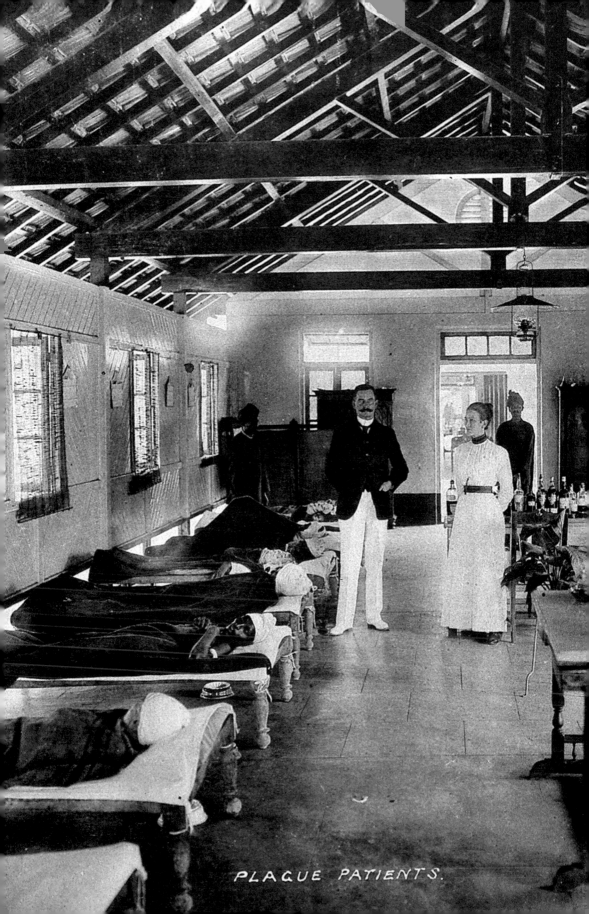

PLAGUE PATIENTS.

19

Epidemics and the Royal Control of Public Health in Lisbon, Portugal, 1480–95

Danielle Abdon

There exists a pervasive view of public health as a modern, 18th-century phenomenon that emerged from factors such as the rise of nation-states, industrialization, democratization, scientific and technological advances, and formal education. Yet, recent publications using case studies of late medieval and early modern cities challenge this narrative.[1] Urban historians Carole Rawcliffe and Guy Geltner have demonstrated prevailing concerns for and interventions in the collective health and sanitation of cities that predate the supposed emergence of public health discourse in Europe during the late 1700s, underscoring the importance of the use of case studies in contesting long-held assumptions in this field.[2] Contributing to this line of inquiry is the example of Lisbon, Portugal, during the 1480s and 1490s—a period when a sequence of epidemics led the Portuguese monarchy to assertively intervene in the public health of the city. These interventions went beyond religious actions meant to purify the city and placate divine wrath, commonly perceived as the source of outbreaks at the time.[3] Rather, they signaled royal preoccupation with three aspects: potential contagion from the arrival of outside peoples, risky behaviors in the city itself, and the maintenance or development of infrastructures crucial to the physical cleanliness of Lisbon. These anxieties and the strategies employed to mitigate them indicate a rising concern for control of public health in the city as Lisbon struggled with the social and sanitary difficulties associated with an emerging global port.

With the ascension of King Dom João I (r. 1385–1433) to the Portuguese throne, which led to the beginning of Portugal's Atlantic explorations, Lisbon slowly transitioned from a medieval city into a global metropolis (Figure 19.1).[4] In 1427, the city had a population of 60,000–65,000 people, a number that would progressively increase in the next century to reach 100,000 in the mid-1500s.[5] This local population growth was driven by an upsurge in transient populations

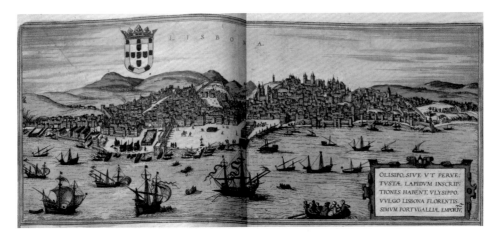

FIGURE 19.1: Detail of *Lisbon*, Georg Braun and Frans Hogenberg, *Civitates Orbis Terrarum*, vol. 1, 1572. (Courtesy of Library of Congress Geography and Map Division.)

connected to the explorations and the arrival of Jewish refugees expelled from Spain in 1492. Yet, the growth also coincided with famines and plague outbreaks to critically deteriorate the public health of Lisbon and its medieval urban fabric.[6] Plague outbreaks in particular reached a critical point in the early 1480s, with the city facing recurring yearly epidemics from 1480 until 1497.[7] Significantly, in the medieval and early modern periods, 'plague' was not understood as a specific disease, such as the bubonic plague, but rather as an umbrella term for pestilential, contagious illnesses.[8] Attempting to reduce and control these outbreaks, the Portuguese monarchy led by King Dom João II (*r.* 1477/1481–95) intensified public health interventions in Lisbon. The commission of the Hospital Real de Todos-os-Santos in 1492 as a large general hospital for the city constituted the most symbolic of these measures. As a result, the institution has garnered scholarly attention for embodying royal control of health care in the city.[9] However, a series of legislative and infrastructural determinations accompanied the hospital commission, indicating a much broader monarchic vision for the public health of Lisbon. Justifying those measures, Dom João II himself explained that "from the city being clean comes much of its health."[10]

Measures deployed by the Portuguese monarchy reflected contemporary medical theory, which at that time relied on a combination of Galenic humoral medicine and the control of six behavioral and environmental factors known as "nonnaturals."[11] While patients could protect or restore their health by regulating most nonnaturals, humoral balance shifted based on the interactions between one's body and the wider environment.[12] The challenge of controlling these interactions gave prominence to miasma theory, fueling authorities' anxieties over air quality since noxious airs were believed to contain miasmatic particles that could poison the lungs, disturb humoral balance, and lead to disease.[13] As a result, early modern medicine was understood to be deeply impacted not only by an individual's agency over their own health but also by their surrounding environment.

Case study: Outbreaks of disease in Lisbon, 1480–95

Scholarship on late medieval and early modern epidemics has emphasized the historical interpretation of outbreaks as stemming from divine wrath, an association also pervasive in 15th-century Lisbon.[14] As outbreaks unfolded in the 1480s, King Dom João repeatedly engaged the Chamber of Lisbon to intervene on the spiritual health of the city. In a royal letter from January 6, 1484, the monarch ordered the Chamber to investigate and punish with penalties all evils and sins being committed in Lisbon.[15] These offenses to God, he argued, explained why the divine had allowed the plague to persist in the city for as long as it had. Dom João's concerns were not new, as illustrated by previous, similar measures attempting to purify Lisbon. On the occasion of a 1437 outbreak, for example, the Chamber ordered masses to be said in every church of the city and a general procession to take place every Friday.[16] The persistence of these measures during the 1480s outbreaks might, at first, frame the king's spiritual concerns and the monarchy's approach to public health as traditional. However, a series of interventions aimed at legislating behavior and infrastructure show the much larger scope of the Portuguese response—one strongly reliant on contemporary medical knowledge.

Rather than attempting to scapegoat or persecute minorities, another common strategy in early modern cities, royal measures signal Dom João's preoccupation with contagion through personal contact between healthy locals and incoming peoples that could carry pestilences from contaminated localities. In a letter dated August 12, 1484, Dom João instructed the Chamber to prevent abuses against Jews in Lisbon, to whom many attributed the plague outbreak.[17] Scapegoating of Jews during epidemics was not new, nor was it restricted to Lisbon, as the spread of the Black Death (1347–51) across Europe had likewise resulted in anti-Semitic discrimination and murders.[18] As the king's instructions indicate, however, Dom João rejected reactionary, faith-based concerns, opting instead for a more practical approach that was further elucidated in later determinations. In the face of the expulsion of the Jewish population from Spain, a royal letter dated September 25, 1492, ordered the Chamber to control their entrance into Portugal. This regulation might suggest religious discrimination at first, but significantly, it did not target all Jews. Dom João deliberately flagged those arriving from Castile since the region was known to be contaminated with the plague at that point.[19] This determination should be seen hand in hand with an order from a month later, which warned the Chamber about potential maritime contagion and instructed the municipality to inspect ships and determine whether their points of origin were contaminated and therefore posed a potential threat of contagion to Lisbon.[20]

When it came to the urban fabric of Lisbon, miasma theory and anxiety over air quality drove administrative interventions. Crucial records to the Lisbon case come from the *Livro das Posturas Antigas* (*Book of Old Measures*), which reports measures by the Chamber to legislate various aspects of urban life and infrastructure.[21] Records that date to as early as 1408 show attempts to control sanitation, including the disposal of trash, manure, and dead animals; the cleanliness of streets; the protection of water fountains against trash and improper use, such as the washing of clothes; and the safeguarding of ditches and pipes from trash accumulation—all scenarios that could lead to the formation of "bad air."[22] In addition to establishing a monetary penalty, the Chamber often granted that those who reported a violation would receive half of the imposed fee, creating a self-monitoring system among citizens to ensure compliance to the municipality's determinations. The office of *almotacé* was established in 1179 to assist with sanitation and maintain Lisbon's public works and salubriousness by paving streets and cleaning public fountains.[23] The precise number of officers, however, remains unknown, and the office's broad purview, which included inspecting weights and measures and controlling various aspects of urban construction, possibly prevented it from prioritizing sanitation.[24]

While public health measures reflected in the *Livro das Posturas Antigas* and the existence of the office of *almotacé* indicate that public health was not a novel concept in the 15th century, the Chamber's strategies were deemed insufficient by the late 1400s. In the same January 1484 letter expressing concern for the evils and sins performed in the capital, Dom João claimed that the epidemic Lisbon was facing derived, in great part, from the bad air formed through the dirtiness of manure and dung heaps in the city, as well as the fact that people were emptying their chamber pots (*camareiros*) at unsuitable locations.[25] Dom João reemphasized his displeasure over the city's hygiene in September 1484, explaining that the Queen and Prince would not remain in Lisbon while he traveled due to the "bad sanitary state of the city."[26] Disagreements between the monarchy and municipal administration over the cleanliness of Lisbon persisted, with the king even threatening to replace elected *almotacés* in 1491 with those of his own choice, if the elected officials did not care for the city as they should.[27] As these examples suggest, acting through the Chamber, the monarchy attempted to legislate not only the behavior of Lisbon's population but also that of elected officials.

Infrastructural interventions, on the other hand, targeted the conditions of the city's ditches and pipes, which were used to move both storm waters and waste matter from Lisbon's urban center towards the Tagus River (see Figure 19.1). Records from the *Livro das Posturas Antigas* signal anxiety over trash accumulation in Lisbon's sewer system. In ditches, debris created unpleasant sights and smells, but the presence of trash at a pipe's opening, designed to guarantee access to the structure for cleaning and maintenance purposes, was even more concerning, as it could result in a burst pipe, causing structural damage to the urban fabric. In both cases, unwanted bad air would ensue.

Lisbon's sewer system centered on an ancient pipeline known as the *rego das imundices*, or ditch of filth—appropriately named for its appearance (Figure 19.2).[28] Indicating an increased monarchic control over Lisbon's main

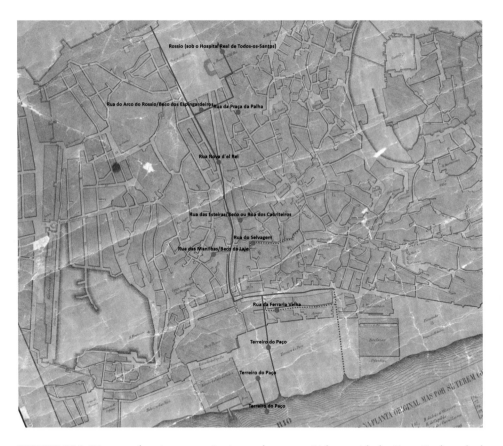

FIGURE 19.2: Diagram showing sewers in sixteenth-century Lisbon, with the Cano Real marked in dark green and pipes of lesser importance in light green and yellow. (Courtesy of Bugalhão and Teixeira, "Os canos da Baixa de Lisboa no século XVI: leitura arqueológica." *Cadernos do Arquivo Municipal* 2, no. 4 (2015): 89–122.)

sewer line, in the 15th century, the *rego das imundices* became known as the Cano Real, or Royal Pipe. The only pipe in the city under royal responsibility when it came to cleaning and repairs, the Cano Real gave the monarchy direct agency in preventing the formation of corrupt air resulting from stagnant and dirty waters in the city itself (Figure 19.3).

Despite monarchic control over the Cano Real, Dom João also perceived the need to expand the city's sewer infrastructure. On January 4, 1483, the king informed the Chamber that additional pipes were needed in several of Lisbon's streets for waste and dirty water.[29] Suggesting that no changes occurred, as epidemics continued into 1486, Dom João once again ordered the Chamber to both create large pipes in the main streets of Lisbon and to add smaller connecting pipes in other streets to facilitate the collection of waste in the city.[30] It is not known how much the existing system was expanded in the late 15th century, but expansion was not the king's only strategy. A letter from Dom João dated October 15, 1489, directed the Chamber to clean but also cover the city's pipes.[31] This built upon an older monarchic strategy, evidenced by records from 1460 and 1472, to sell city lots for the construction of private residences that would cover exposed pipes and sewage.[32] In this case, it was even possible for authorities to specify

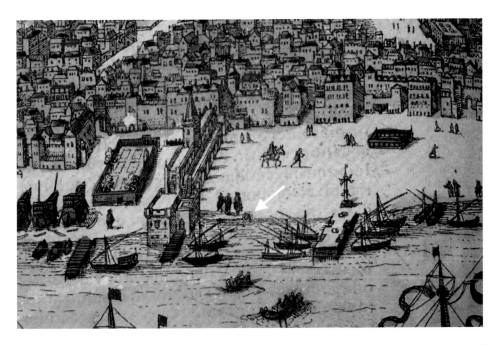

FIGURE 19.3: Arrow indicating the opening of the Cano Real on the Tagus River. Detail of *Lisbon*, Georg Braun and Frans Hogenberg, *Civitates Orbis Terrarum*, vol. 1, 1572. (Courtesy of Library of Congress, Geography and Map Division.)

the type of covering, requiring the new owner to create a vault over the pipe that would prevent bad smells from spreading outside the structure. Significantly, these interventions underscore that, grounded on miasma theory, the king perceived the city's sewer infrastructure as a crucial way to sanitize Lisbon.

Conclusion

Public health interventions implemented by the Portuguese monarchy, either directly by Dom João or indirectly through the Chamber of Lisbon, signal the royal strategy to address the city's collective health by legislating behavior and infrastructure. Dom João's preoccupation with the behavioral purity of Lisbon reinforces historical associations between sin and divine punishment, then believed to be the cause of outbreaks. However, the ways through which the king dealt with the presence and arrival of Jews shows his unwillingness to scapegoat a religious minority, which was instead presented as a problem for authorities under the umbrella of mass migration from contaminated regions. As for residents already living in Lisbon, they became a hazard when risky behaviors promoted the formation of bad air. Finally, in terms of infrastructure, the monarchy concentrated on Lisbon's sewer system as the most efficient way to prevent the formation of bad air in the city, whether by taking control of the Cano Real, expanding the city's system for waste collection, or by covering existing sewage pipes.

This discussion of 15th-century Lisbon not only contradicts the widespread understanding of public health as a modern phenomenon but also serves as evidence of governments' historical reliance on controlling behavior and infrastructure as efficient strategies to prevent or halt epidemics. While behaviors tend to be difficult to see in the historical record, infrastructure permanently shapes the urban development of cities, embodying measures to avoid or revert outbreaks. More broadly, this study underscores the concerted intervention by the monarchy at varying levels of government in order to control the spread of disease.

Acknowledgement: I am grateful to Ann Carmichael and Elizabeth Duntemann for their feedback on this essay. This research was generously supported by the Bibliotheca Hertziana—Max Planck Institute for Art History and the John Carter Brown Library.

NOTES

1. Guy Geltner, *Roads to Health: Infrastructure and Urban Wellbeing in Later Medieval Italy* (Philadelphia: Pennsylvania University Press, 2019), 5–33.

2. Ibid.; Carole Rawcliffe, *Urban Bodies: Communal Health in Late Medieval English Towns and Cities* (Woodbridge: The Boydell Press, 2013).

3. For an overview of religious understandings and responses to plague across cultures and media, see Dean Phillip Bell, *Plague in the Early Modern World* (New York: Routledge, 2019), 72–85.

4. Irisalva Moita, "A imagem e a vida da cidade," in *Lisboa quinhentista: A imagem e a vida da cidade*, ed. Irisalva Moita (Lisbon: Câmara Municipal de Lisboa, 1983), 9–10.

5. This population increase would have been more significant had it not been for the impact of plague outbreaks, shipwrecks, migrations, and wars. As the capital, Lisbon also attracted people on personal business to important governmental bodies, such as the Casa do Cível or the Casa da Suplicação. See ibid., 14–15, and Anastásia Mestrinho Salgado, *O Hospital de Todos-os-Santos: Assistência à pobreza em Portugal no século XVI; A irradiação da assistência médica para o Brasil, Índia e Japão* (Lisbon: By the Book, 2015), 85.

6. For an overview of charitable institutions including but not limited to hospitals in medieval Portugal, see Sérgio Luís de Carvalho, *Assistência e medicina no Portugal medieval* (Lisbon: Elo, 1995), 17–51.

7. See Antonio da Cunha Vieira de Meirelles, *Memorias de epidemiologia Portugueza* (Coimbra: Imprensa da Universidade, 1866), 228–34, for a discussion of sources addressing these outbreaks.

8. These ailments included what modern medicine has identified as bubonic plague, tuberculosis, epilepsy, scabies, erysipelas, anthrax, trachoma, and leprosy. Jorge Prata de Sousa and Ricardo da Costa, "Regimento proveitoso contra a pestilência (ca. 1496)—uma apresentação," *História, Ciências, Saúde—Manguinhos* 12 (2005): 842.

9. Danielle Abdon, "A Plan for the King and the Sick: Portuguese Hospital Architecture during the Age of Exploration," in *Health and Architecture: The History of Spaces of Healing and Care in the Pre-Modern Era*, ed. Mohammad Gharipour (New York: Bloomsbury Press, 2021).

10. Maria Teresa Campos Rodrigues, *Aspectos da administração municipal de Lisboa no século XV* (Lisbon: Imprensa Municipal, 1966), 115. "*Em a cidade ser bem limpa vay muyta parte da saude della.*"

11. The six nonnaturals included sleep, food and drink, evacuation and repletion, motion and rest, passions and emotions, and air quality.

12. The exception was air quality. For an overview of early modern medicine, see Guido Giglioni, "Health in the Renaissance," in *Health: A History*, ed. Peter Adamson (New York: Oxford University Press, 2019), 141–73.

13. Sandra Cavallo and Tessa Storey, *Healthy Living in Late Renaissance Italy* (Oxford: Oxford University Press), 70–112, includes a detailed discussion of the relationship between air quality and health in the early modern period.

14. See, e.g., Richard C. Trexler, *Public Life in Renaissance Florence* (Ithaca, NY: Cornell University Press, 1991), 361–64.

15. Eduardo Freire de Oliveira, *Elementos para a história do municipio de Lisboa*, vol. 1 (Lisbon: Typographia Universal, 1882), 318–19.

16. Ibid.

17. Maria Teresa Campos Rodrigues, ed., *Livro das Posturas Antigas* (Lisbon: Câmara Municipal de Lisboa, 1974), 19395. João also asked for the protection of Jews during non-plague times, as occurred in July 1490. See ibid.

18. Samuel H. Cohn, "Pandemics: Waves of Disease, Waves of Hate from the Plague of Athens to A.I.D.S.," *Historical Research* 85 (2012): 536–37.

19. Campos Rodrigues, *Livro das Posturas Antigas*, 193–95.

20. António Augusto Salgado de Barros, "Lisboa na confluência das rotas comerciais: efeitos na saúde pública (séculos XV a XVII)," *Cadernos do Arquivo Municipal* 2, no. 3 (2014): 253.

21. For an overview of the administration of 15th-century Lisbon, see Campos Rodrigues, *Aspectos*, 31–67.

22. Campos Rodrigues, *Livro das Posturas Antigas*.

23. For a description of this office and its role in the fifteenth century, see Campos Rodrigues, *Aspectos*, 57–62. See also Freire de Oliveira, *Elementos*, 212–18, for a historical overview of the position. Sandra Pinto offers a comparative analysis of this office between Portugal, Aragon, and Castile and how it shaped urban development in "Construir sem conflitos: As normas para o controlo da atividade construtiva em Valência, Sevilha, e Lisboa (séculos XIII a XVI)," *Anuario de Estudios Medievales* 47 (2017): 825–59.

24. Pinto, "Construir sem conflitos," 839–40.

25. Freire de Oliveira, *Elementos*, 318–19.

26. Ibid., 348–49.

27. Campos Rodrigues, *Aspectos*, 115.

28. António Augusto Salgado de Barros, *O Saneamento da cidade pós-medieval—o caso de Lisboa* (Lisbon: Ordem dos Engenheiros, 2014), 18–19; Jacinta Bugalhão and André Teixeira, "Os canos da Baixa de Lisboa no século XVI: leitura arqueológica," *Cadernos do Arquivo Municipal* 2, no. 4 (2015): 89–122.

29. Augusto da Silva Carvalho, *Crónica do Hospital de Todos-os-Santos* (Lisbon: n.p., 1949), 56.

30. António Augusto Salgado de Barros, "Os canos na drenagem da rede de saneamento da cidade de Lisboa antes do terremoto de 1755," *Cadernos do Arquivo Municipal* 2, no. 1 (2014): 86.

31. Arquivo Municipal de Lisboa, Livro III de D. João II, doc. 9.

32. Documentos do Arquivo Histórico da Câmara Municipal de Lisboa, *Livro de Reis*, vol. 2 (Lisbon: Publicações Culturais da Câmara Municipal de Lisboa: 1958), 241. Iria Gonçalves, *Um olhar sobre a cidade medieval* (Lisbon: Editora Patrimonia, 1996), 89.

20

The Guadalquivir River and Plague in Seville, Spain, in the 16th Century

Kristy Wilson Bowers

In the region of southern Spain known as Andalucía, the Guadalquivir River emerges from the mountains in the center of the peninsula and flows westward through Córdoba, bending to the southwest at Seville to drain into the Atlantic Ocean, 87 kilometers away (Figure 20.1). The river anchors Seville and has long been foregrounded in maps and images of the city, although this presentation skews a traditional north-south map orientation (Figure 20.2). While the river runs through the western edge of Seville, depictions of the city most often show the river running across the bottom of the page, so that north is to the left and east is to the top.

The river provided Seville with an international port and linked the city to its hinterland. The city grew significantly after 1503, when Queen Isabel I of Castile (1451–1504) chose Seville as the sole port for the movement of both people and goods between Iberia (Spain) and her New World colonies, establishing the Casa de la Contratación (House of Trade) to manage the flow of traffic. Seville became an important *entrepôt*, absorbing and redistributing a wide range of goods and people from not only the Americas but also Europe. This international traffic inevitably included disease. Seville became a crowded urban center whose population faced frequent epidemics, including deadly outbreaks of influenza (*catarro*), typhus (*tabardillo*), and plague (*mal de peste, mal contagioso, mal de landres*). Most worrisome was plague, which had the highest mortality rates. While some of these epidemics started with the shipping traffic in port, others circulated in from the countryside, spread by overland travelers and merchants. As an urban center, Seville depended upon and held jurisdiction over a *tierra*, a large swath of rural territory dotted with agricultural holdings and small towns and villages, much of which lay to the north of the city (Figure 20.3). Here, the river was both a natural landmark with which to orient oneself and a boundary to be crossed

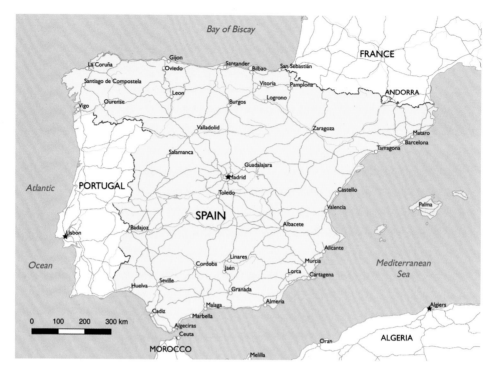

FIGURE 20.1: Map of Spain. (Courtesy of Mapswire.com.)

as people routinely moved about the region, working fields, selling goods, and visiting family. This regional mobility came into stark relief during epidemics as officials sought to track and restrict the movement of both people and goods in an ongoing effort to limit the spread of pestilence.

Case study: Plague along the Guadalquivir River, 1582

Seville's city officials had long-established routines to respond to the threat of plague and an ad hoc approach that repurposed existing structures to meet new needs. The city council itself was restructured to create a temporary health board. The combined council and health board continued to meet several times a week, keeping meticulous records of the decisions reached and orders sent out. These records are still preserved in the city's municipal archive, offering an almost day-to-day view of the unfolding epidemics.[1] Councilmen became health investigators, monitoring and limiting traffic into the city, tracking down individual cases of illness, interviewing doctors, and traveling to outlying towns to investigate and

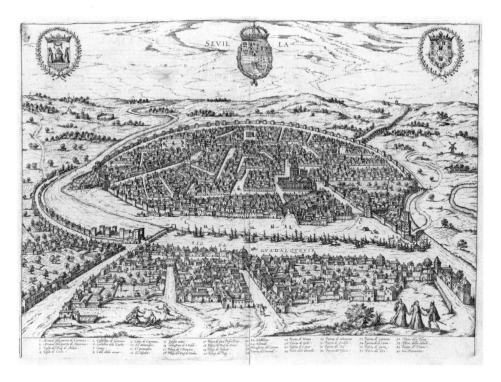

FIGURE 20.2: View of Seville, 1586. Georg Braun and Franz Hogenberg, *Civitates orbis terrarium* (vol. IV, 1588) f. 2v. (Courtesy of University of Seville Library/Biblioteca de la Universidad de Sevilla.)

coordinate responses to pestilence. These responses included securing locations to house the sick and convalescent and jails to hold those found breaking health regulations. City gates were closely monitored. Both people and goods could be quarantined before being allowed into the city or turned away outright if they were believed to be at risk of carrying plague. The old leprosy hospital, the Hospital de San Lázaro, built outside the city in the 13th century, became a way station for quarantining many kinds of goods coming into the city from the countryside.[2] The river was a key focus in these public health interventions, as both the port and numerous upriver crossings were understood to both facilitate the spread of disease and offer a means to limit it.

In 1582, the city faced a significant outbreak of plague, which started in the rural towns of its *tierra*. Officials in Seville moved quickly to begin investigating these rural deaths. After officials put together a list of infected towns to be guarded against, councilmen were stationed at various strategic points inside and outside the city including at city gates, along common roads, in outlying towns, and at

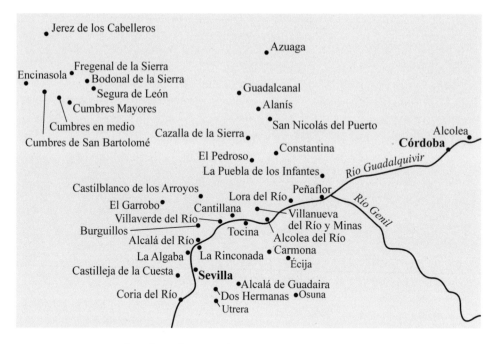

FIGURE 20.3: Map of Seville and towns of its *tierra*. (Courtesy of Kristy Wilson Bowers.)

river crossings. Travelers passing through these official stations had to answer questions and, in many cases, produce paperwork to show where they were traveling from and their destination. While officials did not keep lists of all the people they spoke with, the records from this epidemic do reflect both positive and negative outcomes at the checkpoints: some travelers were investigated and allowed to continue on their way, while others were detained or turned away.

Within the city, the river created two main areas of concern: the port where the ships arrived and the neighborhood of Triana. City councilmen were appointed to monitor incoming ships and to check for signs of infection among crew and cargo. Captains had to provide paperwork confirming the other ports they had visited to prove to officials that they had not been exposed to any contagions. Any sick sailors on board were generally taken to hospitals onshore, while the rest of the crew and goods were quarantined on board; sailors under quarantine were prevented from disembarking until officials could be satisfied that they posed no health threat.[3]

The Triana neighborhood had developed on the west bank of the river, separate from the main city center on the east bank. A floating bridge, the *puente de barcos*, linked Triana to the rest of the city (Figure 20.4). Made of a base of boats roped together with planking on top and anchored to the marshy shore on either side, the bridge was heavily used but prone to washing out in periodic but severe

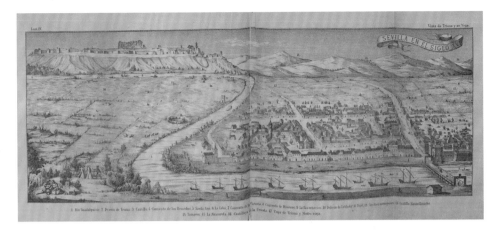

FIGURE 20.4: View of Triana from the east with pontoon bridge in lower right. Note that the river is still foregrounded, though in this view north is to the right. Francisco de Borja Palomo, *Historia crítica de las riadas o grandes avenidas del Guadalquivir en Seville* (Seville, 1878, plate IV). (Courtesy of University of Seville Library/Biblioteca de la Universidad de Sevilla.)

floods. While most of the city was surrounded by walls and gates through which arriving merchants and travelers could be funneled and therefore monitored in times of plague, the neighborhood of Triana had no such walls. City leaders worried a great deal that anyone roaming the countryside could wander unchecked into Triana and from there easily cross the river into the city proper. Because Triana was considered part of the city, there was no effort to shut down or even limit traffic across this bridge. Instead, mounted patrols were sent out to watch for arriving travelers and to warn innkeepers not to allow guests from a list of towns believed to be infected.[4]

Outside the city, people's economic and social lives were enmeshed in networks that stretched throughout the countryside and to other regional cities including Granada, Córdoba, and Carmona. Here the river was a barrier, but a permeable one. The Guadalquivir was another part of the landscape to be traversed, and merchants, muleteers, and other travelers crossed back and forth constantly. Ferries were located at the towns along the river, so river crossings became important choke points where people and goods could be monitored as they moved around. But the river also offered plenty of ways for people to evade the scrutiny of officials.

At the end of January 1582, the city council sent detailed orders to ferrymen up and down the river instructing them not to give passage to any persons or goods without a health license from a judge or councilman. In addition, they were not to give passage to anyone traveling from a list of plague-infected towns.[5] Known cases of plague circulated to the north of the city, so councilmen focused there, visiting ferry crossings at six towns from La Algaba to Villanueva del Río. They worried about the crossing at Coria to the south as well, as people could circle the city to the east, crossing the river to gain entry to Triana unchecked. The councilmen sent to work at these crossings were often accompanied by armed guards.[6] In March, a councilman posted to the tiny village of Bodegon de las Cañas reported news of people traveling from infected towns on the north side of the river.[7] They had avoided the guarded crossings and instead found passage at a secluded spot further upriver. From there, the evaders traveled south to the town of Carmona, which was not part of Seville's territory and reportedly was not guarded against travelers from infected towns. Another councilman, stationed in the town of Alcala del Río, reported back to the full council that he had heard news of an outbreak of plague in the town of Castilblanco and of a group of charcoal-sellers who had traveled in a circuitous route from there to Triana. He therefore advised the council in Seville to check inns in Triana for travelers from Castilblanco.[8] Similar rumors of people evading official scrutiny circulated as fast and as far as the people themselves.

All along the river throughout the spring and early summer of 1582, there was also a steady stream of people caught in official inquiries. Some were found with false papers, others without papers at all, and there were children sent with strangers to find their way to family in the city.[9] There are few hints in the records to tell us what motivated people to take the paths they did as they moved about, to cross the river at a certain point, to visit or avoid towns on their way from point A to point B. Perhaps they moved as they did to evade official scrutiny, but perhaps they did so for innocuous reasons. As Giulia Calvi has shown for Florence, ordinary habits of movement could appear suspicious when seen through the lens of epidemic fears.[10] Officials were entirely focused on the epidemic and stopping its spread, but most of the ordinary people who appear in the records seemed either unaware of the pestilence or unconcerned by it. They moved about as they had always done, both along and across the Guadalquivir River.

Conclusion

Seville's health and welfare depended upon the Guadalquivir River, which acted as both conduit and barrier. The urban infrastructure of port, bridges, and ferry crossings enabled the movement of people and goods, fostering economic and social networks crucial to keeping the city and its surrounding towns running. This also fostered the circulation of pestilential contagions. The port and its shipping traffic brought goods, people, and infections from distant areas where the local officials of Seville had little reach or even communication. Closer to the city, the meandering river and the traffic that flowed along and across it could only be managed at certain points, leaving other stretches unmonitored. The river itself was, therefore, a key public health concern.

The walls of Seville and the river combined the built and natural environments that defined an urban center but did not, indeed could not, separate the city entirely from the surrounding open rural landscape. The circulation of disease did little to stop the circulation of people, and the links between city, river, and countryside were deeply ingrained into many structures and systems. Much of the built environment was created to manage this interconnected terrain. Walls, gates, roads, ports, bridges, and ferries were all means of both enabling and regulating the movement of people across and through a varied landscape. In the effort to control the spread of unseen miasmas or contagions, this architecture and the city employees who monitored it became crucial. Chokepoints regulated movement, creating controlled mobility. At the same time, however, the establishment of official checkpoints at gates and crossings also opened other unmonitored spaces that people utilized to evade official scrutiny, whether they did so intentionally or not. In 16th-century Seville and all early modern cities, managing the intersection of the built and natural environments was a critical part of the response to epidemics.

NOTES

1. The Archivo Municipal de Sevilla (AMS), holds records from the city council in general as well as from various ad hoc health committees, including extensive records for epidemics in 1580, 1582, and 1599–1602. An overview of the city's epidemic history was written in the 19th century by the city's archivist, José Velázquez y Sánchez, *Anales Epidémicos: Reseña Histórica de Las Enfermedades Contagiosas En Sevilla Desde La Reconquista Cristiana Hasta Nuestros Días (1866)* [Chronicle of Epidemics: Historical Review of Contagious Diseases in Seville from the Christian Conquest to Our Times (1866)] (Sevilla: Servicio de Publicaciones del Excmo. Ayuntamiento de Sevilla; Real e Ilustre Colegio Oficial de Médicos de la Provincia de Sevilla, 1996).

2. Kristy Wilson Bowers, *Plague and Public Health in Early Modern Seville* (Rochester: University of Rochester Press, 2013), 58–61.

3. E.g., AMS, sección 13, siglo XVI, tomo 6, fols. 33–34, 144, 155–56, 159.

4. E.g., AMS, sección 13, siglo XVI, tomo 5, fol. 41.

5. Ibid., fol. 31.

6. E.g., the city council minutes in ibid., fols. 103, 109.

7. Ibid., fol. 266.

8. Ibid., fol. 199r.

9. Ibid., fols. 188–91, 192–94, 220–22.

10. Giulia Calvi, *Histories of a Plague Year: The Social and the Imaginary in Baroque Florence* (Berkeley: University of California Press, 1989).

21

Social Inequity and Hospital Infrastructure in the City of Puebla, Mexico, 1737

Juan Luis Burke

In the winter of 1736, the citizens of the city of Puebla de los Ángeles, located in central Mexico, received news of a *matlazahuatl* (plague in the Nahuatl language) outbreak in Mexico City, the capital of New Spain (viceregal Mexico). Mexico City is located just 130 kilometers to Puebla's northwest, so Poblanos knew the epidemic would arrive in a matter of weeks or even days, and it would happen at the worst of times: the city was experiencing an economic downturn, and the year prior had been one of drought, both of which affected the region's grain production and led to corn shortages that were causing hunger among the city's poor.

Puebla, founded in 1531, was New Spain's second-most important urban center. The city is often identified as a settlement that was initially exclusive to Spanish colonizers. However, what is often forgotten is that Indigenous groups migrated to settle in Puebla right from the city's early years, transforming it over a few decades into a thriving agricultural and manufacturing hub that was only overshadowed by Mexico City itself during three centuries of Spanish rule. By the 18th century, the city's diverse demographic consisted of groups of Spaniards, natives, Africans, and *mestizos* (people of mixed ethnic background) coexisting in a society marked by racial hierarchization and an unequal distribution of wealth. Spaniards and *criollos* (people of Spanish descent born in New Spain) accumulated most of the riches. In this context, natives and mestizos made up the bulk of the city's economic labor force. During the city's 18th-century economic decline, reports of rampant unemployment, crime, vagrancy, and alcohol abuse revealed the plight of the city's poor, which was in turn exacerbated by the constant threat of epidemics.[1]

Puebla's urban conditions during the epidemic of 1737 provide an explanation for the reasons the native population was hit hardest during the outbreak and illustrate the role of the city's most important health institution, San Pedro

Hospital. Through the experience of diverse epidemics, the hospital was transformed architecturally, particularly when the understanding that diseases could spread in cramped, unventilated spaces became popular in the late 18th century. San Pedro Hospital, during times of epidemic outbreaks, was forced to simultaneously react to its mission as a religiously sponsored institution while positioning modern medical treatment practice as a central objective of its mandate. In other words, it was forced to tackle two aims: to facilitate spiritual salvation by procuring a good death for plague victims and to provide physical recovery through medical treatment and appropriate health facilities.

Case study: Matlazahuatl or plague epidemic in Puebla, 1737

In colonial Mexico, epidemics accounted considerably for the steep depopulation of the Indigenous peoples of the continent.[2] The most common epidemic-causing diseases were the matlazahuatl, typhus, smallpox (*hueyzahuatl*), measles (*zahuatltepiton*), diphtheria, and pneumonia. Epidemics caused by a variety of diseases were recorded as early as 1521 and became from that time recurring events. Separated by a minimum of a couple of years, there was never more than a decade between one epidemic outbreak and another.[3] The constant presence of these health crises exacerbated the living conditions and lowered the life expectancy of the abundant population living in destitute conditions in Puebla. Extenuating labor regimes, social oppression, poverty, malnutrition, climatic change, and poor hygienic conditions in private and public urban spheres also contributed to the dramatic decrease of the native population.[4]

Puebla's regulations dictated that polluting industries such as tanneries, slaughterhouses, and lime kilns should be placed in the outer peripheries. These urban ordinances were not always enforced, so glass factories, pork slaughterers, bakeries, and many other industries disposed of their waste on the city streets and in its waterways. The sewer and potable water systems were continually being repaired and expanded, with some *barrios* (neighborhoods), particularly those inhabited by Indigenous peoples and other lower socio-economic castes, suffering constant water shortages as a result.

The 1737 matlazahuatl epidemic is one of the best documented in Puebla's viceregal history.[5] The epidemic broke out in Mexico City's Tacubaya neighborhood in late 1736 and spread throughout the entire viceroyalty during the course of a few months. The first of Puebla's barrios to record plague infections in early February 1737 were the impoverished neighborhoods of the city's periphery, like Analco, which were made up of adobe houses where entire families lived in reduced quarters (Figure 21.1). The disease quickly spread to the rest of the city soon thereafter.[6]

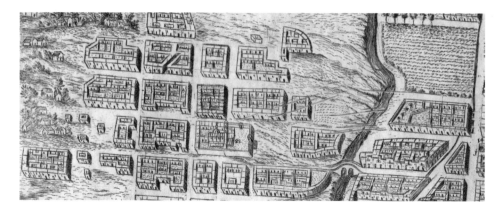

FIGURE 21.1: Detail from a perspectival view of Puebla showing the barrio of Analco, 1754. Analco was mainly inhabited by an Indigenous and mestizo population living in shacks and adobe houses in the 18th century. Analco registered the first deaths during the plague epidemic that broke out in Puebla in 1737. (Courtesy of Fotos de Puebla, fotosdepuebla.org. Image in the public domain.)

The plague waned until October of that year, but deaths were recorded until early 1738.[7] By 1746, the city's total population was just over fifty thousand people, so estimates suggest that about 15 percent of the city's population had died from the plague in the late 1730s; this would mean that about 70 percent of the total deaths took place among the city's native population, despite the fact they made up less than half of the city's population.[8] City authorities responded to the crisis as they could, distributing food to the poorest inhabitants who were already suffering the brunt of food shortages. To worsen matters, the sewage and potable water system, perpetually in disrepair, left various barrios and hospitals waterless for weeks during that year.[9]

San Pedro Hospital was established in 1544 by Puebla's Cathedral Council as part of its mission to fulfill the notion of Christian Caritas. As the largest and most important hospital in the city, San Pedro played an essential role during epidemics like the one in 1737.[10] The Bishop Juan de Palafox y Mendoza (tenure 1640–49) invested considerably in remodeling the hospital. Next, Bishop Manuel Fernández de Santa Cruz (tenure 1677–99) redesigned the adjacent church and added a wing each for the care of Indigenous patients, women, and syphilis sufferers.[11] The hospital acquired its present form in the 1790s. The outstanding reputation of the pharmacy and patient services during their viceregal heyday was primarily due to the rectorship of Dr. Ignacio Domenech. It was Domenech who shifted San Pedro from its heavily religious focus into an Enlightenment-era medical institution that became one of the most efficient and advanced hospitals in New Spain.[12]

Entrenched within the Counter-Reformation Catholic world that existed on both sides of the Atlantic in 1737, San Pedro Hospital continued to be a religiously oriented institution whose foremost objective was to provide its patients with a good, spiritual death, thus procuring their souls' salvation.[13] San Pedro's religious vocation, in other words, remained central to its mandate. The hospital chaplain facilitated a good death by administering the Catholic rites—confession, communion, and extreme unction—to dying patients and performing daily mass on the premises. Deceased patients' bodies were prepared for burial and funeral rites were solemnly conducted in-house.[14] Although it is unknown if this was the case with San Pedro, some hospitals in New Spain employed bedside staff whose mission was to comfort and aid the sick in departing peacefully.[15]

By the first half of the 18th century, the hospital's preoccupation with providing medical care to preserve and rehabilitate the health of their patients can be observed in the way the hospital was staffed by medical professionals. A rector directly appointed by the city's bishop led the hospital and oversaw an administrator. The hospital was also staffed by two physicians, a cohort of nurses and a surgeon-barber who carried out surgeries, bloodletting, leech treatments, and amputations. The doctors, accompanied by a surgeon, nurses, the pharmacist, and sometimes the hospital's rector, would carry out daily rounds of patient visits.

San Pedro's design included the hospital grounds, a large rectangular structure, and a single-vaulted, rectangular church attached to the hospital's south side (Figure 21.2). Cruciform, double-storeyed patient wards divided the complex

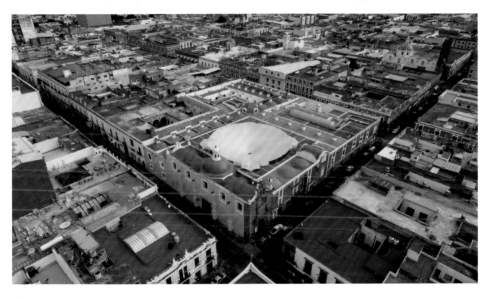

FIGURE 21.2: Aerial view of San Pedro Hospital, showing the domes designed to aerate the patient's wards. The church is seen to the left. (Courtesy of Rubén Olvera, 2020.)

SAN PEDRO HOSPITAL
PUEBLA

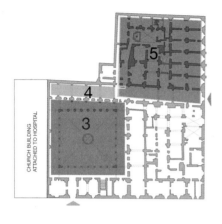
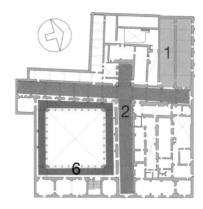

GROUND FLOOR   UPPER FLOOR

1. Twin infirmaries built c.1680, dedicated to patients suffering syphillis
2. Cross-shaped, vaulted patient wards with a dome at the transept
3. Main courtyard with water fountain in the middle
4. Funerary chapel. In 1998, archaeological excavations unearthed mass burials from epidemics
5. Service area with a water fountain courtyard and a service exit
6. Upper floor courtyard corridors, which served as exercise and sunbathing areas for patients

FIGURE 21.3: Plans, ground and second floors, San Pedro Hospital. Plan by Juan Burke, based on Ivan Escamilla González, Julieta García, and Ana María Huerta. *Remedio contra el olvido: Un acercamiento a la arquitectura del ex Hospital de San Pedro* [A Remedy against Oblivion: An Approach to the Architecture of the Former St. Peter's Hospital], ed. Beatriz Mackenzie (Puebla, Mexico: State Government of Puebla, 1999), 19–46.

into four areas (Figure 21.3). The longest ward is 85 meters from north to south, intersecting at their central points, where the transept is marked by a dome. A cruciform typology was common in late medieval and early modern hospitals, as typified by the Ospedale Maggiore of Milan plan by Filarete (1456) and the Spanish Hospital of the Holy Cross in Toledo (1504–15), one of the first buildings in Spain to display Renaissance ornamentation on its façade. The Holy Cross Hospital may have been a precedent for San Pedro. The cruciform model allowed for more efficient surveillance by the medical personnel stationed at the center of the cross, where masses were also officiated.

The notion that diseases were spread by airborne transmission gained popularity in the latter part of the 18th century. San Pedro was remodeled toward the end of the 1700s with tall ceilings and vaulted wards lined with a string of

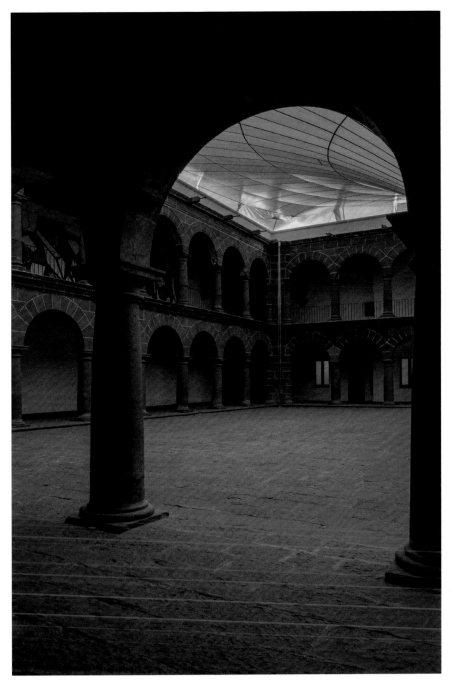

FIGURE 21.4: Interior view of San Pedro Hospital showing the main courtyard. (Courtesy of Rubén Olvera, 2020.)

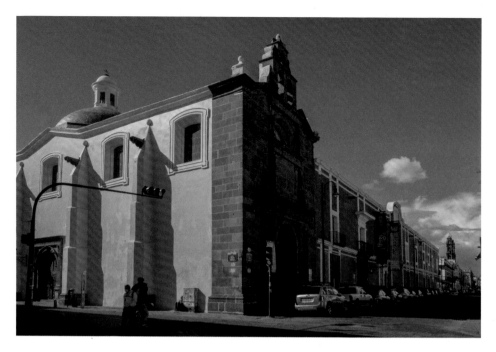

FIGURE 21.5: San Pedro Hospital with the San Pedro church façade in the foreground. (Courtesy of Rubén Olvera, 2020.)

window-pierced lantern domes; this allowed for efficient air circulation and natural sunlight to hinder infections.[16] The southeast quarter was articulated by a large square courtyard that connected the building to the street through its main portal (Figure 21.4).

In 1998, the abandoned San Pedro Hospital underwent massive restoration to adapt it as an art museum (Figure 21.5). Archaeological excavations unearthed a great number of corpses buried beneath the ground floor. In New Spain, it was common practice to bury the dead in the hospital grounds. While Dr. Domenech banned this practice at San Pedro around 1754, making it one of the earliest hospitals to do so in New Spain, the archaeological excavations revealed bodies in shrouds and coffins. This careful preparation is a possible sign that these patients did not die during an epidemic event. Elsewhere, mass graves with layers of bodies placed haphazardly were likely dug during epidemics when the death rate spiked dramatically, and the hospital staff rushed to try to handle the bodies.[17] The archaeological digs also revealed another fact: Spaniards were usually buried in the church building, presumably for a fee, while the dispossessed majority, usually natives and members of lower castes, ended up buried in the hospital grounds.[18] Social class and ethnicity followed plague victims even after death.

Conclusion

Hospitals in New Spain were initially created to exert social control, segregating the ill from the rest of the population and providing caritative assistance to the exploited and exhausted Indigenous and mestizo populations. Hospitals also advanced the mandate of the Catholic Church by serving as religious institutions that facilitated a good spiritual death. Hospitals in this colonial setting also evolved as countermeasures to the constant battering force of epidemics, new forms of labor exploitation, and chronic economic hardship of the native and mestizo populations in cities like Puebla. By the early 18th century, hospitals like San Pedro in Puebla permitted a larger role for medicine and surgery without losing sight of the religious mandate, with physicians and surgeons providing constant medical care. By the end of the 18th century, the constant experience of epidemics and advances in medical architecture prompted improvements to the hospital's architecture. Namely, the tall, vaulted wards improved for air circulation.

The functions of a hospital like San Pedro would be upended during an epidemic event. Archaeological evidence of haphazard mass graves reveals the urgency of body disposal during epidemics. The hospital attempted to control situations that, as in the 1737 epidemic in Puebla, completely overwhelmed the city authorities' capacities at containment. The epidemic was worsened by Puebla's deplorable urban hygiene conditions, poor individual hygiene habits, overcrowding in the peripheral barrios, waste disposal from factories and human defecation on the streets, lack of access to potable water, and the proliferation of rat populations that must have contributed to the spread of fleas and lice, which, in turn, spread the bacteria that caused the plague in humans. The Indigenous populations and poor mestizos who populated the city's peripheral barrios and the tenements scattered throughout the city, where entire families occupied cramped quarters, registered over 70 percent of the deceased during the 1737 outbreak.[19]

NOTES

1. Juan Villa Sánchez, *Puebla sagrada y profana: Informe dado a su muy ilustre ayuntamiento el año de 1746, por el M.R.P. Fray Juan de Villa Sánchez* [Puebla Sacred and Profane: A Report Prepared for Its Very Illustrious City Council on the Year of 1746] (Puebla: Imprenta de José María Campos, 1835), 42; Miguel Marín Bosch, *Puebla neocolonial, 1777–1831: Casta, ocupación y matrimonio en la segunda ciudad de Nueva España* [Neocolonial Puebla: Caste, Occupation, and Marriage in New Spain's Second City] (Puebla, Mexico: El Colegio de Jalisco-Instituto de Ciencias Sociales y Humanidades, Benemérita Universidad Autónoma de Puebla, 1999), 57–58.

2. In central Mexico, some contested but amply cited estimates show a 90 percent decline in the Indigenous population between the start of the colonial period and the early 17th century, from approximately twenty-five million to a little over one million people. See Sherburne Friend Cook and Woodrow Borah, *The Indian Population of Central Mexico, 1531–1610*, Ibero-Americana 44 (Berkeley: University of California Press, 1960), 45–56.

3. Ibid., 49–55.

4. Ibid., 120–33; Gerardo Gutiérrez, "Identity Erasure and Demographic Impacts of the Spanish Caste System on the Indigenous Populations of Mexico," in *Beyond Germs: Native Depopulation in North America*, ed. Catherine M. Cameron, Paul Kelton, and Alan C. Swedlund (Tucson: University of Arizona Press, 2015), 119–45.

5. Miguel Ángel Cuenya Mateos's statistical and archival research in this respect is invaluable, as his work paints the clearest picture of this event.

6. Miguel Ángel Cuenya Mateos, *Puebla de los Ángeles en tiempos de una peste colonial: una mirada en torno al matlazahuatl de 1737* [Puebla de los Ángeles during a Colonial Plague: A Look at the *Matlazahuatl* Plague of 1737] (Puebla, Mexico: El Colegio de Michoacán-Benemérita Universidad Autónoma de Puebla, 1999), 173–75.

7. Ibid., 205.

8. Ibid., 205–7.

9. Ibid., 180–83. Influenced by the dictates of the Council of Trent, Puebla's Bishopric merged San Juan de Letrán Hospital, established *c*.1533, with San Pedro Hospital.

10. The other hospitals in Puebla during the viceregal period were the general and mental diseases Hospital of San Roque, founded in 1593; the Hospital de Bubas (syphilis), established in the second half of the 17th century; the Hospital of Our Lady of Bethlehem (Nuestra Señora de Belém), established *c*.1682, administered by the Order of Bethlemites; and the Hospital of St. Bernard, established *c*.1632, administered by the Order of St. John of the Cross. See Josefina Muriel, *Hospitales de la Nueva España. Tomo II. Fundaciones de los Siglos XVII y XVIII* (Mexico City: Universidad Nacional Autónoma de México -Instituto de Investigaciones Históricas-Cruz Roja Mexicana, 1991), 59–62, 105–8, 444; Josefina Muriel, *Hospitales de la Nueva España. Tomo I. Fundaciones del siglo XVI* (Mexico City: Universidad Nacional Autónoma de México-Instituto de Investigaciones Históricas-Cruz Roja Mexicana, 1990), 238–40.

11. Muriel, *Hospitales de la Nueva España. Tomo I. Fundaciones del siglo XVI*, 180.

12. Ana María Huerta, "La cirugía y sus instrumentos en el Real Hospital de San Pedro de Puebla, 1796–1826," in *El Hospital de San Pedro: pilar de la medicina en Puebla* [St. Peter's Hospital: Pillar of Medicine in Puebla], ed. José Ramón Eguibar, Ma. del Carmen Cortés, and Ma. del Pilar Pacheco (Puebla: Benemérita Universidad Autónoma de Puebla-Academia Nacional de Medicina, 2012), 53–68.

13. Guenter Risse, "Hospitals," in *Europe 1450 to 1789: Encyclopedia of the Early Modern World*, vol. 3 (New York: Charles Scribner's Sons, 2004), 204–6.

14. Muriel, Hospitales de la Nueva España. Tomo I. Fundaciones del siglo XVI, 177–90.

15. In the Spanish language, there is a term to convey the notion of dying at peace with one-self: *bien morir*, literally, to "die well," and some hospitals in viceregal New Spain employed personnel to carry out that task. See María de los Ángeles Rodríguez Álvarez, "La aparición de los muertos," in *El Hospital de San Pedro: pilar de la medicina en Puebla* [St. Peter's Hospital: Pillar of Medicine in Puebla], ed. José Ramón Eguibar, Ma. del Carmen Cortés, and Ma. del Pilar Pacheco (Puebla: BUAP-Academia Nacional de Medicina, 2012), 91–111.

16. Iván Escamilla González, Julieta García, and Ana María Huerta, *Remedio contra el olvido: Un acercamiento a la arquitectura del ex Hospital de San Pedro* [A Remedy against Oblivion: An Approach to the Architecture of the Former St. Peter's Hospital], ed. Beatriz Mackenzie (Puebla: State Government of Puebla, 1999), 33.

17. Ibid., 21.

18. Rodríguez Álvarez, "La aparición de los muertos."

19. Cuenya Mateos, *Puebla*, 255.

22

Colonial Infrastructure, Ecology, and Epidemics in Dhaka, 1858–1947

Mohammad Hossain

It was a sad moment for the people of Dhaka, Bangladesh, when civil surgeon Alex Simpson died from diarrhea in November 1864. Simpson, the first superintendent of the Mitford Hospital, established in 1858, was praised in a eulogy published in the local newspaper, the *Dhaka Prokash*, for his essential role in the treatment of patients with waterborne diseases and in the early growth of the hospital at a time when the mortality of admitted patients for epidemic diseases such as cholera was as high as 60–77 percent.[1] At the same time, Simpson's death necessitated a call to the government to provide another experienced civil surgeon for Dhaka, as many lives depended on it.

The climate and topography of the Bengal Delta, wherein Dhaka is situated, is a suitable habitat for the cholera bacillus and it was believed to be endemic to the region. However, unlike the delta region's historical epidemics such as smallpox, waterborne cholera only began to appear in the 19th century and was closely associated with unsanitary and crowded urban conditions. The first cholera outbreak in the Dhaka district was reported in Sonargaon in July 1817, placing it among the early seats of the first cholera pandemic.[2] During three cholera pandemics from 1817 to 1859, the population in Dhaka grappled with mortality rates as high as 50–60 percent.[3] Although global cholera mortality rates began to subside due to the introduction of public health and sanitation measures, this was not the case in Dhaka and other urban areas of Eastern Bengal until the early 20th century. Prior to the introduction of such measures, cholera prevailed with hyperendemic intensity, with high levels of both disease occurrence and mortality due to a form attributable to deltaic environmental degradation.[4]

Dhaka's population and its associated economic-cum-administrative activity increased by the end of the 19th century, with the city becoming the provincial capital of Eastern Bengal and Assam in 1905. As part of this change, Dhaka acquired better urban health infrastructure that originated with developing colonial responses to cholera epidemics, which ultimately led to reduced cholera-driven mortality in Dhaka. Eastern Bengal and the Dhaka region in particular are of importance for understanding colonial responses to epidemic disease, but there is a dearth of scholarship that evaluates the colonial infrastructural response to the cholera epidemics in the region throughout the 19th and early 20th centuries.

Case study: Epidemics and colonial intervention in Dhaka

Prior to the arrival of the British, hospitals and almshouses (*lungurkhanas*) for the poor and sick were built in Dhaka during the late 16th century, at the time of Mughal Emperor Jahangir (1569–1627). The expenses of these institutions were paid from the income of the *khalsa* lands (those belonging to the Crown).[5] The arrival of British East India Company rule in 1757 brought about an end to such charitable institutions as part of an overall decline in both the population and economic prosperity of Dhaka.

Health-related administrative changes were implemented in the latter half of the 19th century by colonial medical authorities, who often expressed cholera's "special preference" for the Bengal Delta and the alluvial soil found at its river mouths due to the "malarious," low-lying situation of overcrowded urban centers with inadequate sanitation.[6] A keen interest in the relationship between environment and epidemic disease in colonial British India emanated from the fact that the death rate of European troops in India was found to be very high as compared to British troops stationed in other parts of the world.[7] Several essential medico-topographies were published in the early 19th century to this end, among them Dacca civil surgeon James Taylor's *A Sketch of the Topography & Statistics of Dacca* (1840). In this text, Dhaka was described as having grown into "an unhealthy and unsanitary place, a condition accentuated by the physical layout of the city and the uncivic habits and customs of its inhabitants."[8] An unhealthy delta environment consisting of low-lying rice field areas, *char* wasteland, and forests constituted a vital part of Dhaka's colonial narrative (Figure 22.1).

Cholera became a particular public health concern in 19th-century urban centers riddled with poor sanitation and waste management practices, since the disease was generally spread through contamination of drinking water sources by human feces. The bulk of the population in Dhaka—among them artisans, craftsmen, small traders, menials, and laborers—were very poor, making Dhaka especially prone to water contamination. Most of the city's dwellings were haphazardly built and there was a lack of a proper drainage for the discharge of rainwater, sewage, and other liquid refuse. Privies were only cleared of stored waste once or twice a

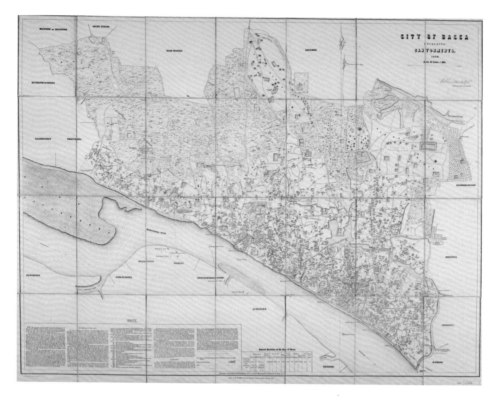

FIGURE 22.1: Map of Dacca, 1859, with newly built Mitford Hospital on the bank of the Ganges River in the south of the city and wetlands and forests to the north of the city. (Courtesy of the British Library.)

year, so sewage often seeped into the drinking water supply from wells that were located dangerously nearby. Household rubbish and collected refuse were discharged into large pits nearby patches of jungle, which were only washed off by overflow during rains.

The chief medical establishments in early 19th-century Dhaka included the Jail Hospital, Native Hospital that provided forty beds and an attached dispensary, Lunatic Asylum, Military Hospital, and a vaccine establishment.[9] They were ill-equipped to deal with epidemic disease. A significant step toward providing health infrastructure for the city came with the founding of the Mitford Hospital in 1858 (Figure 22.2). Mitford Hospital replaced the earlier Native Hospital and became a major health institution in Eastern Bengal in the fight against epidemic diseases such as cholera, malaria, and smallpox. In time, the hospital became the central node of a network of smaller health institutions such as charitable dispensaries set up to provide health care in the rural areas of the Dhaka division (Figure 22.3).

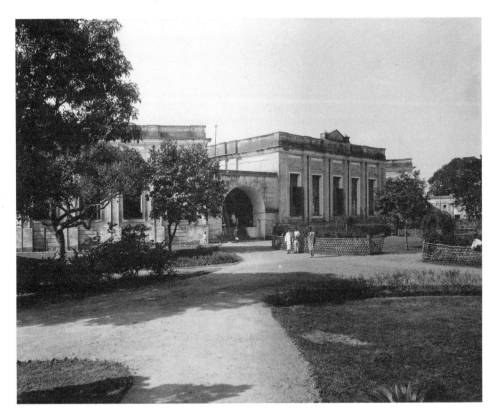

FIGURE 22.2: Mitford Hospital, 1904. (Courtesy of the British Library.)

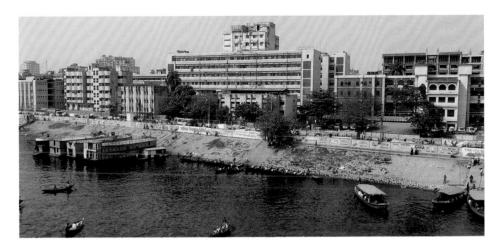

FIGURE 22.3: Sir Salimullah Medical College and Mitford Hospital complex situated on the banks of the Buriganga. (Courtesy of Mohammad Hossain.)

Year	Presidency district (western Bengal)	Dhaka District (eastern Bengal)
1920s	Population: 9,145,321 10 hospitals in urban Calcutta alone (around 1900 beds)	Population: 12,037,649 5 hospitals (around 300 beds)
1940s	Population: 10,108,229 37 hospitals in Calcutta alone (4500 beds)	Population: 13,864,104 Less than 10 hospitals (below 800 beds)

FIGURE 22.4: Tabular comparison of health infrastructure for general populace between Western and Eastern Bengal under British colonial administration. (Drawn by Mohammad Hossain based on census data related to Bengal from 1911 and 1931, and reports on hospitals and dispensaries run under the government of Bengal from 1914 and 1939.)

Amid various phases of expansion and changes in administration, the hospital was converted into a government institution in 1920.[10]

Colonial health infrastructure in Dhaka was often inadequate and disproportionate in terms of coverage throughout the 19th century. Mitford Hospital in Dhaka, with 141 beds for males and 28 beds for females, was the largest among four hospitals in the most populous division of Bengal in the 1920s. However, despite robust population growth in Dhaka, in Eastern Bengal, in the 1920s and 1940s, the number of hospitals and the bed capacity in colonial Calcutta, in Western Bengal, was several times higher. The difference in infrastructure development is attributable to the presence of a large European population in Calcutta (Figure 22.4).

Dhaka's Municipal Committee spearheaded sanitary measures and introduced civic services such as a modern waterworks and a supply of filtered water for residents in 1878.[11] These measures complemented health infrastructure improvements and helped reduce cholera outbreaks in Dhaka. However, outside of later improvements made to the waterworks, the colonial authorities largely neglected aspects of public health for Dhaka, such as city planning and the implementation of a proper drainage system.[12] This may have been partly responsible for the appearance of resurgent hyperendemic cholera in the city later in the 19th and early 20th centuries.

The resurgence of cholera in the Eastern Bengal Delta in the 20th century is attributed to the poor sanitation measures described above, and to regional development-focused activities that adversely affected the deltaic water regime and exacerbated conditions already identified as ideal for epidemic diseases. The construction of dams, railway embankments, and bridges ushered in the invasion of the water hyacinth and the silting of embankments in the choked deltaic river system, which adversely impacted nutrition intake for the people of the region by decreasing fish populations and agricultural output; both factors were significant contributors to the Great Bengal Famine of 1943.[13]

Conclusion

Urban infrastructure development remained integral to the colonial efforts to combat epidemic disease in Eastern Bengal. In Dhaka, this was realized through the development of health and sanitation infrastructure, via the expansion of the Mitford Hospital and the installation of waterworks around the hospital for the provision of filtered water. Such measures undoubtedly played important roles in reducing mortality from epidemic diseases such as cholera. However, colonial policies and responses to disease in Dhaka remained insufficient to eradicate these epidemics, largely due to the inadequate nature of infrastructure development. Sanitation measures and hospital construction were disproportionate to the growth in urban health efforts experienced in other regions within Bengal, such as colonial Calcutta.

The adverse ecological impact of colonial development policies such as railway embankments ultimately contributed to the periodic resurgence of epidemic disease in parts of Eastern Bengal. Urban architectural growth in Dhaka as a response to epidemic disease encompassed health infrastructure development, colonial public health policy, and the built environment's impact on disease ecology. Dhaka's responses to disease, development, and ecological change under colonial governance provide a framework to evaluate the development of urban infrastructure in the period following Eastern Bengal's independence in 1947 in terms of the influence of colonial policies that favored centralized urban development and emphasized progress over environmental sustainability.

NOTES

1. Sharif Uddin Ahmed, *Mitford Hospital and Dhaka Medical School – History and Heritage, 1858–1947 (in Bengali)* (Dhaka: Academic Press, 2007), 48–51.

2. James Jameson, *Report on the Epidemick Cholera Morbus, as It Visited the Territories Subject to the Presidency of Bengal, in the Years 1817, 1818, and 1819* (Calcutta: Government Gazette Press, 1820), 171.

3. William Jones, "First Annual Report of the Sanitary Commissioner for Bengal, for 1868, with Selected Extracts from Forty District Reports; Special Remarks on These; General Observations Regarding the Sanitation In Bengal; Appendices" (Calcutta: Alipore Jail Press, 1869), 103–4.

4. Ira Klein, "Imperialism, Ecology and Disease: Cholera in India, 1850–1950," *The Indian Economic & Social History Review* 31, no. 4 (1994): 510–13.

5. James Taylor, *A Sketch of the Topography & Statistics of Dacca* (Calcutta: G.H. Huttman, Military Orphan Press, 1840), 318.

6. William James Moore, *A Manual of the Diseases of India, with a Compendium of Diseases Generally* (London: J. & A. Churchill, 1886), 76. Many professionals like Moore who were connected with the Indian Medical Service (IMS) during the same period wrote on cholera in colonial India.

7. The death rate of European troops in India was as high as 69 per 1000 troops for the first 50 years of the 19th century. Ibid., 3.

8. Sharif Uddin Ahmed, "The History of the City of Dacca, c. 1840-1885" (Ph.D. diss., School of Oriental and African Studies, University of London, 1978), 235.

9. Taylor, *Sketch of the Topography*, 89.

10. Ahmed, *Mitford Hospital*, 149.

11. Ahmed, "Dhaka under the British Crown - Aspects of Urban History," in *400 Years of Capital Dhaka and Beyond: Politics, Society, Administration*, ed. Abdul Momin Chowdhury and Sharif Uddin Ahmed (Dhaka: Asiatic Society of Bangladesh, 2011), 56–57. The limited area supplied initially covered only four miles in area for the Mitford Hospital, lunatic asylum, jail, and Chauk Bazar.

12. Basil Copleston Allen, *Dacca* (Allahabad: The Pioneer Press, 1912), 79. Allen noted the presence of about five thousand private latrines in the city, which could not be approached and were generally left uncleared from year to year, becoming sources of both stench and disease.

13. Klein, "Imperialism, Ecology and Disease," 497; Iftekhar Iqbal, *The Bengal Delta: Ecology, State and Social Change, 1840- 1943* (London: Palgrave Macmillan, 2010), 168.

23

South American Health Conventions, Social Stratification, and the Ilha Grande Lazaretto in Brazil, 1886

Niuxa Dias Drago, Ana Paula Polizzo, and Fernando Delgado

The Ilha Grande Lazaretto served as the primary quarantine station in Brazil during the second half of the 19th century. It is best understood as the result of a synthesis between the establishment of emerging health guidelines and regional conventions as well as the political and social conditions in the Empire of Brazil (1822–89), namely the persistence of slavery—which, though eradicated elsewhere, remained legal in Brazil—and its associated social and racial hierarchies. This social stratification affected how—and why—Brazil implemented public health interventions. For example, the implantation of lazarettos as the places for quarantine to stem the spread of contagious disease was seen not only in public health terms but also as a means to create an image of healthiness and promote processes of immigration, while planning to substitute the enslaved workforce from Africa with European workers in order to "whiten" the population was promoted as a "civilizing" strategy.[1]

On the other hand, the first South American Health Conventions (1873 and 1887) were a direct consequence of the Paraguayan War (1864–70), one of the greatest armed conflicts in South American history. During the war, more than half of the recorded deaths were caused by communicable diseases, cholera foremost among them. Once the war ended, returning soldiers were the likely carriers of the 1871 Yellow Fever epidemic that struck Buenos Aires, Argentina. The first Health Convention of 1873 intended to unite Brazil, Argentina, and Uruguay in an effort to fight diseases that jeopardized the economies and immigration policies of those countries. Urban sanitation developments were part of the discussion, and the three participating countries committed to build lazarettos and standardizing quarantine policies. The main objective was to avoid the need to shut down ports to foreign ships, with a secondary aim of spreading the idea that warmongering on the continent had come to an end. The Convention sought to deconstruct South America's unhealthy reputation. Although it was not ratified, the 1873 Convention was the first regional public health covenant and was considered the basis for the subsequent development of international economic and political matters.

When a new cholera epidemic appeared in the Mediterranean in the 1880s, the Brazilian Empire's Health Service took action, at last ordering the construction of a model lazaretto on Ilha Grande. The Ilha Grande Lazaretto was to be situated between the two most important ports in Brazil: Rio de Janeiro and Santos. During the same period, the Argentine government built a lazaretto on San Martín Island, on the River Plate. When a cholera epidemic hit Buenos Aires in 1886, the Ilha Grande Lazaretto faced its greatest test, as it was the only port open to ships coming from the cholera-stricken Republic of Argentina. The restrictions imposed on ships from Argentina successfully kept cholera away from Brazilian ports, but the resulting trade crisis threatened peace between the two countries, which necessitated a second Health Conference between Brazil, Argentina, and Uruguay.

The second convention in Rio de Janeiro in 1887 was ratified by the three participating South American countries, contrary to the interests of France, England, and Italy, who did not accept having to submit their ships to the South American inspectors. The 1887 document would become the basis for a similar convention between Peru, Bolivia, Chile, and Ecuador in 1888, and for the continental agreement of the First International Conference of American States in 1889, in Washington, DC.[2] An International Health Regulation was signed between the Empire of Brazil, the Republic of Argentina, and the Oriental Republic of Uruguay during the 1887 convention. As all three began to operate their lazarettos, the regulation determined that each country should "independently develop [...] the provisions that should govern its health facilities."[3] In the case of Brazil, this independent development included provisions that were indicative of the country's entrenched social stratification.

Case study: The Ilha Grande Lazaretto, 1886

In 1884, engineer Francisco Antonio de Paula Freitas and port health inspector Dr. Nuno de Andrade traveled to several islands off the coast of Rio de Janeiro to choose the most suitable place for the construction of the Brazilian Empire's main lazaretto. Their report on their choice of Ilha Grande, presented to the Minister and Secretary of State for Empire Affairs, demonstrated the concern with isolation as well as environmental issues, since sanitary theories were divided between the hypothesis of person-to-person contagion and miasma causes.[4] The report mentions advantages such as the Abraão's cove on Ilha Grande, the distance from urban centers, isolation from the continent, the existence of sources of drinking water, the direction of the winds, and the hillside topography that would allow the separation of pavilions "by levels." The hillside forests were also considered "useful for the hygienic conditions of the establishment."[5]

According to the report, Abraão's cove was adequate to receive the anchorage, as it was sheltered from the tides and currents, provided easy access and safety, and was large enough to contain several ships, which was necessary to allow time for unloading and other purposes. The report also demonstrates the concern with commercial interests, noting the proximity between the island and the railway that would lead to the capital. Ilha Grande occupied a strategic position between the provinces of Rio de Janeiro and São Paulo (Figure 23.1). Its location on the continent demonstrated the importance that these two ports represented for regional trade in South America as well as the immigration policy of the Empire of Brazil.

Engineer Paula Freitas likely had access to European treatises on lazarettos. John Howard's treatise had been translated into Portuguese in 1800 at the behest of King Dom João VI and probably arrived in Brazil together with the Portuguese

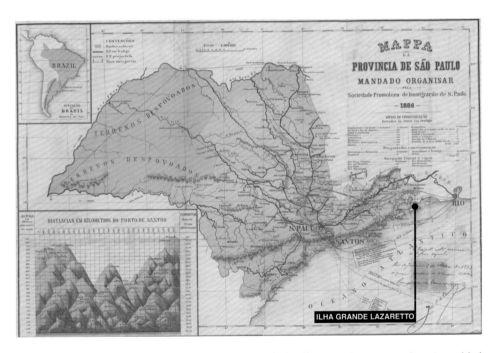

FIGURE 23.1: Map of the Province of São Paulo with the Ilha Grande Lazaretto location added by the authors. Map ordered by the São Paulo Immigration Promotion Society, 1886. (Courtesy of Arquivo Nacional; Fundo Decretos do Poder Executivo – Período Republicano; BR_RJANRIO_23_0_MAP_0001.)

court in 1808.[6] By that time, the first quarantine measures had been implemented in Brazil. Paula Freitas completed his studies at the Polytechnic School of Rio de Janeiro, which exhibited the influence of the French engineering school, the École des Ponts et Chausées. A professor at the École and Director of Public Works in Paris (1809–20), Louis Bryuère, issued judgments on lazarettos that were almost paraphrased by Paula Freitas in his condemnation of the closed, pentagonal composition of the Lazaretto de Ancona in the Adriati.[7] Instead, Freitas mentions the typology of Trompeloup, in Gironde, France, as the ideal.[8] While the Lazaretto of Ancona clustered different services within the same rigid format and did not enable adequate ventilation, the Lazaretto of Trompeloup—built as isolated pavilions with free spaces between them—enabled adequate separation between those being quarantined, according to their arrival date.

In the Ilha Grande Lazaretto project, Paula Freitas adopted two distinct docks, one for luggage and cargo and another for passengers. He provided thorough descriptions of luggage disinfection, as well the "Sanville system" of rails and cranes and the steam disinfection unit, "similar to that at the Moabitt Hospital, near Berlin," all of which demonstrated the important role of technology in the quarantine process.[9] The Ilha Grande anchorage in the neighboring cove provided conditions where "the soil is consistent, dry and elevated, forming different terraces that allow the separate pavilions for quarantine to be placed at different levels, according to the category and date of quarantine."[10] As mentioned above, Paula Freitas's observations indicate the importance he placed on the separation between pavilions and their arrangements on different levels to favor ventilation, but these features were only applied to the buildings constructed for first and second class passengers arriving on the ships.

The lazaretto's regulations clearly stated that different classes of passengers must receive "different accommodations and treatments," so two buildings were constructed for the passenger complex (Figure 23.2).[11] The building intended for third-class passengers featured a closed format and central courtyard. This was similar to the Ancona lazaretto type, which Paula Freitas criticized. Quarantined passengers shared large lounges in the pavilion while the central wing held the dining hall, two courtyards, latrines, and separate washbasins for men and women.[12] The entire building was surrounded by walls, with front and back courtyards that were 10 meters wide. On the slope 300 meters above, the other building was designed with four wings, two for second-class passengers and two for first-class passengers. These had separate dining halls and rooms. The health treatments themselves differed for the passengers of different classes, since the wings for the first- and second-class pavilions were more isolated, with landscaped courtyards between them. The smaller cells of the first-class wings provided greater privacy and health security (Figure 23.3). The attention paid to the details in the

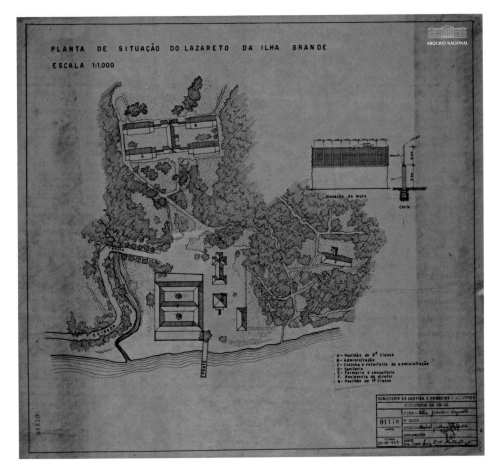

FIGURE 23.2: Site Plan of the Ilha Grande Lazaretto, 1939. (Courtesy of Arquivo Nacional; Fundo Ministério da Justiça e Negócios Interiores; BR_RJANRIO_4T_0_MAP_0563.)

building designs for the first- and second-class passengers, including the roof and façade elements, reinforced the greater concern with how these individuals were treated (Figure 23.4).

In the Brazilian lazaretto, the separation of passengers into pavilions was not intended to minimize contagion but rather to segregate guests according to their socio-economic status. Therefore, the isolation of passengers did not implement scientific criteria to fight against the epidemic. Rather, the proposed separations actually jeopardized the need for quarantined groups to isolate based on the arrival of their ships by offering an architectural arrangement that regrouped them by class. The third-class pavilions were damaged during heavy storms in April 1886, which caused part of the walls to fall. An inspection identified that humidity had

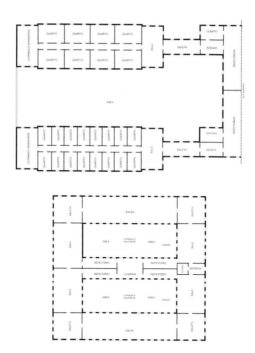

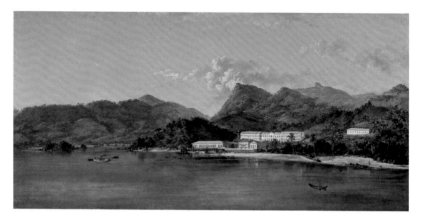

FIGURE 23.3: Floor plans of the Ilha Grande Lazaretto's main buildings, *c*.1909. Redrawn by Júlia Martinelli over plans available in Plácido Barbosa and Cássio B. de Rezende, eds., *Os Serviços de Saúde Pública no Brasil: especialmente na cidade do Rio de Janeiro, de 1808 a 1907 (esboço, histórico e legislação)*, vol. 1. (Rio de Janeiro: Diretoria Geral de Saúde Pública/ Imprensa Nacional, 1909.)

FIGURE 23.4: "Casa de quarentena na Ilha Grande" [Quarantine House at Ilha Grande], by Nicolau Facchinetti, 1887. (Courtesy of Museu de Arte de São Paulo MASP. Photographer: João Musa; MASP.00239.)

jeopardized the recently completed construction, and that there was a need for gutters, ditches, and leveled patios to prevent flooding.[13] This points to the lack of studies on the rain and tidal conditions to which the third-class pavilions on the level of the floodplain were exposed.

The lazaretto received improvements after the proclamation of the Brazilian Republic in 1889. A dam and an aqueduct were constructed in 1893, followed by several renovations. Nonetheless, activity at the site declined after 1913, which saw the emergence of stricter epidemiological methods in the country. A slow and constant process of change and the use of the buildings for new purposes culminated in the 1894 decision to use the facilities as a prison. This was made possible due to the lazaretto's architectural typology, which was based on disciplinary control and surveillance of bodies.[14] In the mid-1930s, Ilha Grande Lazaretto was used as a political prison and was officially transformed into a penitentiary in 1942 under the Getúlio Vargas dictatorship. The site held prisoners until 1954, and was finally demolished in 1962. Ilha Grande became an important tourist destination on the coast of Rio de Janeiro, and the ruins of the complex—with the aqueduct being the only element to remain in its entirety—appear on local maps as the "Ilha Grande Lazaretto."

Conclusion

In 1887, the South American Health Regulation determined that isolation should be carried out "by groups arriving at the facilities," but, at the Ilha Grande Lazaretto, the prevailing criteria divided passengers based on their voyage class. Joaquim Bonastra's extensive work on lazaretto types around the world does not provide similar evidence of significant architectural differences between the pavilions intended for different socio-economic classes of passengers.[15] Although separating individuals according to their class may have been a common practice, the accommodations were similar in regard to their main spatial characteristics, such as the orientation of the pavilions or their language.

Spatial segregation at the Ilha Grande Lazaretto derived from social and racial hierarchies in Brazilian society, where the benefits of social affiliation prevailed against the equitable scientific criteria concerning epidemic control measures. This discrimination against lower socio-economic groups was an overt aspect of the hierarchized structure for within the Brazilian Empire and was directly manifested in the architectural design of the Ilha Grande Lazaretto. This class-based approach to quarantine design was repeated in Brazilian cities a few years later as part of large-scale urban transformations based on social hygiene policies that accentuated social inequalities. Segregationist discrimination measures were subsumed under scientific arguments regarding disease transmission. These conflicts emerge today in real estate issues and a lack of urban infrastructure such as sanitation, the lack of which prevents the entire Brazilian population from benefiting from the minimum health measures recommended by the authorities. These factors also reveal the importance of international agreements when facing epidemics, which has unfortunately been made visible in the South American context during the COVID-19 pandemic.

NOTES

1. Lilia Moritz Schwarcz, *O Espetáculo das Raças – cientistas, instituições e questão racial no Brasil 1870–1930* [The Spectacle of the Races – Scientists, Institutions and Racial Issues in Brazil 1870–1930] (São Paulo: Cia das Letras, 1993).
2. Cleide de Lima Chaves, "As Convenções Sanitárias Internacionais Entre o Império Brasileiro e as Repúblicas Platinas (1873 e 1887) [International Health Conventions between the Brazilian Empire and the Platinum Republics (1873 and 1887)] (Ph.D. diss., Universidade Federal do Rio de Janeiro, 2009), 218.
3. Cap. VI, Art. 50 of the International Health Regulation between the Empire of Brazil, the Argentine Republic, and the Oriental Republic of Uruguay (Rio de Janeiro, 1887); Chaves, "As Convenções Sanitárias," Anexo C.
4. The lazaretto "must be located at a sufficient distance, three miles at least, from the population center [...] to make it difficult for foreign people to access the facilities." In addition, "it must be positioned properly in relation to regional winds, so that the facility has the necessary ventilation." Antonio de Paula Freitas, *O Lazareto do Rio de Janeiro: Relatório Apresentado a S. Ex. o Sr. Conselheiro Dr. Felippe Franco de Sá, Ministro e Secretário do Estado dos Negócios do Império* [The Lazareto of Rio de Janeiro: Report Presented to Your Excellency Mr. Counselor Dr. Felippe Franco de Sá, Minister and Secretary of State for Business in the Empire] (Rio de Janeiro: Typographia Nacional, 1884), 7.
5. Ibid., 11.
6. John Howard, *An account of the Principal Lazarettos in Europe: With Various Papers Relative to the Plague* (London: J. Johnson, C. Dilly and T. Cadell, 1791).
7. Louis Bruyère, *Études Relatives à L'art des Constructions* (Paris: Chez Bance Aîné, 1823).
8. Paula Freitas, "O Lazareto do Rio de Janeiro," 8.
9. Description of the Ilha Grande Lazeretto by Engineer Paula Freitas available in the minutes of the Instituto Polytechnico Brazileiro, September 14, 1887. *Revista de Engenharia* [Engineering Journal], no.170 (September 28, 1887): 221.
10. Freitas, "O Lazareto do Rio de Janeiro," 14.
11. Decree no. 9.554, February 3, 1886. This fact is also reflected in the price of the daily rate for those in quarantine: First Class, 5$000 (5,000 réis); Second Class, 2$500 (2,500 réis); and Third Class, $800 (800 réis).
12. The latrines were placed inside the sleeping rooms and, during the renovation in 1892, they were installed in the central courtyards. Plácido Barbosa and Cássio B. de Rezende,

eds., *Os Serviços de Saúde Pública no Brasil: especialmente na cidade do Rio de Janeiro, de 1808 a 1907 (esboço, histórico e legislação)*, vol. 1 (Rio de Janeiro: Diretoria Geral de Saúde Pública/Imprensa Nacional, 1909), 312.

13. Warning from the Ministry of Agriculture of the Empire to Engineer Antonio de Paula Freitas on April 15, 1886. *Revista de Engenharia* [Engineering Journal], no.136 (April, 28, 1886): 93.

14. The regulation of the Ilha Grande Lazaretto was also the means for order enforcement, a "quarantine police force" that could use military force to repress conflicts. Barbosa and Rezende, *Os Serviços de Saúde Pública no Brasil*, 312.

15. Joaquim Bonastra, "Health Sites and Controlled Spaces: A Morphological Study of Quarantine Architecture," *Dynamis* 30 (2010): 17–40.

24

Plague, Displacement, and Ecological Disruption in Bombay, India, 1896

Emily Webster

In September 1896, Dr. Acacio Viegas was called to Mandvi, a neighborhood in Bombay (Mumbai), India, to attend a series of patients exhibiting unusual symptoms. He arrived at the *chawl* (informal housing) occupied by over six hundred laborers working in the grain trade, to find eighteen people delirious with high fever and tender swelling in the armpit or groin areas. Viegas, aware of the epidemic that had been ravaging Hong Kong for two years, quickly brought word to the municipal government: plague had arrived in Bombay.[1] Within weeks, the disease exploded across the city, infecting thousands. Nearly a third of the population fled to the countryside, carrying pestilence with them.

Many ports across the increasingly connected late-19th century world, from Hong Kong to Hawaii, experienced an outbreak of plague in the subsequent three decades. In Bombay, however, the epidemic took on a cyclical pattern, exacting annual tolls much larger than those experienced by any other urban port. Conservative estimates place the total number of deaths in Bombay City at 175,000, or roughly 20 percent of the city's pre-pandemic population.[2] Bombay suffered so acutely due to the confluence of its local ecology, infrastructure, and position within the British imperial economy.

At the end of the 19th century, Bombay was the British Empire's key shipping link and second-largest port, making it a site of significant economic investment. The city housed grain shipping and cotton production industries, toward which laborers flocked from the surrounding regions in search of work. The population quadrupled to an estimated 816,000 people between 1814 and 1864.[3]

Dramatic population growth invariably led to crowding and the emergence of crowded, informal housing, with up to twenty persons per house. The size and proximity of the houses differed widely by community. While the Fort and central town were organized on a neat grid pattern, areas beyond the European quarter grew informally. The resulting neighborhoods varied in density and organization (Figure 24.1). In 1881, the municipal commissioner, T. S. Weir, marveled over the city's crowding, noting that the "density of population in the most dense section of London is less than the density in any of the 12 most densely population sections of Bombay."[4]

Rats, known to spread the plague bacterium *Yersinia pestis*, largely via fleas, found suitable homes inside crowded and informal housing, neighborhoods plagued by lack of waste removal and especially surrounding the docks. Once the plague struck, hygienic interventions and rat extermination efforts were ineffective against—or even worsened—the epidemic. The Bombay municipal government established an ecological niche for the plague and its rat hosts through physical and social sanitary infrastructures.

Case study: Plague in Bombay, 1896

The city of Bombay in 1896 was a set of multiple ecosystems that facilitated the transmission of plague. Mortality patterns indicated the presence of an "ecology of

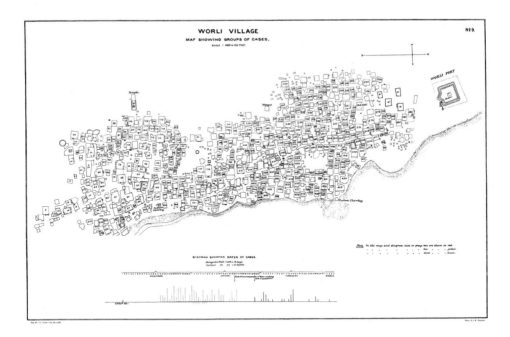

FIGURE 24.1: Map showing the organization of houses of Worli Village in Bombay, 1896. R. Nathan, "No. 9, Worli Village. Map showing groups of cases," in *Plague in India, 1896, 1897*, vol. VI. Medical History of British India Collection. (Courtesy of the National Library of Scotland.)

injustice," an often-pathological intersection of human and nonhuman ecologies resulting from societal structures that created negative effects for people from lower socioeconomic backgrounds.[5] Particularly important to this type of urban ecology, especially in the context of plague, was that its infrastructures (and lack thereof) encouraged rat colonization.

Historically, two species of rat made their homes in Bombay. *Rattus rattus*, the black rat, originated in the tropics and is thought to be indigenous to India. Averse to ground-level harborage, the black rat makes its home primarily within the built structures of human populations and has thus earned the monikers "roof rat" and "ship rat." The Norway rat, *Rattus norvegicus*, is the black rat's main competitor. It prefers ground-level harborage and therefore tends to make its home in sewers, alleys, and in the foundations or basements of houses. The Norway rat is capable of surviving in environments that offer nearly any kind of food (including, occasionally, the feces of other organisms) and seeks any opportunity for cover.[6] Both species will establish small home ranges that are composed of at most a city block and at least a single house. Both rats are responsible for urban infestations, which frequently lead to structural damage, spoiling of foodstuffs, and the transmission of disease. It is likely that living spaces shared with humans meant that the black rat was often responsible for human infections, with the Norway rat acting as a disease reservoir population for both black rats and humans.

The ecological and infrastructural niche of the rat reflects the demographic and structural patterns of plague in Bombay (Figure 24.2). Features of Bombay's built environment at the level of neighborhoods and the city contributed to the long-term persistence of plague. Factors like income and employment levels and race were risk factors for plague incidence and mortality as they altered opportunities for contact with rats and fleas (Figure 24.3). Lower-income persons were more likely to live in substandard housing that was subject to degradation or constructed with ill-fitting materials. This allowed more opportunities for rats to enter living spaces. Sanitary infrastructure was fragmented and the municipal government often neglected the creation of sewers, salubrious housing, and effective waste management. These services were deemed too challenging and thus relegated to individual neighborhoods that often lacked the resources for their implementation. Employment in grain shipping and storage provided close contact between laborers and the rat populations looking for food. Meanwhile, European hegemony provided legal scaffolding to protect white, colonial residents of the city from plague by mandating more stringent sanitary requirements that often insulated them from infected humans and rodents alike. Together, these features provided an urban ecology in which the plague could thrive among rodents and therefore an environment in which incidental human epidemics continued for decades.

Neighborhood	Ward	Density per House	Death Rate per Thousand	Occupational profile
Fort South	A Ward	8.42	4.85	Domestic S (38)
Mandvi	B Ward	23.09	16.68	Manufacturing & Supply (44)
Dongri	B Ward	28.76	16.62	Unskilled Labour (49)
Khumbarwada	C Ward	42.90	18.91	Manufacturing and Supply (40)
Kamathipura	E Ward	23.42	19.06	Manufacturing and Supply (47)
Tarwadi	E Ward	18.36	17.40	Manufacturing and Supply (48)

FIGURE 24.2: Ward, death rate, and occupational profile per five highest mortality districts and the European district of Bombay. Source: Meera Kosambi, *Bombay in Transition* (Stockholm: Almqvist and Wiskell International, 1986), 72; T. S. Weir, Reports of the Health Officer of Bombay, 1896–1909, IOR/V/25/840/23, African and Asian Studies Collection. (Courtesy of the British Library.)

While the numerous sanitary organizations that emerged in Bombay around the outbreak of plague identified many of these risk factors, efforts intended to ameliorate these conditions achieved little as the epidemic gained strength. Despite increasingly interventionist measures of plague control and a growing number of medical doctors, bacteriologists, and sanitary officials who struggled to understand the disease, mortality rates remained high for Bombay and the Indian subcontinent. As the plague gained imperial notice, it is likely that plague responses worsened the epidemic by neglecting the relationship between infrastructure, health, and ecology.

While urban infrastructure played a significant role in the spread and persistence of plague across Bombay, interventions from the municipal government perpetuated racialized ideas of hygiene and cleanliness or focused on rat extermination. Less than a month after the first case of plague, the Bombay Municipal government significantly extended its powers to address the epidemic.[7] Almost immediately, these measures changed the relationship of the imperial government to the private spaces and bodily sovereignty of Bombay's citizenry. Municipal officials could order the thorough disinfection of the interior of any citizen's home and forcibly remove residents to the hospital

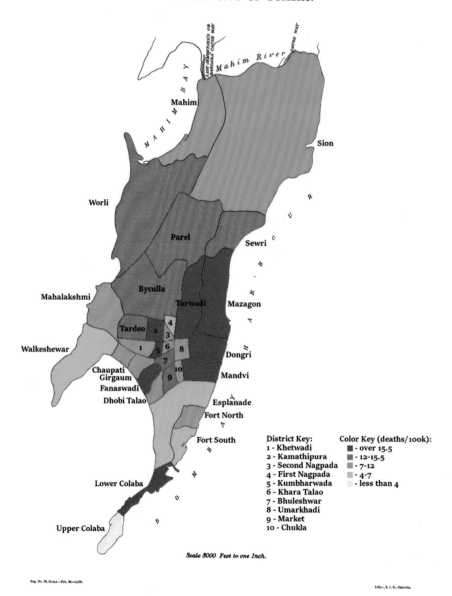

INCIDENCE OF PLAGUE IN DIFFERENT QUARTERS
OF THE CITY OF BOMBAY.

District Key:
1 - Khetwadi
2 - Kamathipura
3 - Second Nagpada
4 - First Nagpada
5 - Kumbharwada
6 - Khara Talao
7 - Bhuleshwar
8 - Umarkhadi
9 - Market
10 - Chukla

Color Key (deaths/100k):
■ - over 15.5
■ - 12-15.5
■ - 7-12
■ - 4-7
- less than 4

Scale 8000 Feet to one Inch.

FIGURE 24.3: Map of plague mortality per 100,000 by district, Bombay, 1896–1910. James Campbell, *Report of the Bombay Plague Committee on the Plague in Bombay for the Period Extending from the 1st July 1897 to the 30th April 1898*, vol. 2 (Bombay: Times of India Press, 1898). Medical History of British India Collection. IP/13/PC.5. (Courtesy of the National Library of Scotland.)

upon the discovery of illness.[8] The Epidemic Diseases Act, passed in early 1897, extended these controls, detailed the measures legally allotted to the newly established Plague Medical Officer, and conferred special powers upon local authorities to control epidemic disease. The government was thus granted the right to inspect all persons traveling into or out of the city and to detain those suspected of plague contamination. More ominously, the legislation claimed that "the state may take, or require or empower any person to take some measures and by public notice prescribe such temporary regulations to be observed by the public."[9] Within months of the first case, government officials had near-total license to alter the relationship of Bombay's residents to their city in the name of plague control.

Plague interventions, which largely consisted of evacuations, whitewashing of laborers' housing, and burning of their belongings, may have exacerbated the spread of plague in the city. Urban rat mobility is largely determined by access to food and harborage, so rats range further and into alternate burrows if their principal burrow is compromised or destroyed.[10] The whitewashing and sanitizing practices of the Bombay municipal government, including washing down houses and adjacent areas with boiling water and carbolic acid, likely disturbed the local rat population and exacerbated this behavioral tendency to relocate.[11] Sanitary measures would have effectively destroyed rodent burrows in infected houses and flushed the resident rats into adjacent homes or neighborhoods, as would efforts to burn or raze huts and temporary housing. Plague officials noted these altered spatial geographies in the wake of forced removals. The Plague Committee, for example, reported in 1898 that "experience had shown that plague passed from house to house, and that neighbours living several doors off a plague house were frequently attacked after the inmates of the plague house and been removed."[12] Other measures, like the suggested punching of holes into the roofs and walls of homes to allow adequate ventilation and sunlight, made it easier for rats to enter.[13]

Occupational dynamics continued to be an important risk factor for the development of plague in Bombay, even as the etiology of the disease shifted to the rat-flea theory. This clarification of transmission dynamics led to very little local sanitary change. Despite avid documentation of rat movements, the monitoring and research of rat populations further exacerbated class dynamics and exposure risk. As the city became a major site of research, the municipal government largely employed Indian lower-caste men to work as ratcatchers and rat handlers. Even the creation of knowledge thus contributed to the overarching "ecology of injustice" present in Mumbai, as members of lower socio-economic groups were more frequently exposed to rats, fleas, and plague through this work (Figure 24.4).

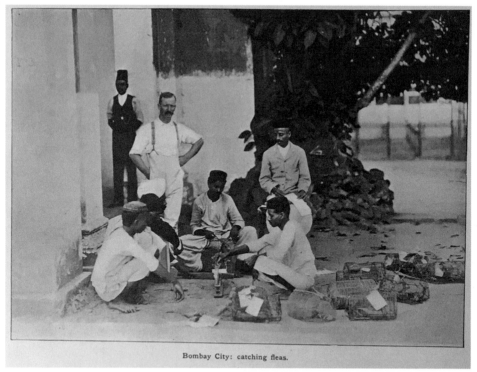

Bombay City: catching fleas.

FIGURE 24.4: Employees of the Bombay Bacteriological Laboratory combing rats for fleas. "Miscellaneous Photographs: Reproductions of Photos of the Bombay Plague Investigation." SA/ LIS/R.197. Box 15, Archives and Manuscripts Collection. (Courtesy of the Wellcome Library.)

Conclusion

Urban infrastructure defines the interactions and experiences of a city's human and nonhuman residents. Infrastructure enabled disease in imperial Bombay by altering ecologies and determining the risk of exposure. Bombay's position in the British imperial economy as a grain and cotton shipping port influenced its rapid growth, so, when combined with racialized public health practices and infrastructural neglect from the municipal government, the expanding city became a haven for rats. Once plague emerged in Bombay, the city's grain workers and ratcatching research assistants faced exposure in the name of global commercial and information regimes. Such dangerous jobs offered the highest risk of plague exposure because of the racialized social structure perpetuated by the city and the colony as a whole. Socially determined risk factors like house size, crowding, neighborhood infrastructure, and location compounded mortality risk.

At the end of the 19th century, global agricultural trade, industrialization, and the mass relocation of laborers to urban centers shaped disease environments.[14]

During Bombay's acute struggle with the third plague pandemic, changes in the city's disease environments were highly specific to the confluence of global and local forces in urban space. Bombay in the 19th century blossomed around systemic inequality, encouraged the movement of goods and people at a pace that corresponded with the life cycle of plague bacterium, and experienced rapid and dramatic alterations of its ecosystems as the city was incorporated into global commercial networks. Bombay holds important material similarities with other large urban centers, but the specificities of its infrastructure reveals the operation of the pandemic on multiple scales.

NOTES

1. H. M. Fernando, "Report on Bubonic Plague in Bombay," April 1897, Nos. 119–120, Simla Records, Sanitary [Plague] Branch, Home Department, National Archives of India, New Delhi, India.

2. Ira Klein, "Urban Development and Death: Bombay City, 1870–1914," *Modern Asian Studies* 20, no. 4 (1986): 744.

3. Teresa Albequerque, *Bombay: A History* (New Delhi: Promilla, 1992), xiv; and Miriam Dossal, *Imperial Designs and Indian Realities: The Planning of Bombay City, 1845-1875* (Bombay: Oxford University Press, 1991), 22.

4. He added that "in London the average is about 49 persons to each acre, in Bombay 52; but the extreme pressure in London is 222, whereas in Bombay it rises to 759." T. S. Weir, "Abstract of Report of the Bombay Municipality for 1889-1890 in Report on the Sanitary Measures in India for 1889-1890," General Department, vol. 174 (Mumbai: Maharashtra State Archives, 1891).

5. Gregg Mitman, *Breathing Space: How Allergies Shape Our Lives and Landscapes* (New Haven, CT: Yale University Press, 2008), 134.

6. Alice Y. T. Feng and Chelsea G. Himsworth, "The Secret Life of the City Rat: A Review of the Ecology of Urban Norway and Black Rats (*Rattus norvegicus* and *Rattus rattus*)," *Urban Ecosystems* 17 (2014): 159.

7. Papers Regarding Plague Operations in Bombay for the Secretary of State in Connection with the Questions Asked in the House of Commons by Mr. Maclean, March 1898, Nos. 398–411, Simla Records, Home Department, Sanitary Plague Branch, National Archives of India, New Delhi, India.

8. M. E. Couchman, Account of the Plague Administration in the Bombay Presidency from September 1896 till May 1897, IP/14/PC.4, India Papers Disease Collection. National Library of Scotland, Edinburgh, Scotland, United Kingdom; and David Arnold, *Colonizing the Body: State Medicine and Epidemic Disease in Nineteenth-Century India* (Berkeley: University of California Press, 1993), 201.

9. Couchman, Account of the Plague Administration, 55–56.

10. Kaylee A. Byers, Michael J. Lee, David M. Patrick, and Chelsea G. Himsworth, "Rats about Town: A Systematic Review of Rat Movement in Urban Ecosystems," *Frontiers in Ecology and Evolution* 7 (2019): 3.

11. Couchman, Account of the Plague Administration, 122; Myron J. Echenberg, *Plague Ports: The Global Urban Impact of Bubonic Plague, 1894–1901* (New York: New York University Press, 2007), 76; Revised Plague Rules Issued by Local Governments and Administrations, April 1901, Nos. 233–247, Sanitary Plague Branch, Home Department, National Archives of India, New Delhi, India.

12. Couchman, Account of the Plague Administration, 101.

13. Report of the Indian Plague Commission, Chapter VI, 1900, Plague Branch, General Department, Vol. 1008, No 628, Maharashtra State Archives, Mumbai, India.

14. Mark Harrison, *Contagion* (New Haven, CT: Yale University Press, 2013), xii.

25

French Urbanism, Vietnamese Resistance, and the Plague in Hanoi, Vietnam, 1885–1910

Michael Vann

The city of Hanoi, located on the Red River in Tonkin, Vietnam, sits on land continuously inhabited since prehistoric times. Hanoi's location at the center of a delta provides access to the region's numerous rivers. This abundance of water is both a blessing and a curse for the region. The delta contains numerous canals that facilitate trade, and nutrient-rich effluent makes the delta an extremely fertile for rice production. Yet the region is cursed with annual floods (Figure 25.1). Regularly destroying crops, roads, and villages, these inundations often threatened Hanoi itself. The city became Hà Nội (Inside the Rivers) in 1831 and maintained its role as a commercial center with the vernacular name Ké Cho (Great Market).

The city's political importance fluctuated. When the French occupied Tokin in the 1880s, Hanoi was merely a provincial capital. At the turn of the 20th century, Governor General Paul Doumer made Hanoi the capital of the federation of French Indochina, reviving the city's importance and setting off a demographic explosion and a building boom. Within a few years, the city's Vietnamese population grew to over one hundred thousand people, while the French population remained small. Including troops stationed in the barracks, the Europeans never constituted more than about 5 percent of the city's total residents. The European quarter occupied roughly one-third of the city's land, leaving another third for the so-called native quarter and the remainder for the administrative offices and the military. Hanoi's growth was fueled by a steady influx of Vietnamese peasants fleeing rural poverty and a small Chinese community with connections to several provinces in China's mountainous south and coastal ports.

The colonial state viewed the predominantly Vietnamese city with suspicion, deeming it unhealthy and in need of modernization. French administrators held that the newly developed science of urbanism would solve a host of Hanoi's public

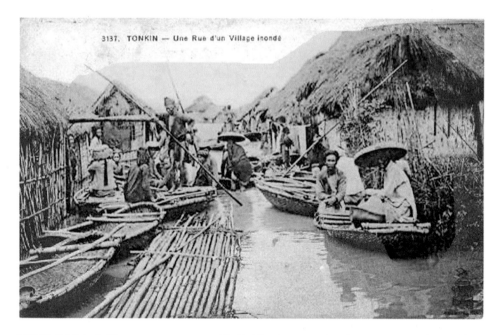

FIGURE 25.1: A Vietnamese water world. (Public domain: "Tonkin – Une Rue d'un Village Inondé" postcard by Pierre Dieulefils, n.d.)

hygiene issues. Urban growth during the colonial era and the establishment of railways and shipping lines to ports in South China and Southeast Asia had created conditions that facilitated the spread of plague and cholera in the early 20th century. Although sewer construction figured prominently in the plans of the technocrats, the sewer system created an unprecedented health crisis, forcing the colonial state to recognize the limits of what urban infrastructure could achieve. Instead, they turned toward robust public health measures, but the Vietnamese population resisted the invasive nature of these policies, which induced a new conflict.

Case study: Colonial urban infrastructure and the third bubonic plague pandemic in Hanoi

Hanoi is a very wet city. As is common in Southeast Asia, the local population developed semiaquatic ways of life. Precolonial Hanoi contained lakes, fishponds, and canals and was a natural hub for waterborne trade. Merchants brought their wares to the nearby riverbank or into the city itself in small boats. The citadel contained wet rice paddies, and, with unclear city limits, Hanoi quickly transitioned into farming villages. While there were a few small roads and paths leading to the city, most Vietnamese and Chinese moved about Tonkin on the water. On market days, which occurred several times per week, agricultural producers from the surrounding region would swarm into the city in the early hours of the morning to set up impromptu stands in the streets or sell their goods out of baskets. With thousands of shoppers, beggars, street urchins, stray dogs, and the noise of merchants crying out their wares and haggling with customers, the phantasmagoria of colors, sounds, and smells horrified early French observers.[1]

When the French conquered Hanoi in 1883, they took a disdainful view of its water-based urban culture and the lurking threat of nature.[2] Interpreting the indigenous market system as a sign of native inferiority and oriental chaos, the French "civilizing mission" sought to bestow the order and reason of modern methods of social organization upon Asia.[3] The French believed they could make Vietnamese cities more efficient, reflecting a positive faith in colonial progress and a racist contempt for Vietnamese urban life.

A contemporary observer suggested that precolonial Hanoi was not a city but a collection of dozens of villages (Figure 25.2).[4] To create a modern urban center, the colonizers drained the city, filled in ponds, and closed up canals. The fight against waterborne diseases such as cholera further justified these urbanizing moves. In the 1890s, the French built state-of-the-art sewers and a fresh water system (Figure 25.3).[5] Donald Reid's study of Paris shows how sewers, serving both as case study and metaphor, were crucial to French conceptions of modernity.[6] In contrast to the French capital, colonial Hanoi was a classic dual city. The racial divide between Europeans and Asians determined access to the benefits of the city's new urban infrastructure, so while French villas had running water and flush toilets, most of the Vietnamese and Chinese residents of the Old Quarter collected water from public fountains and human waste was removed in buckets by pre-dawn night-soil collectors. This Old Quarter had gutter drains, not proper sewers, so during heavy rain or typhoons, backflow fouled the streets with sewage. Nonetheless, colonial propaganda praised Hanoi's fifteen kilometers of sewers as a modernist triumph, which may have helped in the fight against cholera, brought by the French expeditionary forces from Algeria. Governor General Doumer's memoirs showed his enormous pride in this urban infrastructure project (while ignoring the racially determined structural inequalities and shortcomings) (Figure 25.4).[7] But the sewers created a new health crisis.

In 1902, medical authorities realized that the bubonic plague was headed toward Hanoi. The third plague pandemic began in Yunnan, China, in the 1850s and reached Canton and Hong Kong in the 1890s. From there, the new global network of steamships and railways spread the disease to ports in the Pacific, Indian, and Atlantic Oceans, creating a true pandemic on six continents. Working in Hong Kong in 1894, the Swiss researcher Alexandre Yersin of the Institut Pasteur

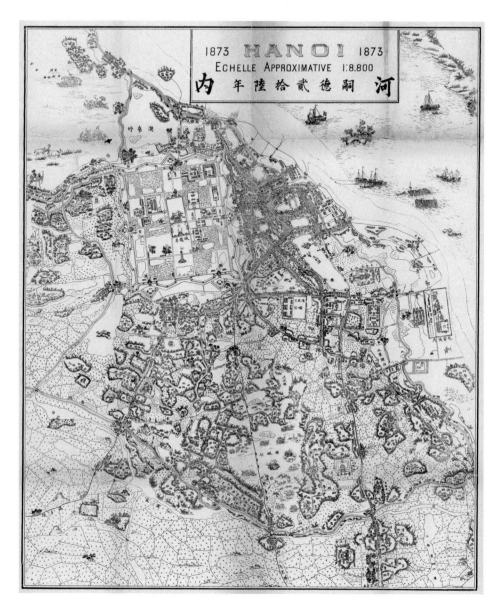

FIGURE 25.2: Pre-French Hanoi. (Public domain: Map of Hanoi in 1873 drawn by Phạm Đình Bách in 1902.)

identified the bacterium that spread the disease, although his rival, the German-trained Japanese doctor Kitasato Shibasaburo, initially claimed credit.[8] Four years later, another Pasteurian, Paul Simond, identified rat fleas as the vector that spread the plague, adding a degree of visceral repulsion to the collective anxiety about

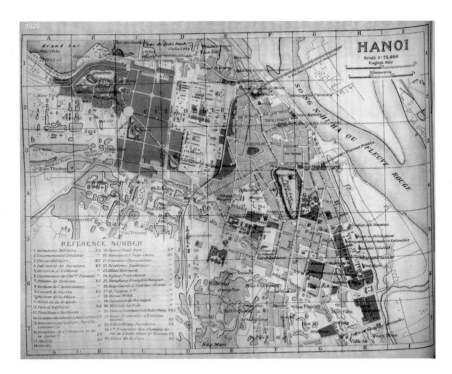

FIGURE 25.3: Hanoi after Doumer's building boom. (Public domain: *An Official Guide to Eastern Asia: Easy Indies*, vol. 5. Tokyo: Department of Railways, 1920, 139.)

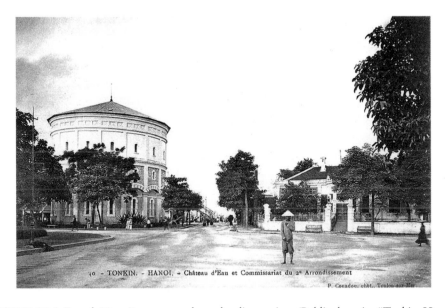

FIGURE 25.4: French Hanoi's water works and police station. (Public domain: "Tonkin. Hanoi. Château d'Eau et Commissariat de 2eme Arrondissement." Postcard by P. Couadou, Toulon sur Mer.)

the disease. An understanding of transmission mechanisms led to public health measures and public health officials in cities from Rio de Janeiro to San Francisco experimented with various rat eradication programs.[9] The plague, associated with the Middle Ages, incited an energetic response from the French technocrats so wedded to their conception of modernity.

French authorities in Hanoi feared the eventual arrival of the disease:

> Because of the [Vietnamese] population density, the closeness of the houses in the native quarter, the carelessness of the Annamites [of the central Vietnamese French protectorate] in regards to even the most basic rules of hygiene, the capital of Tonkin, as well as the other population centers of the colony, could quickly become a wonderful field test for the plague, if— as certain persons, whose competence in this matter is indisputable, predict— the illness reappears and invades the country.[10]

Citing the ubiquitous presence of rats in shops and in transported goods, French health experts singled out the Chinese in the spread of plague throughout Southeast Asia.[11] Tonkin was particularly at risk because of its proximity to China and the movements of Hong Kong merchants.[12] Hysteria over the plague fused with existing Sinophobia, resulting in openly racist policies against members of the Chinese diaspora.[13] The colonial administration initially blamed the indigenous population, within their urban geography of the Other, for creating conditions that could cause an epidemic. It soon became clear that Hanoi's new urban infrastructure was contributing to the problem.

With industrialized transportation moving rats around the world and urban growth leading to a global explosion in rat populations, rats were the "totem animal for modernity."[14] Transportation infrastructure brought the disease into the city via enterprising brown rats stowed away on the new Hanoi-Yunnan railway and ships moving between Chinese ports and Haiphong. Once in Hanoi, this invasive species discovered a new ecosystem, quickly colonizing the colonizer's sewers. Sheltered from predators and with access to plentiful food, the rats began to multiply. Soon, they were seen coming out of manholes in the French neighborhoods and there were reportedly climbing up sewer pipes and out of toilets in some of Hanoi's poshest addresses.[15] Municipal health authorities swung into action and tried to eliminate all the rats in the city but were faced with a series of failures. First, Vietnamese sewer workers viewed work as rat killers as beneath them. Then, after a bounty of a few pennies was placed on dead rats, the officers at the city's two police stations, which served as collection points, complained that they did not want piles of rodent corpses in the commissariat. When the bounty was modified to a cash payment for just the tails of dead rats, it seemed to work well for a few months. Between April and July 1902, French officials recorded daily rat kills regularly over fifteen thousand and sometimes topping twenty thousand.[16] But then the administration received some bad news. While on the edge of town, a French official saw a rat run past with no tail. He discovered that enterprising Vietnamese were catching rats, cutting off their tails, and letting them go to make more rats. Further investigations discovered rat farms in Hanoi's suburbs and a rodent-smuggling network bringing rats from all over Tonkin to Hanoi. It turned out that some of the tails were not even rat tails, but had come instead from mice and voles.[17] The great Hanoi rat hunt was a spectacular catastrophe.

Faced with this dramatic failure, the colonial authorities acknowledged that their modern urban infrastructure had created a long-term health crisis. With no quick fix, they turned to aggressive public health measures.[18] A new medical service was to establish the cause of every death in the city. The system would require the family of the deceased to notify a Vietnamese street chief, who would notify the police. Each police station would have a European agent and Vietnamese translator tasked with investigating deaths. To determine the potential threat of contagion, the white officer was authorized to inspect the home of the deceased and to interview family and neighbors. Once the agent submitted a report, a municipal doctor (also French) would conduct a postmortem with an eye to establishing the presence of a contagious disease. If the cadaver showed signs of cholera or plague, there would be further interviews and police agents would disinfect the residence and dispose of the body in a manner to prevent the spread of the disease. Homes of the deceased were to be sterilized with lye or other solutions, but the poorer victims lived in wood and thatch huts that had to be burned. Even in homes that could be sterilized, furniture, bedding, and other possessions were burned by the authorities to stop the spread of the plague. Family members or others who might have been exposed to the disease were sent to lazarettos outside the city.[19] By the end of the first year, the new energetic measures seemed to be working effectively.[20] However, many Vietnamese viewed Western medicine and colonial policies with suspicion and the invasive sterilizations provoked a series of conflicts over the destruction of homes and personal possessions and the quarantining of families. The French seizure and incineration of Vietnamese corpses disregarded the importance of traditional Vietnamese burial rites, which in turn provoked public displays of hostility toward the colonial authorities.[21] Despite the advancement policies of public health officials, French changes to Hanoi's infrastructure and urban culture became a flash point for anti-colonial movements.

Conclusion

Engineers and state administrators hoped that technocratic fixes would make colonial cities safer, healthier, and more prosperous. Yet, Hanoi's sewer projects went awry. While undertaken with the goal of combatting epidemic disease in Hanoi, French urban infrastructure and public health measures had serious unintended consequences, which included new health crises and increases in anti-colonial sentiment. The colonial state not only failed to eradicate cholera but also inadvertently created conditions for a bubonic plague outbreak—modernizing urban infrastructure was not necessarily a panacea. Indeed, the increase in the scale of large cities and growth of industrialized networks of global transpiration made urban centers vulnerable to epidemic diseases. When faced with cholera and the challenge of the plague, it became clear that Hanoi required invasive public health measures.

French colonial Hanoi's draconian public health policies proved profoundly unpopular and exacerbated tensions between colonizer and colonized in Vietnam. Mistrustful of the French occupiers to begin with, Vietnamese residents of Hanoi were pushed to the breaking point by the plague-driven destruction of personal property, burning of homes, quarantining potentially exposed people for weeks on end, and the seeming disappearance of loved one's bodies. A series of letters signed by "the people of Hanoi" protested the colonial state's public health measures. These were followed by demonstrations at some of the city's most important pagodas.[22] What started off as the implementation of French policies to improve the material conditions of the city quickly became a security crisis for the colonial regime. Epidemics are always stress tests for sociopolitical systems. In French Hanoi, a series of crises linked to the third bubonic plague pandemic revealed the multiple weaknesses of the colonial order.

NOTES

1. Gaston Bonnefont, *Aventures de Six Français aux Colonies: Ouvrage Illustré de Deux Cent Cinquante Garavures* (Paris: Garnier Frères, 188?), 719.

2. Hanoi National Archives I (HNA), Mairie de Hanoi (MdH), dossier 35, "Rapport sur le fonctionnement de la Municiplaité de Hanoi," (1891).

3. Centre des Archives Outre-Mer (CAOM), Fonds de Agence Economique de la France d'Outre-mer (AGEFOM), carton 236, dossier 294, "Hanoi hier et aujourd'hui," (1938).

4. Luycien Heudebert, *L'Indo-Chine Francaise* (Paris: G. Dujarric, 1909), 195–201.

5. CAOM, Fonds de Gouverneur Général d'Indochine (GGI), dossier 6365, "Programmes des travaux à réaliser sur les fonds de l'emprunt de 1.500.000 F. 5 plans joints," (1897).

6. Donald Reid, *Paris Sewers and Sewermen: Realities and Representations* (Cambridge, MA: Harvard University Press, 1991).

7. "Le développement de la Ville de Hanoï (Janvier 1897–Janvier 1901)," *La revue Indo-Chinoise*, no. 126 (March, 1901): 227; L. Fayet, *Avant projet sur les Égouts de Hanoï* (Hanoi: Imprimerie d'Extrême-Orient, 1939).

8. CAOM, AGEFOM carton 237, dossier 296, "Les médicins français en Indochine" (n.d.).

9. Myron J. Echenberg, *Plague Ports: The Global Urban Impact of Bubonic Plague, 1894–1901* (New York: New York University Press, 2007).

10. CAOM, GGI, dossier 64174, "Tonkin" (1903).

11. Laurent Joseph Gaide and Henri Désiré Marie Bodet, *La Peste en Indochine* (Hanoi: Imprimerie d'Extrême-Orient, 1930), 5, 27.

12. Ortholan, "La peste en Indo-Chine. (Historique)," *Annales d'Hygiène et de Médicine Coloniale* 11 (1908): 633–38.

13. Robert Peckham, ed., *Empires of Panic: Epidemics and Colonial Anxieties* (Hong Kong: Hong Kong University Press, 2015).

14. Jonathan Burt, *Rat* (London: Reaktion Books, 2006), 18.

15. CAOM, Fonds de Résident Supérieur du Tonkin (RST), dossier 34580, "Santé Publique. Mesures à prendre contre la peste et le cholera" (1903); V. Rouffiandis, "La peste bubonic au Tonkin," *Annales d'Hygiène et de Médincine Coloniale* 8 (1905): 609–30.

16. CAOM, GGI, dossier 6675, "Destruction des animaux, Hanoi-Ville" (1902); CAOM, GGI, dossier 6725, "Destruction des rats- Tonkin" (1904).

17. HNA, MdH, dossier 44, "Rapport annuel du 1er juillet 1930 au 30 juin 1931" (1931).

18. CAOM, GGI, dossier 64174, "Tonkin" (1903); CAOM, RST, dossier 34580, "Santé Publique. Mesures à prendre contre la peste et le cholera" (1903); CAOM, AF, carton 9, dossier 54, "Situation politique et économique du Tonkin" (1906).

19. Le Roy des Barres, *Rapport sur la mortalité à Hanoï en 1903* (Hanoi: Imprimiére Express, 1904), 1.

20. CAOM, AF, carton 9, dossier 54, "Situation politique et économique du Tonkin," (1906).

21. Buu Hiep, *La Médicine française dans la vie annamite* (Hanoi: Imprimiére Le-van-Phuc, 1936); Le Roy des Barres, *Rapport sur la mortalité à Hanoï*, 1; CAOM, GGI, dossier 6739 (1906).

22. CAOM, GGI, dossier 6739 (1906).

26

Building a Community on Leprosy Island in the Philippines, 1898–1941

Mary Anne Alabanza Akers

The Philippines is a Southeast Asian country that has experienced the long-term impact of Spanish colonization and of the indelible imperialism forced upon it by the United States of America. An archipelago of more than 7,100 islands with abundant natural and mineral resources, the Philippines garnered the interest of Spain in 1521, and of the United States in 1898, when the country was acquired as an outcome of the Spanish American War. Early records of Spanish missionaries reveal that leprosy was found among the Indigenous tribes prior to colonization. At that time, the local dialect contained terminology referring to skin diseases like *buni* (ringworm), *butlig* (skin eruptions), *aliponga* (fungal skin infection), and *nacnac* (fester with pus).[1] However, the accounts of how leprosy reached the archipelago are scarce.

The Spanish used leprosy to evangelize, telling the Filipinos to convert to Catholicism to be healed.[2] Their focus was on bolstering spiritual well-being, an aim that was placed above the medical treatment of the people. Of course, religion did not heal leprosy. The disease continued to spread as the Spanish colonizers lacked a systematic approach to containment. Eventually, the Franciscan Order established hospitals in Manila and other areas, but this did not diminish the numbers of Filipinos infected with leprosy.[3]

The slow-growing leprosy bacterium *Mycobacterium leprae* was first identified under a microscope in 1873 by Norwegian scientist Gerhard Hansen. The origin of leprosy—a germ, rather than hereditary genes—was revealed by Hansen's research, which showed a chronic infection that manifested in damage to the body's peripheral nerves, skin, and mucous membranes. As a contagious disease, the way to stop its spread was to isolate those who were infected and to eradicate the germ through treatment.

When the United States occupied the archipelago in 1898, they were confronted by deplorable sanitary conditions, which led to constant outbreaks of disease, left behind by centuries of Spanish neglect. To fulfill their civilizing mission, the Americans constructed health and sanitation infrastructure and inculcated American ideals. The high incidence of leprosy and the unchecked drifting of diseased individuals between communities required a segregation plan. In 1901, Culion Island was conceived of as a leper colony in the Philippines. Culion Island became a world center in the early 20th century for research and effective practices to alleviate leprosy. Culion Island exemplifies how a community can emerge through physical, social, economic, and political infrastructural development.

Case study: Leprosy and site segregation on Culion Island

In the early 1900s, an American report estimated that approximately five thousand Filipinos were afflicted with leprosy.[4] Of course, leprosy also posed a threat to thousands of American military troops deployed to the Philippines, and the Americans were fearful that the disease would overwhelm the country if its spread were not contained. The geographical advantage of the archipelago was its abundance of islands, forming potentially isolated paradises for the afflicted. The healthy climate with sea breezes, rich soils for cultivation, abundant grazing land, and suitable harbors convinced the Americans that the lepers would lead quality lives in healthy homes and freely enjoy the outdoors, rather than enduring confinement with other afflicted people within city hospitals. After a comprehensive survey of the Philippines, the American colonial government recognized the beneficial features of Culion Island as the ideal place for a leper colony.[5]

An Executive Order in 1904 sealed the sale of Culion Island. Under Act 389, the American government appropriated $50,000 to develop the site by constructing a network of roads, water lines, and sewer systems. The Americans built the superintendent's dwelling, a hospital, and vernacular houses made of bamboo and nipa palm. By May 1906, the first 370 leper patients were transported to Culion Island (Figure 26.1). As the Director of Health in the Philippines, physician Dr. Victor Heiser pushed for legislation to isolate people who tested positive for the *Mycobacterium leprae* bacterium. The so-called Leper Law (Act 1117) was passed in 1907 as "An Act Providing for the Apprehension, Detention, Segregation, and Treatment of Lepers in the Philippine Islands."[6]

While some Filipinos with the disease willingly agreed to be transported to Culion Island, others were captured by the provincial police and forcibly sent. Word that Culion was a miserable place was a deterrent to voluntary segregation, as were deep family ties—the thought of family separation led to great anguish. To counteract negative impressions, an educational campaign was launched using movie reels to show the beauty and bounty of the place. Culion Island was

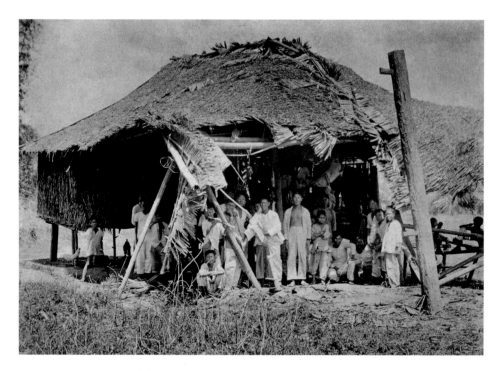

FIGURE 26.1: Men with leprosy who were isolated prior to their transfer to Culion Island. (Courtesy of the Science Photo Library.)

described as a place of unusual beauty with the most appealing harbor, attractive hillsides, and abundant trees and flowering shrubs (Figure 26.2). The films showed the new inhabitants happy and contented as they received treatment, with their daily needs for food, water, and clothing provided for. Arable land to cultivate and a weekly gratuity were also given.

Culion Island was envisioned as a leper colony that served as a laboratory for curative health and citizenship. However, upon arrival, the first afflicted settlers were greeted with the terrifying sight of ten-foot barbed wired quarantine fences, so unlike the scenes depicted in the educational films. The Americans believed the Filipino settlers eventually took delight in their surroundings because of their constant expressions of gratitude.[7] As the settlement expanded, additional infrastructure including a freshwater system from an inland mountain stream with distribution connected to bath houses, latrines, and laundries was laid out. The hilly topography allowed the drainage system to flow downhill toward the sea. The local government renovated a large dining hall that served meals for approximately three hundred people. An amusement hall was built to distract the residents from boredom and loneliness. The concrete one-storey tropical hospital was designed

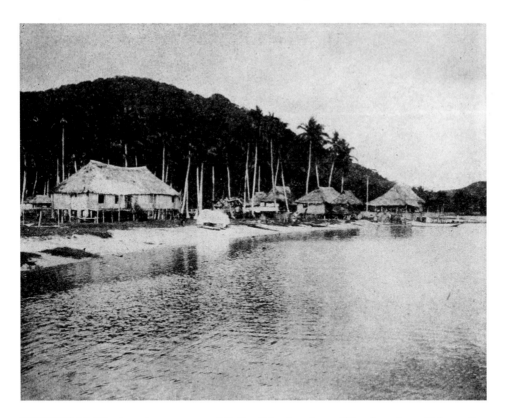

FIGURE 26.2: The Americans promoted Culion Island to those afflicted as a beautiful paradise with native huts, fruit trees, and health facilities. (Courtesy of The Reading Room at Alamy Stock Photo.)

with an open plan and large windows to ensure maximum ventilation and circulation from sea breezes. Residents were assigned to individual huts during the early stages of leprosy. These homes were designed with wide windows that propped open to make the rooms "practically part of the outdoors."[8] Buildings, outdoor spaces, and community services were installed, including a town hall with a post office and library, a gymnasium, a playground, schools, and an open-air theater.

The Americans resocialized the inhabitants while performing experiments to heal the symptoms of leprosy. Instruction included domestic hygiene training and the encouragement of healthy behaviors, such as regular bathing, the washing of clothes, and calisthenic exercise. To indoctrinate the Filipinos into American culture, the hospital introduced baseball and basketball, Hollywood films and popular songs. The residents sang the Star-Spangled Banner under the American flag and celebrated the Fourth of July, American Independence Day. To instill civic pride, a band, organized with instruments and uniforms, was paid to perform in the plaza every week. The residents organized their own government, consisting of a president and ten councilors based on the American model of democracy. Voting in the Island's elections was strongly encouraged. Women enjoyed full suffrage, and although a minority, they often decided the elections.[9] A police force of residents was formed to maintain order.[10]

The colonial government intervened in the sexual lives of Culion inhabitants by segregating the men and women through the construction of separate dormitories. This arrangement prevented natural physical relationships, yet the residents continued to seek each other for love. They complained to the Catholic priest and nuns and to the superintendent, who took their concerns to Dr. Heiser.[11] As the result of their discontent, the regulations were relaxed and marriage between patients was permitted in 1910.[12] However, the population ballooned and in 1928 officials again revoked the permission to marry. Threats and violent incidents erupted, and the girls' dormitory was burned in protest. After five years, this prohibition on marriage was rescinded.

Despite the Island's isolated location, the local economy developed. The elected government encouraged residents to farm, fish, garden, and make things to sell in the community market and store. Residents created their own currency, supported by a weekly allowance of 10 cents provided by the United States government to keep the economy alive. The training of young nursing aides and schoolteachers was not only a health and education strategy but also a source of employment. When additional roads were later constructed to connect various parts of the Island, the leper community supplied the construction labor.

Eventually, the Island was segregated into districts designated for the *leprosos* (patients) and the *sano* (non-patients), including healthy families and staff (Figure 26.3). In 1915, a Children's Home was established in the *sano* section to serve as a nursery for babies and young children who were removed from their parents before they could be exposed to leprosy. These infants were cared for in the Children's Home building and reared away from their families. Parents could visit, but interaction was only permitted through a glass partition.[13] Approximately ten years after the Children's Home was founded, a process began under which healthy children under two years of age who had not contracted leprosy from their parents were sent to the Welfareville Institute in Manila for possible adoption.[14]

Conclusion

The American governors of the Philippines envisioned Culion Island as more than a segregation exercise, investing in a research and training center in the 1920s that purported to be the foremost experimental hub with "any promise of finding the

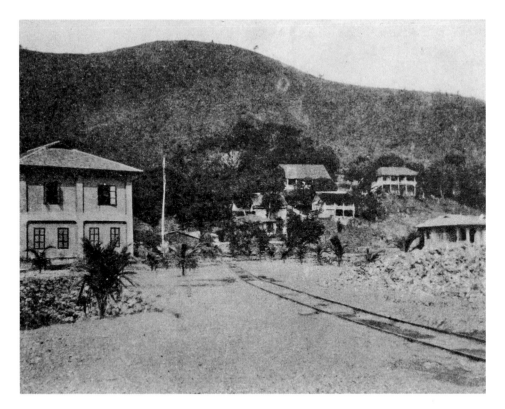

FIGURE 26.3: The Island developed into a thriving community with its own government, economy, transportation network, and community life. (Courtesy of The Reading Room at Alamy Stock Photo.)

ultimate solution of this age-old curse of the human race."[15] Dr. D. W. Wade was hired to establish The Leonard Wood Memorial for the Eradication of Leprosy, named after the governor general of the Philippines, who persuaded the Philippine Legislature to appropriate exorbitant funds for Dr. Wade's research program.[16] The granted funds amounted to one-third of the health budget for the entire Philippines and almost 3 percent of the government's total budget.[17]

Culion Island gained worldwide recognition as the model for leprosy patient segregation and treatment. The Island's popularity soared in the 1920s during which time the population reached more than four thousand people to become known as the world's largest leper colony. A decade later, budget deficits and the establishment of additional provincial leprosy treatment centers around the country decreased admissions to the Island. The development of Culion Island can best be described as an organic, international process: the Americans laid out the physical and medical infrastructure for health and healing, but real Filipino community building emerged from the intersection of the social, economic, and political lives of the afflicted. The stories of the residents and accounts of staff and visitors tell of the collective agency of Culion Island residents. Despite painful segregation from their families, they used their collective experience to persevere and survive. What started as a place of segregation developed into a community with strength and resilience that allowed it to hold its own against strict intrusions over the private lives of the residents. It was indeed a model for the world.

NOTES

1. Lorelei D. C. De Viana, "Early Encounters between the Spanish Religious Missionaries and Leprosy in the Philippines," in *Hidden Lives, Concealed Narratives: A History of Leprosy in the Philippines*, ed. Maria Serena I. Diokno (Manila, Philippines: National Historical Commission of the Philippines, 2016), 24.

2. Maria Eloisa G. Parco De Castro, "Rediscovering a Paradigm: The Fransciscan Order's Response to Leprosy and the Afflicted in the Philippines, 1578–1898," in *Hidden Lives, Concealed Narratives*, 41.

3. The established Hospital de San Lazaro became the center for leprosy care, although it also provided medical services for other illnesses.

4. Wataru Kusaka, "Discipline and Desire: Hansen's Disease Patients Reclaim Life in Culion, 1900-1930s," *Social Science Diliman* 13, no. 2 (2017): 6.

5. Located about 600 miles southwest of Manila, Culion Island, with a total land area of 150 square miles and about 40 acres of suitable land for habitation, was one of a cluster of islands referred to as the Calamianes Group. Prior to the occupation of the island for the afflicted, a small town was already situated there but they were resettled to nearby Basunga.

6. Maria Serena Diokno, "Fear of Contagion, Punishment, and Hope," in *Hidden Lives, Concealed Narratives*, 6.

7. Philippine Commission, *Seventh Annual Report of the Philippine Commission to the Secretary of War, 1906* (Washington, DC: Government Printing Office, 1906), 17.

8. Perry Burgess, *Who Walk Alone* (New York: Henry Holt, 1940), 121.

9. Treatments included doses of chaulmoogra oil, initially given as a drink and later as an intramuscular injection. Margaret Marion Wheeler, "The Culion Leper Colony," *The American Journal of Nursing* 13, no. 9 (June 1913): 664.

10. Arthur A. Weiss, S.J. *Woodstock Letters* 77, no. 1 (February 1, 1948): 38.

11. When Culion Island was conceived, Secretary of the Interior Dean C. Worcester approached the Catholic Church leadership in the Philippines, Apostolic Delegate, and the Archbishop of Manila, to seek assistance and support. Jesuit priest Father Valles and Four Sisters of Charity of the St. Vincent de Paul Order were assigned to the Island to care for the afflicted.

12. Thirteen couples married in 1910. This jumped to 100 couples in 1911.

13. Such a strategy was the result of ongoing observations of the spread among young members of the community because of their contact with the afflicted residents. E. Muir, "Report on a Visit to the Leper Island of Culion and on the Anti-Leprosy Work in the Philippine Islands," *Indian Medical Gazette* 60, no. 6 (June 1925): 261–64.

14. Jose A. Arcilla, "The Culion Leper Colony, 1900s–1970s," *Philippine Studies* 57, no. 2 (2009): 312. The Culion administration decided on such a drastic measure because the data showed that 50 percent of non-afflicted children who stayed with their diseased parents developed leprosy by their fifth birthday.

15. Esmond R. Long, "Forty Years of Leprosy Research History of the Leonard Wood Memorial (American Leprosy Foundation) 1928 to 1967," *International Journal of Leprosy* 35, no. 2 (1967): 239.

16. Dr. Wade was a professor of pathology and bacteriology in the College of Medicine and Surgery of the University of the Philippines in Manila. His research interest was the pathology of the disease and the extent to which the chaulmoogra oil treatment at that time was effective in treating and mitigating the symptoms.

17. Ronald F. Chapman, "Leonard Wood and Leprosy in the Philippines: The Culion Leper Colony, 1921–1927. A Review," *Journal of the History of Medicine and Allied Sciences* 38, no. 4 (1983): 469.

27

Shifting Health Paradigms and Infrastructure in Australia in the 20th Century

Karen Daws and Julie Willis

Following colonization by Great Britain in 1788, Australia was seen as a healthy place with the advantage of physical isolation from the rest of the world providing its primary defense against disease.[1] Early colonial records show that disease was characterized by accidents, childhood fevers, and conditions related to poor sanitation and nutrition. The first epidemic outbreak, the exact nature of which remains the subject of controversy, devastated the Aboriginal population near Sydney in 1789. The impact of this epidemic on the culture of the colony was significant, diminishing the Aboriginal peoples' capacity to resist the colonial invasion and disrupting cultural and healing practices, thereby impacting relationships with the colonists.[2]

Infectious diseases introduced by the colonizers such as diphtheria, scarlet fever, whooping cough, measles, and influenza eventually became more or less endemic. These illnesses occasionally occurred on such a scale that an epidemic would be announced. For example, a measles outbreak in Sydney in 1867 elicited official concern; scarlet fever and diphtheria epidemics were declared in multiple locations in the Australian colonies between 1858 and the 1890s; and further outbreaks of infectious diseases such as smallpox in Sydney in 1881 and in Melbourne in 1857, along with bubonic plague in 1900, were also classed as epidemics. These diseases were endemic in Europe but did not become so in Australia. There were also several outbreaks of influenza that culminated in the 1919 epidemic, which caused an estimated fifty million deaths worldwide and some fifteen thousand deaths in Australia.

Concern for public health shaped the urban environment in Australia. The very earliest town plans were laid out on rising ground in gridiron patterns with wide streets to encourage ventilation.[3] Public health authorities in towns and cities directed their attention toward ventilation, waste disposal, appropriate locales for noxious industries, and overcrowding, reflecting the origins of this discipline.

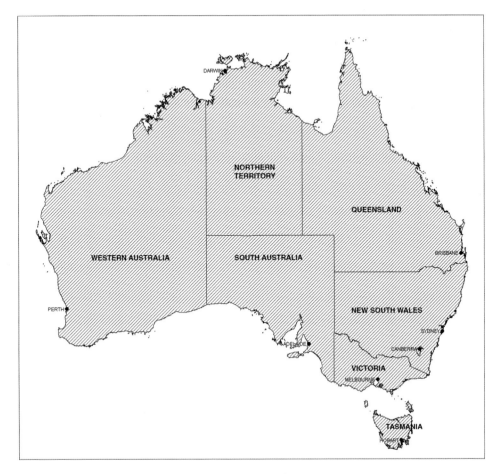

FIGURE 27.1: Map of Australia, showing colonial (later state) boundaries. (Courtesy of the University of Melbourne.)

These ideas were rooted in the sanitarian paradigm of public health, a political and social movement of the 19th century that linked health to the environment where people lived, especially the poor. The movement advocated for widespread improvements in sanitation and in building practices to mitigate disease.

Case study: Public health, urban environment, and the influenza epidemic in Australia, 1919

In the 19th century, the public health disciplines of nosology (the classification of diseases), bacteriology, and epidemiology developed, but did not challenge, the sanitary essentials of the field. Nosology, based on the system developed by English epidemiologist William Farr (1807–1883), was adopted in the Australian colonies of Victoria in 1855, New South Wales in 1858, and Tasmania in the 1850s. Diseases such as diphtheria, scarlet fever, whooping cough, measles, and influenza were initially classified as zymotic, and later as miasmatic, an understanding of disease causation and transmission that implicated putrefaction processes. Miasma was understood as the presence of decomposed organic matter in the air. Both these conceptions implicated air, water, and place as vectors for disease. The term "zymotic" was used in Australian statistical reports of death until 1907, after which these diseases were reclassified as "general," along with cancer, diabetes, and thyroid diseases.[4] It was not until 1920 that a classification was adopted to describe infectious, endemic, and epidemic disease as a separate category. By conceptualizing a disease as zymotic within the sanitary paradigm, it was implicit that it was preventable through hygienic measures. This was a fundamentally social and cultural construction of infectious diseases that framed such illnesses as aberrations. Infectious diseases were thus increasingly identified, differentiated, and described as distinct entities over the course of the 19th century.[5] Within hospital buildings in Australia, treatment for generic zymotic fevers occurred in wards that were called "fever wards," which were not specially designed or constructed. As infectious diseases were increasingly named and differentiated, specially designed infectious diseases wards were developed.

In the colony of Victoria, the Central Board of Health (CBH) consistently requested that responsible local authorities provide infectious disease wards to be made available for use in disease outbreaks, beginning in the 1850s. However, these demands were qualified with suggestions for temporary constructions. In 1876, the CBH published a design for an infectious disease ward, which according to their report was "available for any emergency [but] being only for occasional and temporary use, need be only of the simplest description" (Figure 27.2).[6] The design showed a one-room building of lightweight timber construction, with provision for ventilation and raised from the ground, to avoid damp. The use of panels was to allow for it to be dismantled when it was no longer needed, revealing a belief in the temporary, passing nature of epidemics.[7]

Despite the influence of public health on the urban environment, public health authorities in Australia were almost always ambivalent about the need for permanent infectious disease wards. Australian hospital administrators and medical practitioners also resisted including infectious disease wards on hospital grounds based on the perceived risk to other patients. The structure of the colonial health administration meant that local municipal councils were responsible for funding buildings for infectious diseases, and hospitals sought to avoid paying for new facilities. As a result of the ambivalence of public health authorities, demands for

PLAN

Scale, 8 feet to the inch.

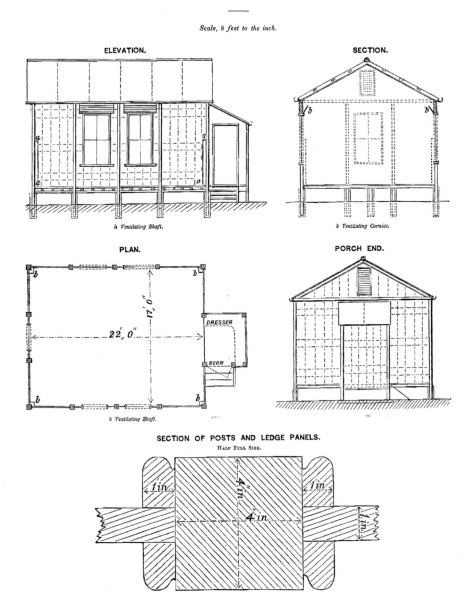

FIGURE 27.2: Central Board of Health temporary building for contagious diseases, Melbourne. The building included ventilation tubes in its corners. From Central Board of Health, *Sixteenth Report of the Board*, Victorian Parliamentary Paper no. 55 (Melbourne: John Ferres, Government Printer, 1876), 38.

treatment and the lack of facilities came into conflict at the hospitals themselves. Demand for hospitals to treat diseases such as diphtheria and scarlet fever rose; most infectious disease wards were used almost exclusively for these cases.

The infectious disease wards that were eventually, albeit reluctantly, provided at hospitals in Victoria and other Australian colonies were often temporary, rudimentary, and subject to alternating periods of neglect and agitated attention that were dictated by the cyclical nature of infectious disease outbreaks. These buildings were sited at stipulated distances from hospital buildings, reflecting the idea that buildings and places themselves could harbor diseases. This was expressed at the Queen's Memorial Infectious Diseases Hospital, built in 1904 near Melbourne, where two sets of roads directed the movement of people and things through the site. By designating "noninfected" routes as distinct from the "infected" roads, place was implicated as a source of disease (Figure 27.3). By extension, this plan offered the idea that the noninfected—the rest of Australia—was disease-free.

The very terms "endemic" and "epidemic" derive from the Greek root "demos" (δεμοσ) in reference to the populace, which is linked to the concept of place. The

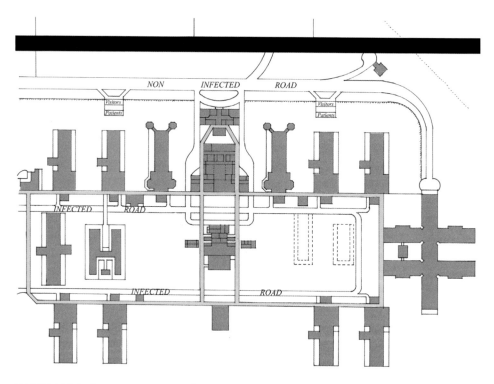

FIGURE 27.3: Queen's Memorial Infectious Diseases Hospital, Anketell & K. Henderson, 1916 plan. (Courtesy of Department of Health Victoria Archives; redrawn by Julie Willis, 2020.)

19th-century sanitarians believed a place (and by association its populace) could be intrinsically healthy or unhealthy. Australian scholar Alison Bashford links the concept of the healthy place to certain foundational ideas about Australian culture and geography that influenced public health, immigration policies, and Australian nationalism in the early 20th century.[8] The idea that infection could be embedded in place was extended to construction materials. Non-permeable materials that could be readily cleaned were often used for infectious disease wards in permanent buildings to reduce the risk of contagion lingering within the fabric. Tents (as all canvas-clad structures were known) were widely used for patient care even prior to the influenza epidemic as they provided good ventilation and could be incinerated or otherwise disposed of once the outbreak had passed. Such a tent was used for patients with diphtheria in a town in Victoria in 1910 (Figure 27.4). This pattern of tent use and disposal further reinforced the notion of disease as a temporary concern.

In 1919, troops returning to Australia from the war in Europe (1914–18) provided a conduit for influenza and introduced the unprecedented dislocation, illness, and death that was being experienced on a global scale due to the epidemic. When

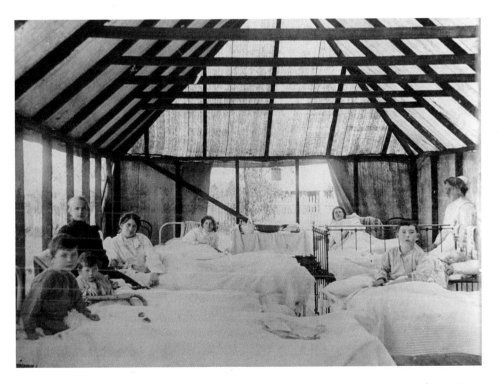

FIGURE 27.4: Swan Hill Hospital, diphtheria tent. Photograph by George Hamilton, 1910. (Courtesy of the Swan Hill Regional Library.)

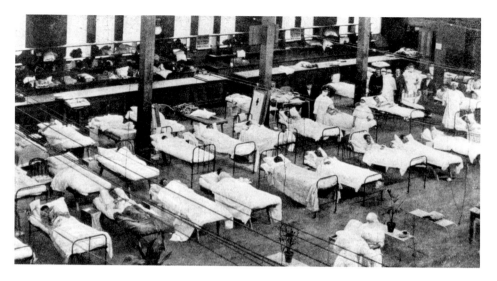

FIGURE 27.5: Royal Exhibition Buildings, Melbourne, used as hospital wards, 1919. (Courtesy of Museums Victoria.)

news of influenza first arrived from Europe, the Australian government responded with strict quarantine measures. John Howard Lidgett Cumpston (1880–1954), Australian Director of Quarantine, credited maritime quarantine with substantially reducing the spread of influenza to the continent.[9] Quarantine stations were built at the entrances to major Australian ports beginning in the early 1830s and had proved very successful in quelling or limiting disease outbreaks.[10] Australia resisted British trends that de-emphasized the role of quarantine in preventing epidemic diseases and maintained perceptions of disease as something alien to the Australian continent that could be prevented from entering.

Despite the hopes placed in the quarantine system, cases of influenza appeared within Australia. However, there were, as yet, no infectious disease facilities with the capacity to cope with the incoming case numbers. Rudimentary hospitals were made ready, which meant the appropriation of public spaces or public buildings as makeshift facilities. In Melbourne, where the epidemic first appeared, tents were erected on the grounds of the Queen's Memorial Infectious Diseases Hospital and army barracks were appropriated as wards for the ill. The Royal Exhibition Building was also converted into a hospital (Figure 27.5). In Sydney, existing hospitals were entirely reconfigured as influenza hospitals, and tents and schools were also used as temporary infirmaries. In smaller towns, it was common for the local school, closed because of the epidemic, to be used as a hospital. Small halls were also put into service and tents were set up on common grounds and parks.

By September 1919, less than eight months from the first case in Victoria, these facilities were dismantled and the beds and equipment sold.[11]

The belief in the intrinsic healthfulness of Australia resulted in temporary infrastructural responses to the influenza epidemic in 1919. Following the end of the influenza epidemic, public health authorities continued to request that isolation facilities be maintained at the ready in the event of another outbreak. There was a small increase in the number of dedicated healthcare buildings for infectious diseases after 1919, but these were often sited at the rear of hospital grounds and ultimately left to fall into disrepair. Australia's responses to the influenza epidemic of 1919, in terms of hospital infrastructure, were temporary in nature. This official reaction may be attributed to Australia's geographical isolation and the accompanying notions about the inherent healthiness of place and the ephemerality of disease. The 19th-century sanitarian paradigm influenced how infectious diseases infrastructure was mobilized, designed, and viewed in response to the influenza pandemic of 1919.

Conclusion

The appearance of infectious disease in colonial Australia impacted urban infrastructural responses both before and after the influenza epidemic of 1919. The belief in Australia as a healthy, isolated place contributed to the perception of epidemic disease outbreaks as temporary urban aberrations rather than an expected part of life. Infectious disease wards themselves were often temporary and never achieved the same level of administrative and institutional regard as quarantine policies or urban public health strategies. Despite the global scale and ferocity of the influenza epidemic, Australian infrastructure responses did not deviate fundamentally from the established colonial pattern of rudimentary infectious disease wards and hospital tents.

Scientific development of ideas about disease and the emergence of the disciplines of nosology, bacteriology, and epidemiology in the 19th century changed the way that infectious diseases were conceptualized in Australia. The Australian response to the influenza pandemic was influenced by the health care changes occurring within a sanitarian paradigm that held on to ideas regarding the intrinsic healthfulness of place and the ephemerality of illness. These factors were often tacitly understood but were rarely made explicit in policy or documents. The urban health infrastructure in Australia revealed the influence of these ideas at the practical level, in cases where tents and temporary structural responses to epidemic disease demonstrated the sanitarian paradigm. Deeply embedded social and cultural ideas about disease in Australia influenced the nature of health care infrastructure.

NOTES

1. Alison Bashford, *Imperial Hygiene: A Critical History of Colonialism, Nationalism and Public Health* (Basingstoke: Palgrave Macmillan, 2014), 126.

2. Grace Karskens, *The Colony: A History of Early Sydney* (Crow's Nest, Australia: Allen and Unwin, 2010), 376.

3. The earliest street layout for Sydney by Surveyor General Baron Alt demonstrates this, although it was not put in place. The layout of Hobart and Perth also demonstrate these ideas, which were codified in 1829 with the drawing of the Darling Regulations that governed the setting-out of new towns. The width of streets was regularly cited as a health requirement. See Miles Lewis, *Melbourne: The City's History and Development* (Melbourne: City of Melbourne, 1995), 26–28.

4. This reflected the widespread adoption of the Bertillon system of nosology.

5. William F. Bynum, "The Evolution of Germs and the Evolution of Disease: Some British Debates, 1870–1900," *History and Philosophy of the Life Sciences* 24, no. 1 (2002): 53–68.

6. Central Board of Health, *Sixteenth Report of the Board*, Victorian Parliamentary Paper no. 55 (Melbourne: John Ferres, Government Printer, 1876), 37.

7. Ibid. The building still included elements seen as necessary for the accommodation of patients, with ventilation tubes in each corner and a large vent in the rear gable.

8. Alison Bashford argues the influence of the concept of the "healthy place" on practices of "enclosure, segregation and classification" that shaped foundational racial, nationalistic, and public health policies in Australia in the 20th century. These were played out in quarantine practices, selective immigration policies, and the enforced isolation of people with leprosy, in particular Aboriginal people. Bashford, *Imperial Hygiene*, 187.

9. John Howard Lidgett Cumpston, *Influenza and Maritime Quarantine in Australia* (Melbourne: Commonwealth of Australia Quarantine Service Publication 18, 1919), 37.

10. The first was at North Head, at the entry to Sydney Harbour, established in 1832. Some of the quarantine stations were in continuous operation until the mid-1980s and played important roles in epidemics.

11. "Influenza Hospitals Dismantling Begun," *The Argus*, September 18, 1919, 8.

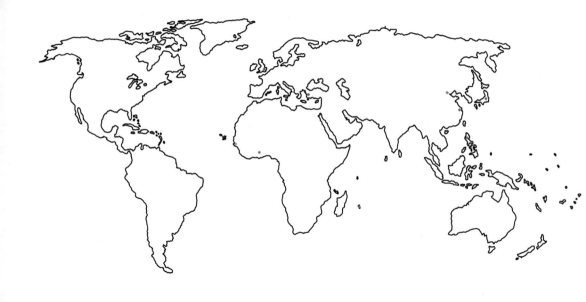

PART 4
Urban Design And Planning:
Interventions and Implications

Case Studies for Urban Design and Planning

Present-day cities and countries

This page: Map indicating the locations of case studies in this section of the book. (Map in the public domain, with annotations drawn by Andrew Bui.)

Left page: Quarantine in Marsa, Muscat. Photograph by Francis Frith, January 1, 1870. (Public Domain, courtesy of Wikimedia Commons.)

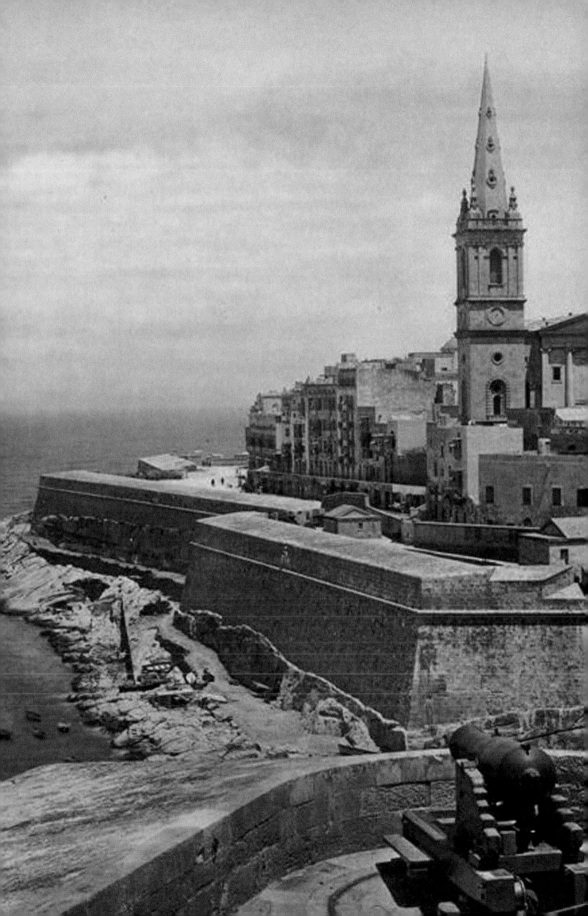

28

Urban Design, Social Epidemiology, and the Bubonic Plague of Palermo, Italy, 1575–76

Carlo Trombino

During the last quarter of the 16th century, the Mediterranean was characterized by intense naval warfare. Following the battle of Lepanto in 1571, in which a coalition of Catholic states defeated the Ottoman fleet, the sea remained a theater of continuous clashes and assaults. Sicily, a viceroyalty of Spain, struggled to maintain spaces of self-government amid the wider Spanish control over its religious, political, and economic life. As a result of Sicilian efforts, customs, trade, public health, and the defensive corsair fleet were governed by Sicilian authorities. At the end of the 16th century, however, these conditions in Sicily and the Mediterranean would introduce a deadly enemy. In 1575, a Sicilian corsair galley that had been out preying on ships from Islamic ports returned to sell the stolen goods in Sicily's markets, not realizing that some of the cargo was carrying rats infected with the bubonic plague. When the ship was unloaded and the goods taken to the Sicily's port cities to be sold, the plague spread across the island.

One of the most important Sicilian scientists of the modern era, Giovan Filippo Ingrassia (1510–1580), was instrumental in the early responses to the plague. Ingrassia implemented isolation measures and supervised a set of new health worker protocols and a renewed urban planning scheme, working with a pool of medical experts to tackle the disease. The contagion theory, which correctly identified germs for the spread of disease, had been recently proposed by Italian scientist Girolamo Fracastoro (1478–1553), but prior to advancements in microbiology, the exact nature of the bubonic plague was not yet understood. Ingrassia's book, *Informatione del pestifero, et contagioso morbo il quale affligge et haue afflitto questa citta di Palermo, & molte altre città, e terre di questo Regno di Sicilia, nell'anno 1575 et 1576* [Information on the Pestiferous and Contagious Disease that Afflicts and Has Afflicted This City of Palermo, and Many Other Cities and Lands of this Kingdom of Sicily in the Years 1575 and 1576] written during the pandemic in 1575 and published in 1576, became one of the most important studies on epidemic disease control of the period.

Ingrassia's *Informatione* offers a complete report of his plague interventions, with maps carefully detailing his epidemic urban planning. The text can be seen as a medical treatise and a philosophical dissertation through its five books that describe the nature of the plague, the first steps taken to detect it, the scientific committee set up to curb the contagion, the health measures inscribed into urban planning and organizational strategies, the treatment of plague patients, and hygiene and medical protocols.[1]

Ingrassia implemented one of the first historical examples of public health-driven urban intervention, which ultimately reshaped the built environment of the city of Palermo. One of the most populated cities of the Mediterranean, Palermo had a population of almost one hundred thousand people at the end of the 16th century. Ingrassia's plan utilized preexisting urban spaces and partially completed building projects to accelerating the construction of new facilities. He showed how lawmaking informed by science was essential to curbing the contagion rate. He also demonstrated the importance of reducing the crowded conditions in the city, thereby leading to the expansion of the urban plan outside the historic walls.

Case study: Urban pandemic intervention in Palermo, 1575

Giovan Filippo Ingrassia was born in Regalbuto, Sicily, and graduated from university in Padua. He was regarded as an accomplished anatomist and as one of the first theorists of forensic medicine for "getting the physicians inside courtrooms."[2] Ingrassia pushed to leave behind old theories on the astral influx on epidemics.[3] After publishing several books during his tenure at the University of Naples between 1545 and 1553, he came back to Sicily to teach anatomy and was appointed as Protomedico del Regno di Sicilia (Public Health Official of the Kingdom of Sicily) from 1563 until his death in 1580. This role of Protomedico was created at the end of the 14th century by Sicilian ruler King Martin of Aragon. In that same period, he worked with the Spanish Inquisition and was an advocate of torture as a decisive juridical tool.[4] He was a man of the ideologically intransigent Viceroy De Vega and was possibly inspired by his political sponsor.[5] The powers invested in the Protomedico position thus enabled Ingrassia to create a network of public health laws.

In 1575, the first plague cases reported from Palermo and other cities prompted Ingrassia to investigate by interrogating the attending physicians. An emergency committee composed of the mayor, judges, and deputies known as the Deputatione di Sanità was headed by Viceroy Carlo D'Aragona.[6] Ingrassia, as the Protomedico, was appointed as the expert for public health. Several trusted medical sources on the ground helped him to detect the exact nature of the disease.[7] It soon emerged that the captain of the galley carrying the plague-infected goods had gone to "sleep, or, better, to stay awake," as Ingrassia ironically remarked, with a prostitute.[8] Those who had come into contact with the woman were tracked down in order to trace the spread of the contagion. Contemporary reports by medical sources from other Mediterranean cities like Palazzo Adriano made it clear that the situation could have escalated quickly without rapid and appropriate responses.

Ingrassia intended to scare the population into "the most fear and incitement to obedience" regarding the new health policies.[9] Yet, law and order were not enough to keep the death toll low. Ingrassia soon noted that the impoverished segment of the population was suffering far more than the wealthiest members of society.[10] Subsequently, Ingrassia developed a class-based approach to isolation policies, with a substantial intervention to reshape Palermo's urban space. Initially, the swamps and bogs were drained to reduce unhealthy conditions for the community. This was followed by an urban waste removal program and the installation of safe storage for municipal debris. Ingrassia crafted strict protocols to be followed by health workers that spanned from nursery to burial needs. The emergency laws advocated quarantine, isolation, forced lockdown (*barreggiamento*), confinement, the burning of infected goods, the closure of schools, and the cessation of processions and public spectacles.[11] Severe measures were taken against transgressors. The pirates who stole and sold plague-infected goods were punished by having their hands cut off before being hung or thrown from the top of the Inquisitionist's headquarters at the Steri Palace. Ingrassia was able to set a benchmark for the realization of a new, unprecedented way for legislators to imagine, shape, and dictate life within the urban space.[12]

Ingrassia established *lazzaretti*, public hospitals. This integrated network of emergency outposts both inside and outside the walled city of Palermo was founded as "first one, then two, then eight and then ten, as we thought it was needed, [were] equipped with surgeons and medical staff."[13] The 12th-century Arab-Norman palace of La Cuba was adapted to serve as a hospital with surgeons, physician's residences, and male and female barracks for hospital day care. Infringements of the emergency laws were heavily sanctioned and gallows and other instruments of torture were also present (Figure 28.1).[14] Ingrassia had a deep understanding of the Sicilian social environment he lived in and he intervened to solve the structural problems faced while attempting to isolate inside one's own houses. He ordered that those who could not safely distance from others at home should be transferred to the newly built and renovated households in Borgo Santa Lucia, where he had ordered the draining of the nearby swamps as a health precaution. A project for a new neighborhood in that same area outside of the walled city was

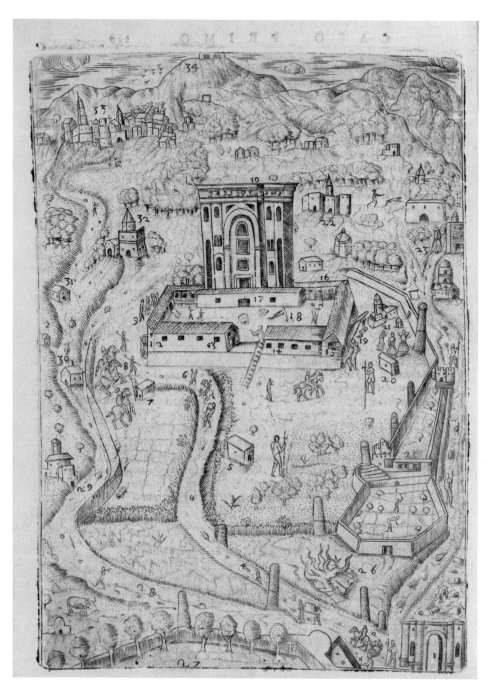

FIGURE 28.1: A detailed description of La Cuba Palace in Palermo during the 1575 epidemic. Giovan Filippo Ingrassia, *Informatione del Pestifero et Contagioso Morbo* [The Information of the Pestiferous and Contagious Disease] (Palermo, 1576). Photo by Jessica Rossi. (Courtesy of Archivio Centrale dello Stato Italiano, Palermo, RML0158166.)

under consideration for an allotment of land made by Guglielmo Fornaya in 1567 near the site of the new port.[15] Ingrassia's epidemic urban planning was a decisive factor in the urbanization of the area near Borgo Santa Lucia that allowed for new households outside the city walls to be used to isolate the relatives of those who had died of the plague. This epidemic urbanization scheme eventually became an extension to the north of Palermo, as part of an expansion process that continued until recent times (Figure 28.2).

Ingrassia convinced the Duke of Bivona to allow his garden to be used for the cleaning, sanitization, and burning of infected goods. New and previously available water sources were used more effectively. Newly built and renovated houses were occupied by suspected plague victims who were forced to isolate but could not afford to safely quarantine at home. This focus on the treatment of disadvantaged groups is constant in Ingrassia's work.[16] He obliged physicians to offer pro bono aid to the *poueri* (poor) for common ailments during the emergency, yet he

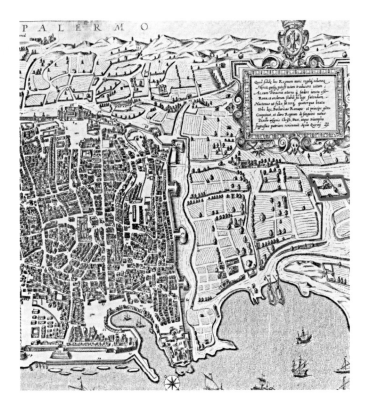

FIGURE 28.2: Map of Palermo, 17th century, Matteo Florinij. On the right, the northern borough of Borgo Santa Lucia, selected by Ingrassia to host plague patients. (Courtesy of Archivio Centrale dello Stato Italiano, Palermo, XI G 16400001.)

managed to maintain the social order by permitting only "deserving members" of the city's elite plague victims to be buried within churches. In general, he advocated for a public effort and public funding to fight the pandemic.

Informatione is both a plague diary and a *pastiche*, intertwining the author's observations with the transcription of the decrees he promulgated during the emergency (Figure 28.3). The book is filled with quotes from scientists, religious excerpts and literature, and sharp remarks made about contemporary Sicilians.[17] Ingrassia focuses on the details of public health management, from a recipe for chicken soup to advising "disorderly youth" on how to reduce their risk of contracting syphilis

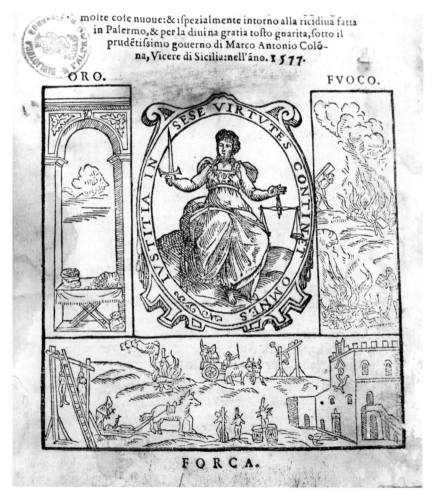

FIGURE 28.3: The book cover of Giovan Filippo Ingrassia's *Information del Pestifero et Contagioso Morbo* [The information of the Pestiferous and Contagious Disease] (Palermo, 1576). Photo by Jessica Rossi. (Courtesy of the Biblioteca Centrale della Regione Siciliana.)

by citing the means of its spread.[18] In this sense, the book is a yet-unexplored source for everyday life in the period.

Conclusion

Ingrassia's groundbreaking epidemic policies were characterized by a long-term vision, in which emergency laws were embraced as an opportunity to improve the city of Palermo. Urban design was indeed part of a new, integrated public health system, with a specific focus on class and gender that safeguarded the whole of Sicilian society, regardless of economic and social status. By doing so, Ingrassia shifted from efforts to contain an epidemic to an approach that intended to prevent urban epidemics, with *Informatione* becoming a fundamental source for the study of biopolitics in the 16th century.[19] Ingrassia used urban planning as a tool to prevent the spread of the plague: the establishment of *lazzaretti* along with quarantine and public health measures had been implemented for centuries in the Mediterranean world, but the need to reorganize the city in order to be ready for a possible future epidemic was one of the main innovations of Ingrassia's thought. He used this military metaphor for his policies: "Castles and fortresses are prepared in times of peace to find themselves ready for the time of war."[20] This of course meant that an effective public health network was needed in non-epidemic times as well as during plague years.

The reshaping of the urban environment of Palermo influenced the way the city evolved in the following centuries, and the way it appears in the 21st century. The proposed covering of the Papireto River and water-flow management were long-term projects enacted in the decades after Ingrassia's death. His book, *Informatione*, was probably the most important study of epidemic outbreaks to emerge from the period. It was translated into Latin and was widely diffused throughout Europe, setting a benchmark for future emergency responses to urban plague outbreak and prevention, including a reemergence of bubonic plague in Palermo itself in 1624.[21]

NOTES

1. The first-edition cover depicts Gold (*Oro*), Gallows (*Forca*), Fire (*Fuoco*), and Justice (*Giustizia*). This allegory is intended to present to the reader the main themes of Ingrassia's public health strategy: public funding, contagion-curbing health measures, and the strong fist of the law against transgressors of the emergency protocols.
2. Rosamaria Alibrandi, "Ut Sepulta Surgat Veritas. Giovan Filippo Ingrassia e Fortunato Fedeli sulla Novella Strada della Medicina Legale" [Ut Sepulta Surgat Veritas. Giovan

Filippo Ingrassia and Fortunato Fedeli on the New Path of Forensic Medicine], *Historia et ius rivista di storia giuridica dell'età medievale e moderna*, no. 2 (November 2012): 1–18.

3. Renato Malta, Alfredo Salerno, and Aldo Gerbino, *"L'Informatione del pestifero et contagioso Morbo*: Processi diagnostici" [*The Information of the Pestiferous and Contagious Disease*: Diagnostic Processes], *Atti Convegno Primaverile Società Italiana di Storia della* (June 2010): 48–52. This paper is useful also in the understanding of Ingrassia's use of the terms "Plague" and "Epidemic."

4. Alibrandi, "Ut Sepulta," 5.

5. Giovan Filippo Ingrassia, *Informatione del pestifero et contagioso morbo* [The Information of the Pestiferous and Contagious Disease], ed. Luigi Ingalisio (Milano: Franco Angeli, 2005), 15.

6. Rossella Cancila, "Salute Pubblica e Governo dell'Emergenza: la Peste del 1575 a Palermo" [Public Health and Government of the Emergency: The Plague of 1575 in Palermo], *Mediterranea – ricerche storiche*, no. 37 (August 2016): 242.

7. He later complained in his book about those who criticized their slow response, always defending the right of scientists to interrogate and to accept doubt: "The laws is in *dubijs pro amico*, and there is no better friend than life, not one's own, but the community's." See Ingrassia, *Informatione*, Book I, 119.

8. Ibid., Book IV, 30.

9. Giovan Filippo Ingrassia, *Bando et ordinationi fatte per l'Illustri Spettabili Signori Offitiali della Felice Città di Palermo conchiuse e terminate nell'accoglienza la Deputatione della Sanità sopra il morbo contagioso che corre nella detta città* [Announcement and Orders on the Contagious Disease That Runs in This City Made for the Distinguished Gentlemen Officials of the City of Palermo Accepted by the Health Administration] (Palermo: Giouan Mattheo Mayda, 1575).

10. Ingrassia cited the plague epidemic in Padua as a case in which the richest part of society was suffering more from the disease. In Palermo, Ingrassia's contract-tracing study demonstrated a similar pattern at the beginning of the outbreak, but later he observed that plague was affecting the poorest inhabitants to a greater extent.

11. For public health politics of quarantine for ships, goods and people, see Paolo Calcagno and Daniele Palermo, *La quotidiana emergenza – I molteplici Impieghi delle Istituzioni Sanitarie nel Mediterraneo Moderno* [The Daily Emergency – The Multiple Uses of Health Institutions in the Modern Mediterranean] (Palermo: New Digital Frontiers, 2017).

12. Extreme measures were taken, such as the killing and burial of 20,000 dogs considered carriers of contagion. See Francesco Maggiore-Perni, *Palermo e le sue grandi epidemie, Dal XVI al XIX Secolo* [Palermo and Its Great Epidemics, from the 16th to the 19th Century] (Palermo: Stabilimento Tipografico Virzì, 1894), 138; Ingrassia, *Informatione*, Book V, 42.

13. Ingrassia, *Informatione*, Book II, 144.

14. See maps in ibid., 140, 204.

15. Maurizio Vesco, "Un piano di espansione per Palermo nel secondo Cinquecento: Guglielmo Fornaya e la fondazione del borgo di Santa Lucia" [An Expansion Plan for Palermo in the Second Half of the 16th Century: Guglielmo Fornaya and the Foundation of the Village of Santa Lucia], in *Storie di Città e Architetture – Scritti in Onore di Enrico Guidoni*, ed. Giuglielmo Villa (Roma: Edizioni Kappa, 2014), 151–64. Vesco recalls in this article that the Fornaya venture was ill-fated, suffering from a lack of funding and bureaucratic hindrances.

16. Corrado Dollo, *Modelli Scientifici e Filosofici nella Sicilia Spagnola* [Scientific and Philosophical Models in Spanish Sicily] (Napoli: Guida, 1984).

17. Malta, Gerbino, and Salerno, "L'Informatione del pestifero." For example, he accuses the Mastri di Mondezza (street sweepers) of being idle being there only "to wait for their salary." Ingrassia, Informatione, Book I, 41–42.

18. Ingrassia orders specifically to enforce the lockdown and confinement of male and female prostitutes, see Ingrassia, *Informatione*, Book V, 42.

19. Dollo, *Modelli Scientifici*. See also Nicola Cusumano, "Fetal Monstrosities: A Comparison of Evidence from Sicily in the Modern Age," *Preternature: Critical and Historical Studies on the Preternatural* 2, no. 2 (2013): 156–87; Guido Panseri, "La nascita della polizia medica" [The Birth of the Medical Police], in *Storia d'Italia: Annali 3: Scienza e tecnica nella cultura e nella società dal Rinascimento a oggi*, ed. Gianni Micheli (Turin: Einaudi, 1980), 157–96.

20. Ingrassia, *Informatione*, Book V, 17. Rossella Cancila, "Ingrassia, il medico che nel 1575 sconfisse la peste a Palermo" [Ingrassia, the Doctor Who in 1575 Defeated the Plague in Palermo], *L'Identità di Clio*, February 18, 2020, https://www.lidentitadiclio.com/peste-palermo-ingrassia; Malta, Salerno, and Gerbino, "*L'Informatione del pestifero*."

21. Cancila, "Salute Pubblica," 236. Ingrassia's book was translated into Latin by Joachim Camerarius in 1583. The entry "*Sicile*" for the *Encyclopedie* by Diderot and D'alembert largely focused on Ingrassia, underlining his pivotal discoveries in the field of anatomy and epidemiology. Two centuries after his death, the enlightened encyclopedists described him as the pinnacle of Renaissance medicine throughout Europe.

29

Cholera and Housing Reform in Victorian London, England, 1850–1900

Irina Davidovici

Few cities illustrate the link between public health, urban planning, and housing reform more clearly than 19th-century London. Its deadly 1832 and 1854 cholera outbreaks belonged to the succession of pandemic waves that, during the century, changed the public health landscape worldwide. The repeated, indiscriminate spread of cholera across social classes led to the political momentum behind previously unthinkable public measures: the adoption of stringent health policies, the assumption of government responsibility for the laborers' living conditions, and the rise of housing expertise in architecture and urban planning. The war for public health was fought in the built fabric of the metropolis.

Up until the middle of the 19th century, it was widely believed that cholera was transmitted through miasma, a poisonous vapor caused by rotting organic matter. London's colloquially named "King Cholera" spread outward from the city's overcrowded, malodorous slums, thereby associating the miasma theory with the dire living conditions of its rookeries (Figure 29.1). These nodes of poverty, insalubrity, and disease created a widespread suspicion of slum inhabitants and an association between physical decrepitude and moral dissolution. Friedrich Engels's harrowing mid-century description of St. Giles, the infamous rookery on the site of the current-day London neighborhoods of Soho and Covent Garden, was typical in this respect. In a place where "filth and tottering ruin surpass all description" and "heaps of garbage and ashes lie in all directions, and the foul liquids emptied before the doors gather in stinking pools," the residents seemed inevitably doomed to a contagion of immorality.[1] Engels observed that "those who have not yet sunk in the whirlpool of moral ruin which surrounds them, [are] sinking daily deeper, losing daily more and more of their power to resist the demoralizing influence of want, filth, and evil surroundings."[2] In a similar vein, Reverend Thomas Beams likened 1850s St. Giles with a "sink of filth and iniquity," whose built fabric was

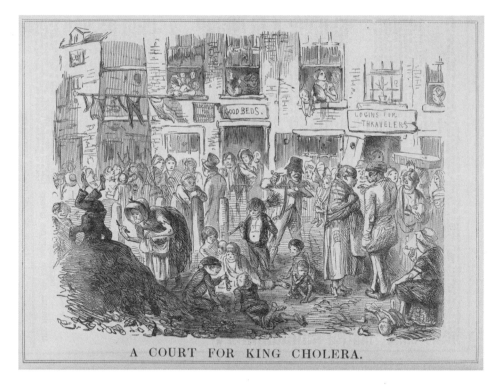

FIGURE 29.1: "A Court for King Cholera," illustration by John Leech, *Punch*, London, September 25, 1852. (Courtesy of Wellcome Collection, Attribution 4.0 International CC BY 4.0.)

ominously described as "a honeycomb, perforated by a number of courts and blind alleys, cul-de-sacs without any outlet other than the entrance."[3]

The identification of poverty, immorality, and contagion was made visible in Charles Booths's *London Poverty Maps*, which concisely described the typical slum inhabitant as "vicious, semi-criminal."[4] The Booth maps enacted a "moral geography" for London, according to which the poorest, densest areas doubled as foci of criminality and infectious disease.[5] The maps also revealed the distribution of wealth on the west side of the city, determined—among other considerations—by the direction of prevailing winds. Concentration of capital, clean air, and moral respectability were thus the prerogative of the rich west, while pollution, disease, and the associated miasma congregated in dangerous and impenetrable working-class areas, near the River Thames and in the industrialized East End.

Case study: London housing as a matter of disease and care

The evidence that undermined the steadfast Victorian association between social and spatial inequality eventually came from medical science. English physician John Snow (1813–1858), in his work *On the Mode of Communication of Cholera*, refuted the widely held assumption that the disease was transmitted, as miasma, through the air.[6] Using data compiled during the 1854 outbreak, Snow correlated a cluster of cholera deaths in St. Giles to a public water pump in Broad Street, which was found to have been infiltrated by the cesspit of a neighboring house. The revised edition of Snow's essay included a map of his findings, connecting the concentration of deaths to the location of the infected water supply (Figure 29.2). This discovery had momentous implications. By refuting the miasma theory and correctly identifying the transmission of the disease as caused through the ingestion of infected matter, Snow attacked the commonly made connection between cleanliness and virtue: hygiene had never been a matter of morality. At the same time, by showing cholera to be waterborne, Snow's mapping firmly embedded the contagion within London's densely built fabric of tightly packed alleyways, inadequate sanitary infrastructure, and overcrowded housing.[7]

This connection between bodily disease and decaying urban tissue cannot be underestimated, for in it the aim of public health converged with a main aim of social reform at the time: the improvement of working-class life conditions through better housing. It is well known that public health agendas—incorporating the typological evolution of the modern hospital—have long been encoded in the discipline of urban design.[8] In the 1970s, sociologist Blandine Barret-Kriegel drew parallels between the hospital's inner spatial organization and principles of modern city planning. The spatiality of the 18th-century hospital was based on two interconnected codes: first, the dispersion of people, beds, rooms, and hospital pavilions; and second, the flow of circulation, understood both as the functional connections between the dispersed "islands" of people and spaces, and the free movement of air.[9] Similarly, as the site of contagion and healing, the city was preventively subjected to an equivalent organization.

The rationalization of urban structure that prefigured the principles of modernist planning by more than a century was animated by principles of dispersion (of buildings) and circulation (of air and material). If the demands of capitalist expansion led to unsustainable urban growth and densification embodied by the slums, their corrective manifested as a systematic attempt to erase slums and plan new districts along these guidelines. The same principles were therefore employed in the planning of reform housing, which was closely connected with public health policies. In 19th-century London, where housing reform was enabled by the Public Health Acts of 1848 and 1875, the pioneering architecture of emerging residential

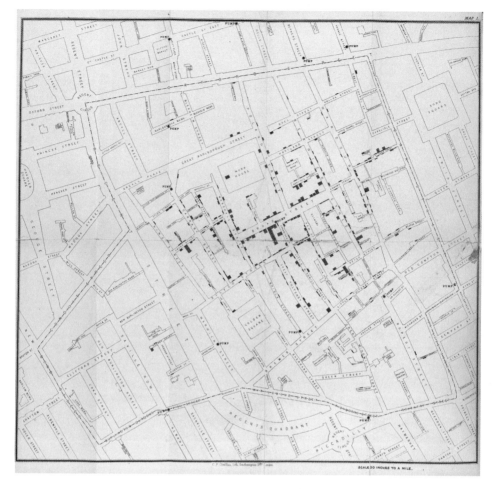

FIGURE 29.2: Map 1 showing St. Giles's cholera deaths. John Snow, *On the Mode of Communication of Cholera*, 1855. (Courtesy of Wellcome Collection, Attribution 4.0 International CC BY 4.0.)

typologies was organized around tenets of dispersal and flow.[10] Snow's findings of cholera as a waterborne disease were eventually addressed by the creation of a modern sewer system, designed by Joseph William Bazalgette, under the aegis of the Metropolitan Board of Works. Independently, however, the design responses in the fields of housing and overground urbanism remained firmly associated with strategies of aerial circulation—arguably as a device available to architects and building entrepreneurs.

Exhibited in London in 1851, Henry Roberts's Model Houses for Families demonstrated the hold of dispersal and circulation principles upon domestic

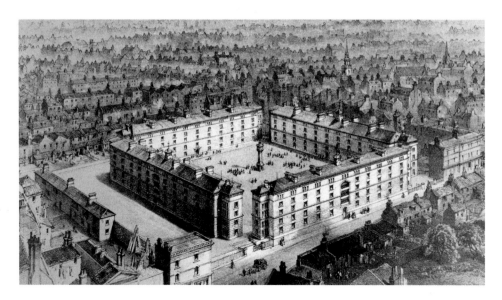

FIGURE 29.3: Henry Astley Darbishire, Peabody Square, Islington, from *Appleton's Journal of Literature, Science and Art,* New York, July 31, 1869. (Courtesy of London Metropolitan Archives.)

architecture. The compartmentalization of personal space into individual rooms was complemented by the natural ventilation of the central circulation and toilet core, which brought fresh air into the deepest crevasses of the plan.[11] On an urban scale, similar codes structured the planning of estates for the Peabody Trust (est. 1862), London's largest working-class housing provider during the 19th century (Figure 29.3).[12] The Trust's first architect-surveyor, Henry Astley Darbishire, was responsible for the standardized design of some twenty estates dotted through central and East London, built in proximity to some of the direst slums. As gated communities surrounded by railings and locked up at night, the Peabody estates were isolated from the surrounding streets, a characteristic that was doubled by a sense of moral distancing. Peabody residents were accepted according to the ambiguous criterion of respectability and were required to prove a regular income, as well as to adhere to strict norms of behavior and hygiene under the control of superintendents.

Darbishire set out the characteristics for the Trust housing at the Peabody Square in Greenman Street, Islington, in 1865. The design consisted of four long blocks organized around a quadrangle. On the variously shaped sites of the subsequent estates Darbishire designed up until the late 1880s, he implemented standardized layouts of modular blocks between four and six storeys high, arranged around recreation courtyards. Derived from the urban typology of the aristocratic

Georgian square, the recognizable design illustrates the emergent concept of the residential precinct as an island of regularity, order, light, and air. The principles of compartmentalization and distancing were applied across scales, from individual rooms and family dwellings to city blocks and the urban spaces between them. Early Peabody squares were open at the corners to allow for the natural ventilation of the quadrangles, which clearly defined them against the surrounding labyrinthine urban fabric.

A continuous row of shorter blocks at the south of the Islington square was added in the early 1870s, as continued demand for housing led to the densification of the site. Darbishire first used this compact block typology at the Blackfriars estate in 1871 after the earlier, longer blocks had proven both impractical and unpopular. The newer version, derived from Henry Roberts's Model Houses for Families, minimized the social interactions of compartmentalized nuclear families through the reduction of common circulation areas. Five dwellings on each floor opened onto a central, naturally ventilated core where both the staircase and communal bathrooms were located. The semi-external staircase served an explicitly hygienic purpose to implement natural ventilation and efficient quarantine conditions as well as an implicitly moral purpose to create a public, neutral buffer zone between dwellings, thereby reducing the potential for dubious encounters. Roberts's model introduced privies as a daring departure from the usual cesspits, but the Peabody Trustees opted for so-called associated dwellings, with common toilets that were regularly inspected for cleanliness. The compact plans also proved more efficient for an urban scale by allowing for easier distribution of the blocks in the nooks and crannies of irregular sites. Ironically, it was a stipulation by the 1875 Artisans' and Laborers' Dwellings Act that relocated at least the same number of new residents as the displaced slum dwellers and compromised Darbishire's standard planning by resulting in a demand for increased densities. The blocks of the Peabody Estate in Great Wild Street, Covent Garden, were one storey higher than usual and fused together around a narrow court, which created conditions that resulted for the first time in a higher rate of infant mortality than in the surrounding streets.[13]

The dominance of the Peabody Trust in the affordable housing scene was challenged in the 1890s as a policy matter. For the first time, the 1890 Housing of the Working Classes Act empowered the newly founded London County Council (LCC, established in 1889) to build and manage housing for the working classes, thus paving the way for state agencies to take the lead over philanthropic and market ventures. The Boundary Street Estate, the first development of the LCC, was representative of the "maturing of responsibility" demonstrated by the intervention of local government in the provision of social housing (Figure 29.4).[14] A truly progressive urban model, this landmark estate, built on the cleared site of

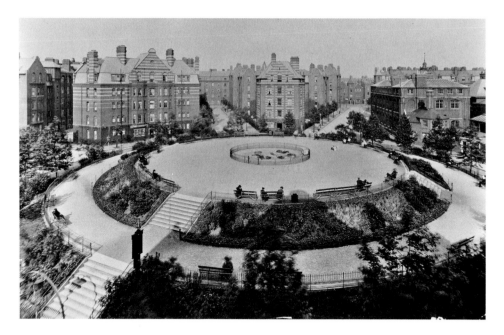

FIGURE 29.4: Arnold Circus, London County Council Boundary Street Estate, 1893, photographed in 1903. (Courtesy of London Metropolitan Archives.)

the Jago slum, was planned to a radial layout that signaled a new urban order for a dignified class of artisans. Designed and detailed in the ideological framework of a late Victorian socialism, Boundary Street Estate illustrated a shift in the architect's attitude toward the resident, a newfound deference for the laboring classes that persisted in the work of 20th-century avant-garde designers.

Conclusion

The modern discipline of urban design can be directly correlated with a defensive impulse against unsanitary living conditions. The cholera crises of 19th-century London claimed thousands of lives across the social spectrum, resulting in political momentum for far-reaching social and planning reform. While cholera was addressed through Bazalgette's sewer underground system, representing the city authorities' centralized response to outbreaks, its impact on London's overground built environment was paradoxically met by distancing strategies to aid aeration. In inner-city rookeries, the narrowness of streets and dark, overcrowded houses were most readily addressed, resulting in revised typologies of workers' housing. The aim to eradicate disease led to metropolitan programs of slum clearance, contributed to the adoption of new building standards and instigated new housing typologies. Epidemiological findings integrated air-circulation strategies into urban design, contributing to new types of socially and physically distanced dwellings. Efforts to curb the spread of disease thus helped to crystallize modern housing policy and configured early typologies of mass housing as a matter of disease and care.

The indiscriminate spread of disease across social classes added to the urgency of identifying and eradicating its causes. Yet, even cholera was insufficient to uproot the firmly entrenched social prejudices and the geography of inequality encoded in the Booth maps of the city. As the slums were forcefully cleared, the improved housing that replaced them was occupied by more prosperous classes of artisans. The original and often most vulnerable inhabitants were pushed out, first contributing to overcrowding in adjacent neighborhoods and eventually disappearing into unwritten histories.

NOTES

1. Friedrich Engels, "The Great Towns," in *The Condition of the Working-Class in England in 1844: With Preface Written in 1892*, trans. Florence Kelley Wischnewetzky (Cambridge: Cambridge University Press, 2010), 27.

2. Ibid.

3. Thomas Beames, *The Rookeries of London: Past, Present, and Prospective* (London: Bosworth, 1852), 32.

4. See Iain Sinclair, *Charles Booth's London Poverty Maps: A Landmark Reassessment of Booth's Social Survey* (London: Thames & Hudson, 2019), 19.

5. Robin Evans, "Rookeries and Model Dwellings," in *Translations from Drawing to Building and Other Essays* (London: Architectural Association, 1997), 98.

6. John Snow, *On the Mode of Communication of Cholera*, 2nd ed. (London: John Churchill, 1855).

7. "Cholera was not morally borne but waterborne. And those roads and alleyways, and the pipes laid beneath them and the buildings built among them, were causing disease." Michael Murphy, "In Search of the Water Pump: Architecture and Cholera," *Harvard Design Magazine: Architecture, Landscape Architecture, Urban Design and Planning*, no. 40 (Spring–Summer 2015): 151.

8. Blandine Barret-Kriegel has argued that the transformation of the historical hospice into the modern hospital extended to the outside of buildings, resulting in a "medicalization of the urban space." Blandine Barret-Kriegel, "L'hôpital comme équipment" [The Hospital as Equipment], in *Les Machines à guérir: aux origines de l'hôpital moderne* [The Healing Machines: The Origins of the Modern Hospital], ed. Michel Foucault (Bruxelles, Liège: Pierre Mardaga, 1979), 25.

9. Ibid., 26.

10. See, e.g., Nicholas Bullock and James Read, *The Movement for Housing Reform in Germany and France, 1840–1914* (Cambridge: Cambridge University Press, 1985); John Nelson Tarn, *Five per Cent Philanthropy; An Account of Housing in Urban Areas between 1840 and 1914* (London: Cambridge University Press, 1973).

11. Evans, "Rookeries," 108.

12. See Irina Davidovici, "Recoding Reform: Ideology and Urban Form in London's Early Housing Estates, 1865–1900," in *Recoding the City: Thinking, Planning, and Building the City of the Nineteenth Century*, ed. Britta Hentschel and Harald R. Stühlinger (Berlin: Jovis, 2019), 82–94; and Irina Davidovici, "The Depth of the Street," *AA Files*, no. 70 (2015): 103–23.

13. Tarn, *Five per Cent*, 84.

14. Ibid., 123.

30

Public Health, Urban Development, and Cholera in Tokyo, Japan, 1877–95

Susan L. Burns

Over the course of the late 19th century, Japan was wracked by a series of devastating cholera epidemics. These occurred in 1877, 1879, 1882, 1885, 1886, 1890, 1891, and 1895 and resulted in more than 360,000 deaths nationwide. Tokyo was hit particularly hard. In the 1882 epidemic, more than 11 percent of all cases were in Tokyo, although the city's population constituted only 3.2 percent of the country's total population. The percentage of cases in Tokyo in subsequent epidemics was lower, between 5 and 7 percent of the national total, but continued to be disproportionate in relation to the city's population.[1] This alarmed officials at all levels of government. Tokyo's population in 1886 reached 1.2 million, making it the most populous city in the country. In addition, the city was intended to showcase the accomplishments of the new "imperial" government centered on the Meiji Emperor both as Japan's capital and as the epicenter of the project of modernization that had been undertaken by a government that had only come to power in 1868.

Over the course of two decades, local and national officials sought to understand why cholera flourished in the city and to develop policies to control the disease. Cholera is caused by *Vibrio cholerae*, a comma-shaped bacterium that originated in the warm waters of the Ganges Delta. When ingested by human beings, *V. cholerae* causes explosive diarrhea and vomiting, and these fluids contain large amounts of the bacteria. Poor hygiene and lack of sanitation allow the (re)contamination of water, which can be a vector for transmission and allow the disease to spread widely and easily. Washing one's hands in infected water or eating raw fruits and vegetables cleaned in contaminated water can transmit the illness, as can handling the soiled clothing or bedding of an infected person. Although it was recognized early on that the city's aging water supply system and inadequate sanitary provisions contributed to the spread of the disease, the government was slow to act on improving the city's infrastructure.

Instead, public health measures targeted the city's residents, who confronted a host of new regulations that intervened in their everyday lives and domestic spaces.

Not only were the police authorized to inspect and disinfect the homes and toilets of residents during cholera outbreaks, but they also could compel those dwelling in the city to clean streets and drains. All traffic around homes with an identified case of cholera was to be stopped and a sign that proclaimed "cholera here" was to be posted outside. Nothing proved more contentious, however, than a new regulation that allowed cholera victims to be forcibly transferred to new quarantine hospitals and disproportionately targeted the city's poor.

Case study: Cholera in Tokyo, 1877–95

Cholera first struck Edo, as Tokyo was known before 1868, in the summer of 1858. Officials of the Tokugawa shogunate were all but helpless in their efforts to deal with the then-unfamiliar disease, and by the end of the 1858 epidemic, at least thirty thousand people had died, although the death toll may in fact have been as high as two hundred thousand. Contemporary accounts describe how crematoria in the city and local temple graveyards were overwhelmed by the unprecedented number of deaths (Figure 30.1).[2] When cholera returned to the city in 1877 after an outbreak in the

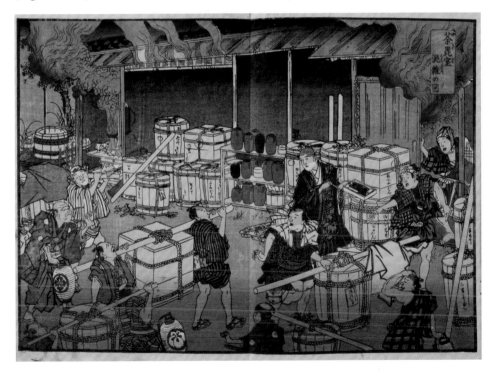

FIGURE 30.1: An overwhelmed crematorium during the 1858 cholera epidemic in Edo. The barrel-like containers are caskets. (Kanagaki Robun, *An Account of the Ansei Cholera Epidemic* (*Ansei korori ryūkōki*) [NP: Tenjudō, 1858]). (Courtesy of Fujikawa Digital Collection, Kyoto University Library.)

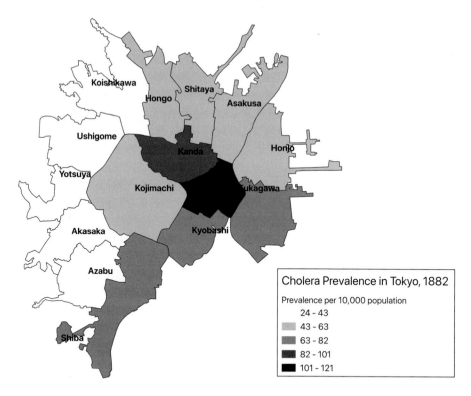

FIGURE 30.2: Cholera prevalence in Tokyo during the 1882 epidemic. The map reveals a pattern that would be seen in subsequent epidemics: rates were highest in wards that had both high population density and high levels of water contamination. (Map by Susan L. Burns.)

nearby port of Yokohama, Japan's new government mustered new techniques—including the compilation of statistical data—to confront the disease. As a result, it became clear that the disease was far more prevalent in some of the city's fifteen wards than in others. In repeated epidemics, the four wards of Nihonbashi, Kanda, Kyōbashi and Fukagawa had rates of cholera that were three to five times higher than other parts of the city, and these four wards accounted for more than 50 percent of the total number of cholera cases in Tokyo between 1882 and 1895 (Figure 30.2).

British physician John Snow demonstrated the spread of cholera via water contaminated by human waste in 1854, although it was some years before this understanding of its transmission was generally accepted in Europe and elsewhere. The role that water and waste played in spreading cholera was known in Japan by at least 1871. In that year, Ishiguro Tadanori, an army doctor, published a translation of a European text under the title *Korera ron* (On Cholera). It explained that human waste spread the disease, and it emphasized the need to keep toilets clean and to dispose of the excrement of the infected with care.[3] Public health officials in

Japan were quick to embrace this understanding of the disease.[4] In 1880, the Home Ministry informed the Tokyo Metropolitan Police Bureau and the Tokyo prefectural government, who shared responsibility for public health in the city, that "the disease poison is contained in the vomit and diarrhea of the sick person [...] and if it enters into dirty and polluted water or soil, its propagative power increases as it moves."[5] The Ministry added that, from there, it "enters drinking water and from there into the human body where it multiplies, causing the symptoms of explosive diarrhea and vomiting."[6] The notion that the virulence of "disease poison" that could increase due to exposure to other forms of contamination was, to be sure, mistaken, but the new knowledge that cholera was spread via the water supply reinforced growing concerns about Tokyo's drinking water and sanitation.

In the late 19th century, Tokyo's water supply continued to rely upon an antiquated system of aqueducts created in the mid-17th century. The first of these, known as the Kanda aqueduct, moved water from Inokashira Pond, located twenty kilometers outside of Tokyo, through a system of canals and bamboo and wooden pipes to the city itself. This aqueduct provided water to Koishikawa, Ushigome, Kanda, and Nihonbashi wards. Several decades later, construction began on the Tamagawa aqueduct, which moved water from the Tama River over 43 kilometers into the city, where it supplied water to Akasaka, Azabu, Shiba, Kōjimachi, and Kyōbashi wards. A branch of the Tamagawa aqueduct, known as the Senkawa aqueduct, supplied water to some parts of Hongō and Shitaya, but these wards, as well as Honjō and Fukagawa, relied primarily on ground water and water delivered by vendors.[7]

The first water-quality tests of the modern period were performed in 1874 by Georg Martin, a German scientist hired by the Japanese government to teach at Tokyo's new Medical College. He found the water sourced from the Tamagawa River to be "incredibly pure" and of far better quality than the headwater of the Kanda aqueduct. However, water supplied by both aqueducts was contaminated by high levels of organic matter by the time it reached city residents due to waste that entered via the open canals and decaying pipes lying beneath the city (Figure 30.3). The first plan for improving the water supply was developed in that year when the Home Ministry ordered Cornelius Johannes van Doorn, a Dutch civil engineer employed by the Ministry, to draw up a plan for modernizing Tokyo's water supply. He estimated that the necessary improvements would cost $1.5 million (approximately 1.47 million yen) and with an additional $185,000 required per year to maintain it.[8] Tokyo prefecture's total tax revenue in 1879, the first year for which there is data, was 268,939 yen.[9] It was impossible then for the prefecture to undertake improvements without funding from the central government.

Studies of water quality continued. In 1877, Robert Atkinson, a British scientist hired in 1874 to teach at what would become Tokyo University, carried out the first analysis of the groundwater in wells around the city and found that "the number

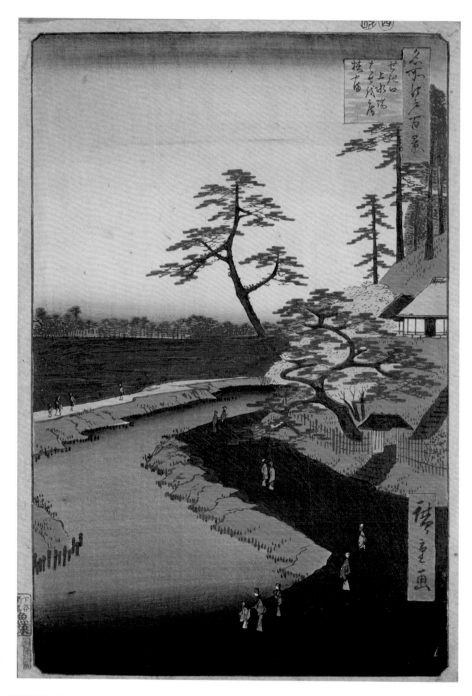

FIGURE 30.3: Sekiguchi, where the Kanda aqueduct enters the city. By the 1870s, it was no longer as pristine as it appears here. (Utagawa Hiroshige, *One Hundred Famous Views of Edo* (*Meisho Edo hyakkei*), 1857. (Courtesy of Tokyo Metropolitan Library Digital Collection.)

expressing 'the previous sewage contamination' is very high."[10] He concluded that "most of the surface waters are dangerous, and some are exceptionally bad."[11] In 1885, Tawara Ryōjun, an employee of the Home Ministry's Bureau of Hygiene, carried out further extensive testing of groundwater. He found that, of the 106 wells tested, 73 had water with dangerous levels of sewage contamination.[12] Public health officials recognized that the wards that consistently had the highest rates of cholera received water at the end of the aqueduct system or relied upon ground water.

The contamination of Tokyo's water supply was intimately connected to other aspects of the city's urban infrastructure. Japan's farmers had long utilized human waste as fertilizer, but as the population in Edo swelled over the course of the 17th and 18th centuries, villagers living near Edo increased food production to meet consumer demand through intensive agriculture. When waste produced locally was no longer sufficient to meet their needs, farmers turned to the city itself for this resource and the "human manure" produced by urban residents became a valuable commodity.[13] Agents from agricultural villages forged contracts with specific city residents that gave them the right to remove the waste from their toilets, for a price.[14]

As was the case with the water supply, concern about cholera did not lead to efforts to modernize Tokyo's waste removal system. In this period, the Japanese government prioritized spending for the military and industry over investment in social welfare. Unable to pursue infrastructure improvements without funding from the central government, public health authorities in Tokyo responded to cholera by targeting aspects of the everyday life of the city's residents. Edicts issued beginning in 1877 addressed the human manure trade by restricting the extraction and removal of waste to nighttime hours and requiring covers on the waste buckets. Other directives addressed the state of the city's toilets: residents were ordered to inspect toilets and replace decaying subterranean wooden waste receptacles with ceramic containers. Residents were also regularly required to dredge drains, clean streets, and clear garbage dumps. Public urination was forbidden, as was the washing of clothes and dishes near public wells.

During cholera outbreaks, strict rules governed the disposal of human and other waste from infected households. In 1886, the police were empowered to issue fines for noncompliance to these regulations. It was forbidden to dispose of potentially infected waste in toilets, drains, or garbage dumps; instead, it was to be burned under police supervision at designated sites around the city.[15] Though essential, these measures were greeted with considerable resistance. Those involved in the human manure trade argued that the restrictions interfered with their early-morning routine of bringing produce to market and then collecting waste; travel and work by lamplight supposedly created a fire hazard. Ordinary residents balked at the requirement to clean up after neighbors, much less strangers.[16]

Public health officials were particularly concerned with two types of toilets: the 1,300 "public" toilets that lined the city's streets and the shared communal toilets used by residents in so-called *ura nagaya* (a typical form of tenement housing). The often poorly constructed and notoriously filthy street-side toilets were typically established by human manure dealers on private land, with the agreement that the property owner would be paid for the excrement retrieved from the waste receptacles. Public health authorities were quick to order the removal of any toilets deemed problematic, so over the course of a decade their number was reduced by half.[17] Typically five or six families shared each of the communal toilets of the *ura nagaya*, single-storey wooden tenement structures divided into one-room apartments (Figure 30.4). As early as 1878, public health officials expressed concern about the proximity of these toilets to communal wells, which might be only a meter or two distant. In spite of extended discussions, no new building regulations were established until the 20th century.[18]

Unwilling to undertake expensive public works projects and unable to enforce complete compliance with the burdensome regulations, Tokyo authorities relied primarily on another strategy to control the spread of cholera: the isolation of the infected in hastily constructed and often inadequately staffed quarantine hospitals. The first quarantine hospitals were established in 1877, utilizing "public" property that the police and prefectural officials could easily repurpose. Such properties included prison grounds and so-called police hospitals, all sites that contributed to the growing stigma surrounding the disease. Public health officials

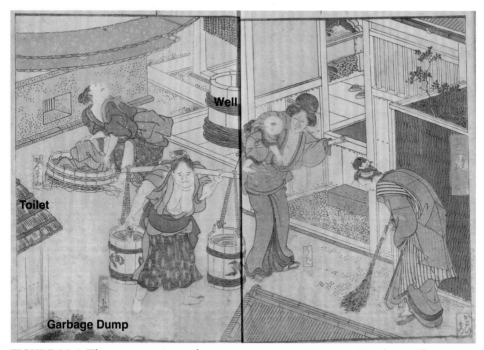

FIGURE 30.4: The common areas of a *nagaya* tenement. (Utagawa Toyokuni, *Ehon imayō sugata* [NP: Kansendō, 1802]). (Courtesy of National Diet Library Digital Collection.)

experimented with the placement of the quarantine hospitals, which were typically burned together with their furnishings and supplies at the end of an epidemic.[19] Nearby residents rose up in protest when quarantine sites were placed in densely populated urban neighborhoods out of concern that the crowded hospitals threatened their own health.[20] Yet, when the hospitals were placed on the less populated periphery of the city, many of the infected died while being transported on stretchers.[21] In 1889, the city authorities abandoned the unpopular temporary quarantine hospitals in favor of a system of "infectious disease hospitals" with improved facilities and trained staff.[22] Significantly, these were likewise located on the periphery of the city in a spatial arrangement that reflected urban anxieties and the discrimination against cholera victims (Figure 30.5).

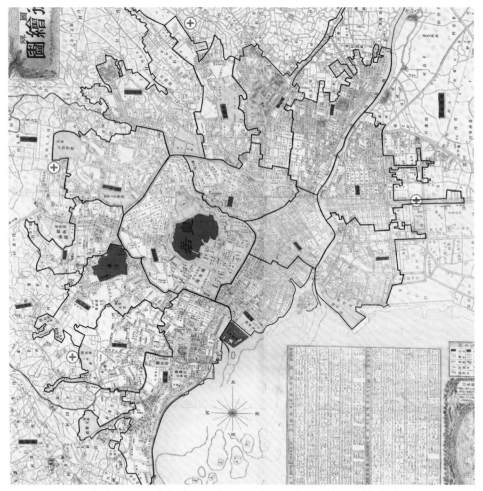

FIGURE 30.5: The location of the four infectious disease hospitals established in 1889. Detail from Itō Seisai, *Tōkyō Onezu: Zen meishō zukai* (Tokyo: Kodama Yashichi, 1881). (Courtesy of the International Center for Japanese Studies Digital Collection.)

Quarantine hospitals were intended for the city's poor and working-class residents, which further contributed to popular animosity toward their patients. Government policy required doctors to notify local police in the case of a diagnosis. The police held the authority to determine whether a patient could remain at home or should be removed to a quarantine hospital. The rules for at-home quarantine were elaborate: the patient needed to be isolated from the rest of the household in a private room with access to separate toilet facilities and a dedicated nurse, who would have no contact with anyone but the patient.[23] It was, of course, impossible for those living in the city's tenements to abide by such rules. By the late 1880s, people of means had the option to seek treatment in the "infectious disease wards" of the new private hospitals in Tokyo, in which they could quarantine in relative comfort without disrupting the rest of the household.[24] The growing association of poverty and cholera was thus reinforced by the class-based approach to quarantine and hospitalization.

Conclusion

As a series of cholera epidemics ravaged Tokyo in the late 19th century, local and national officials soon recognized the relationship between the disease, the water supply, and sanitation in the city. In other cities, including New York, London, Paris, and Hamburg, fear of cholera propelled expensive infrastructure projects, most notably the construction of underground sewers. However, although studies repeatedly exposed the contamination of Tokyo's water supply, no sustained efforts were made to address the city's infrastructural problems until the 1890s and change came slowly. In 1911, 70 percent of Tokyo residents still relied upon the old aqueduct and ground water for their drinking water.[25] The cash-strapped government funded other priorities, including industrialization and military expansion, leaving Tokyo's public health officials to attempt to control the spread of the disease by regulating the behavior of urban residents. The people of Tokyo were subject to a host of onerous rules and regulations that disrupted the fabric of everyday life. They were also made responsible for sanitary improvements, including the cleaning and disinfection of streets, wells, and drains and the renovation of toilets.

Cholera exposed more than the problematic priorities of the government. It also revealed the social, economic, and material inequities that shaped urban life. Poor and working-class residents who lived in Tokyo's eastern wards were disproportionately vulnerable to cholera because of circumstances beyond their control, such as their lack of access to clean water and sanitary facilities. Workers and the poor were also disproportionately affected by onerous quarantine policies. Although the middle-class and wealthy Tokyoites were permitted to quarantine at home or in the infectious disease wards of new hospitals, the poor could be forcibly removed to quarantine hospitals, where seven out of ten patients died. Notably, it remains unclear whether the quarantine hospitals that proved so divisive played a meaningful role in controlling the spread of cholera in Tokyo. Epidemics continued into the 20th century, until the construction of a modern water supply and improvements to sanitation proved effective at stopping the spread of the disease.

NOTES

1. Raw statistical data on cholera and population referenced here and below come from three sources: *Naimushō tōkeisho hōkokusho* [Home Ministry Statistical Reports], *Dai Nihon Naimushō tōkeisho hōkokusho* [Statistical Reports of the Home Ministry of Great Japan], and *Tōkyō-fu tōkeisho* [Statistical Reports of Tokyo Prefecture]. National Diet Library Digital Collection, Japan.

2. Kanagaki Robun, *Ansei korori ryūkōki* [A Chronicle of the Cholera Epidemic of the Ansei Era] (NP: Tenjudō, 1858), Fujikawa Digital Collection, Kyoto University Library, Kyoto Japan. On the difficulty of calculating the number of deaths, see Yamamoto Shun'ichi, *Nihon korera shi* [A History of Cholera in Japan] (Tokyo: Tōkyō Daigaku Shuppankai, 1982), 19–23.

3. Ishiguro Tadanori, *Korera ron* (Tōkyō: Shimamura Yarisuke, 1871).

4. On Snow, see Sandra Hempel, *The Strange Case of the Broad Street Pump: John Snow and the Mystery of Cholera* (Berkeley: University of California Press, 2007).

5. Naikaku Kirokukyoku, ed., *Hōki bunrui dai taizen* [A Complete Compilation of Laws and Regulations, Classified], *vol. 32: Eisei* (Tokyo: Hara Shobō, 1981), 51.

6. Ibid.

7. Itō Yōichi, *Edo jōsuidō no rekishi* [The History of Edo's Water System] (Tokyo: Yoshikawa Kōbunkan, 2010).

8. Moniwa Chūjirō, *Nihon suidōshi* (Tokyo: Nakajima Kōgaku Hakushi Kinen Jigyōkai, 1927), 267.

9. Naimubu Shomuka, ed., "Zeikin" in *Tōkyō-fu tōkeisho Meiji 15-nen* (Tokyo: Tōkyō-fu, 1882), 10.

10. R. W. Atkinson, "The Water Supply of Tokio," *Transactions of the Asiatic Society of Japan* 6, part 1b (1878): 95.

11. Ibid. 98.

12. Tōkyō-fu Suidō Kaisei Iin, ed., *Tōkyō suidō kaisetsu gairyaku* [An Outline for the Reform of Tokyo's Water Supply] (Tokyo: Tōkyō-fu, 1877), 312–18; Atkinson, "Water Supply," 87–98; Eiseikyoku Shikenjo, ed., "Tōkyō-fu jōgesui shiken seiseki" [The Results of Testing of Drinking and Waste Water in Tokyo Prefecture], *Eisei shiken ihō*, no. 3 (nd): 1–24.

13. Kayo Tajima, "The Marketing of Urban Human Waste in Edo/Tokyo Metropolitan Area, 1600-1935" (Ph.D. diss., Tufts University, 2005), 38–39, 69–74.

14. Ibuchi Reiji, "Kinsei toshi no toire to shinyō shori no genkai" [Toilets in Early Modern Cities and the Limits of Waste Disposal], *Rekishi to chiri*, no. 484 (1995): 46–59.

15. Tōkyo-to, ed., *Tōkyō-shi shikō* [A Draft History of Tokyo], vol. 62: *Shigaihen* (Tokyo: Tōkyō-to, 1970), 60–61; *Tōkyō-shi shikō*, vol. 66: *Shigaihen* (Tokyo: Tōkyō-to, 1974), 768–77; *Tōkyō-shi shikō*, vol. 67: *Shigaihen* (Tokyo: Tōkyō-to, 1975), 533.

16. Andō Yūichiro, "Tōkyō shiku kaisei izen no shinyō shori taisaku: Ushigome-ku gaitō benjo sojinin Nakamura Kametarō no dōkō wo chūshin ni" [Waste Disposal Measures before the Tokyo Urban Reforms: With a Focus on Nakamura Kametarō, a Toilet Cleaner in Ushigome Ward], in *Kankyō to rekishi*, ed. Ishi Hiroyuki and Kabayama Kōichi (Tokyo: Shinseisha, 1999), 207–8.

17. Andō Yūichiro, "Shuto Tōkyō no kankyō eisei gyōsei: Shinyō shori shisuteme no henben to jōyaku kaisei" [The Administration of the Environment and Public Health in the Capital City Tokyo: Changes in the Waste Disposal System and Treaty Revision], *Hikaku toshishi kenkyū* 22, no. 1 (2003): 48.

18. Tanaka Yoshio, "Meiji 19–20 nen Tōkyō-fu ni yoru nagaya kenchiku kisokuan no fuseiritsu ni owaru keii to sono riyu ni tsuite" [The Process and Reasons for the Failure to Establish Regulations for Tenement Housing in Tokyo prefecture in 1886–1887], *Nihon kenchiku gakkai keigakakari ronbun hokokushū*, no. 390 (1988): 86–94.

19. Tōkyō-fu, ed., *Tōkyō-fu shi: Gyōsei hen* [The History of Tokyo Prefecture: Administration], vol. 6 (Tokyo: Tōkyō-fu, 1937), 662–63, 666, 670, 673, 674.

20. See, for example, the 1882 petition by residents of Atago-cho in Shiba Ward asking for the nearby quarantine hospital to be closed. Item ID: 000117824. File number: 612. A6. 03. Tokyo Metropolitan Archives.

21. Isogai Hajime, *Meiji no hibyōin: Komagome Byōin ishikyoku nisshishō* [Quarantine Hospitals in the Meiji Period: Doctors' Journals from Komagome Hospital] (Tokyo: Shibunkaku, 1999), iii.

22. Tōkyō-fu, ed., 679–86.

23. Yamamoto, *Nihon korera shi*, 431–32.

24. Kudō Tetsuo, *Tōkyō iji tsūran* [A Report on Medical Affairs in Tokyo] (Tokyo: Nihon Iji Tsūran Hakkōjo, 1901), 94–95, 107, 111–12. Tokyo-fu, *Tōkyō-fu shi*, vol. 6, 682–84.

25. Ishizuka Hiromichi, "Tōkyō no toshi suramu to kōshū eisei mondai" [Urban Slums in Tokyo and Public Health Problems], in *Kokuren Daigaku Ningen to shakai no hatatsu puroguramu kenkyū hokoku* (Tokyo: United Nations University, 1981), 22.

31

The Hong Kong Plague and Public Parks in the British Settlements of Shanghai and Tianjin, China, 1894

Yichi Zhang

A French merchant ship sailed from Shanghai, arriving in Hong Kong on May 13, 1894. Although this was a commercial enterprise, and the ship sailed to many countries, the ship's operators refused to accept any cargo or passengers in Hong Kong, despite the economic loss their refusal incurred.[1] The reason was simple: a plague was rampant in Hong Kong. Initially breaking out in Guangzhou in February of the same year, this plague killed 60,000 people in a few weeks and rapidly spread to the nearby city of Hong Kong, causing a further 80,000 deaths there.[2] Consequently, although the operators of this French ship were keenly aware of the gravity of the threat, their ship, like many others that docked at the quaysides of these seaports, created the pathway of transmission of the disease to other cities in China and Southeast Asia.

The administration of the British settlements in Shanghai and Tianjin soon concluded that their cities had also been touched by this plague that began thousands of kilometers away. The reason was their close trade links with Hong Kong. As key nodes of the British trade network in East Asia, Shanghai and Tianjin's British settlements served as the economic engines of their respective cities and drove the modernization of China. The British settlement in Shanghai, founded in 1845, was the first foreign settlement in modern China; it later amalgamated with the American settlement to form the British-dominated International Settlement. The British settlement in Tianjin, founded in 1860, continually expanded its territory, eventually becoming the largest independent British settlement in China by the start of the 20th century.

British consuls administered these Chinese territories, meaning that British settlers could impose their urban planning ideas on the settlements. In response to the plague, the urban authorities of these settlements attempted to strengthen protection of their own health by importing public health and infrastructure ideas from Europe. This, in turn, reshaped their urban landscapes in both the short and long terms. Public parks, as significant outdoor urban landscapes, provided ideal places in which to embed such protection measures into the daily life of the masses and to publicize these ideas and the associated infrastructure. Indeed, the establishment, design, and use of public parks in the British settlements of Shanghai and Tianjin offer a compelling view of the response of foreign communities to the 1894 plague, the comparative history of epidemic urbanism, and British post-colonial influence in East Asia.

Case study: The park system in British settlements in China, 1894

The creation of public parks in Europe was motivated by the desire to improve the physical and mental health of the working classes during the Industrial Revolution.[3] However, this designed landscape in China emerged from the needs of European settlers to expand their settlements. This is exemplified by the foundation of the Public Garden in Shanghai in 1864 by the Shanghai Municipal Council. Arguing that a new public park was for public usage, they occupied land outside of their settlement boundaries for the project. British residents in Tianjin argued that a public park would beautify the city and constructed Victoria Park in honor of Queen Victoria's Golden Jubilee in 1887.[4] The parks of the early settlement period were just green squares of lawn with simple garden furniture that failed to function other than as decorative social spaces and tools for expansion.

The outbreak of the Hong Kong Plague in 1894 changed the purpose of these parks, which were reimagined as places for the inhabitants to access fresh air and prevent illness. Popular ideas about public health in Britain at that time suggested that illness was caused by the environment, so residents took measures to renovate and maintain that environment, including, among other things, the regular, thorough cleansing of the streets and drains.[5] During this process, settlers recognized that wastelands, such as rubbish dumps and swamps, were potential breeding grounds for pests and diseases.[6] Authorities began to transform wasteland into public parks. The Shanghai Municipal Council filled in the pond in front of Quinsan Terrace to form Hongkew Park in 1896. The administrators of the Public Recreation Ground in Shanghai filled in puddles near the Cricket Club Pavilion to convert the land into a garden in 1898. Residents lauded the public parks for their perceived key role in improving public health. For example, a resident of the settlement in Shanghai wrote of these benefits that they were especially noticeable "in the summer season when disease [was] rifest and the benefits of the Public Garden the greatest."[7] In 1902, when the plague was still a fresh memory, a settler in Shanghai noted that transforming derelict land into public parks helped to "protect against what is a menace to all the Settlements in common."[8]

Urban authorities also employed parks as a tool to change social practices that could endanger public health. In Chinese cities at the end of the 19th century, many people disposed of human waste by dumping it directly into the streets. In 1894, an observer writing to the *Shen Pao* newspaper noted that "the city filled with human waste in the summer, as there were no lavatories."[9] To prevent the spread of plague, the municipal councils sought to improve habits by enforcing new regulations that forbid people from relieving themselves in the streets, and encouraging residents to use the lavatory infrastructure newly provided for this purpose. As highly significant public spaces of the settlements, public parks became a nexus where this infrastructure could be accessed by the urban residents. In Shanghai, the municipal council constructed lavatories in the Public Garden and Public Recreation Ground—the two main public parks of the International Settlement. Thereafter, these facilities were promoted in other parks, such as Chinese Park in 1906 and Hongkew Recreation Ground and Wayside Park in 1914.[10] The British Municipal Council in Tianjin constructed a multifunctional building known as Gordon Hall in Victoria Park in 1890, which not only served as the town hall, ballroom, and library of the settlement but also provided lavatories for park visitors.[11]

It was well known that an "adequate supply of clean water would play a key role in urban health" and that "unclean water had a certain relationship with 'plague,' as well as dysentery, diarrhea, hepatitis and cholera."[12] Consequently, the urban authorities introduced a public water system in Shanghai in 1883 and Tianjin in 1898 with the goal of improving public health. Once in place, the system provided public drinking fountains, the earliest of which appeared in public parks (Figure 31.1). In 1895, the Shanghai Municipal Council constructed a drinking fountain in the Public Garden and then at Quinsan Square in 1912; the British Municipal Council in Tianjin provided the same facilities in Victoria Park at the end of the 19th century.

New ideas relating to public health arising from the Hong Kong Plague had a long-term effect on public parks in the settlements of Shanghai and Tianjin. Originally installed in the parks to combat the plague, lavatories and drinking fountains gradually became standard features, improving the overall design of public parks in all the settlements. Public parks were increasingly seen as an essential element of maintaining public health and well-being by providing pleasant open space and an opportunity to enjoy fresh air and abundant sunshine.

The rapid development of the settlements in Shanghai and Tianjin in the early 20th century alarmed residents who had experienced the effects of the Hong Kong Plague, as they believed good sanitary standards and ventilated environments would effectively stem the spread of sickness and make their settlements "plague-proof."[13]

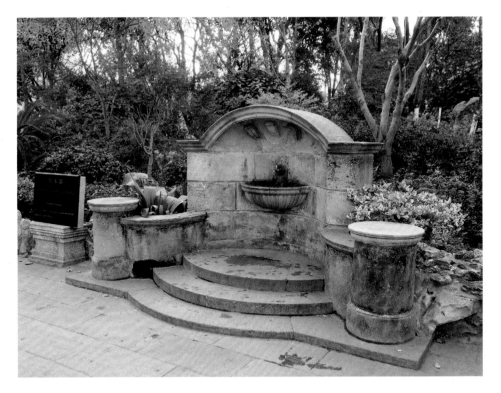

FIGURE 31.1: Drinking fountain, built in 1929, in the historical Hongkew Park of Shanghai. (Photograph by Yichi Zhang.)

The extensive growth of new urban construction could therefore see the plague return in new areas characterized by restricted airflow, overcrowding, and the inability of residents to isolate. Public parks would facilitate the flow of breeze and fresh air, and thus contribute greatly toward the health of the city dwellers. The municipal councils of the settlements actively promoted the construction of public parks in the rapidly growing districts. Hence, the Shanghai Municipal Council opened Wayside Park in the Eastern District in 1908 and Jessfield Park in the Western District in 1914.[14] The Work Committee in the British settlement in Tianjin developed the old nursery garden in the triangle between Elgin Avenue, Race Course Road, and the Dyke, transforming it into Elgin Park in 1920.[15]

As urban construction within the settlements intensified during the next decade, land prices increased beyond the reach of municipal councils. It became impossible to acquire large fields to create parks within the settlements. The construction of parks outside the settlements would have required securing the consent and cooperation of the local Chinese government. Thus, the finite size of the settlements

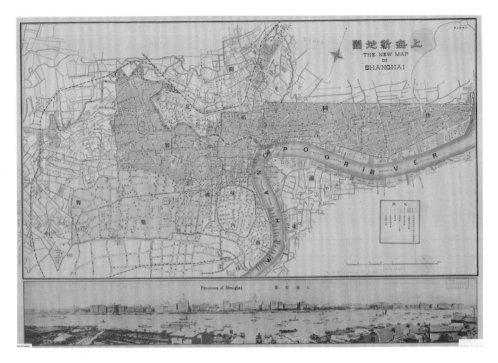

FIGURE 31.2: Layout of public parks (in green) in Shanghai International Settlement (in pink and orange) in the 1930s. Fusazō Sugie, *The New Map of* Shanghai (Shanghai: Shanghai Nihondō Shoten, 1931), 1. (Courtesy of the Geography and Map Division, Library of Congress.)

resulted in the introduction of a version of the European "park system." In 1930, in order to "facilitate the daily use by urban citizens," the municipal councils used the park system strategy to connect small open spaces and large parks into a network and thus reshaped the urban landscape of the settlements.[16]

To maximize access to open space and improve public health, the authorities suggested that each resident should be no more than half a mile away from a small park of twenty to forty *mou* (about three to six acres) in area—that is, parks should be spaced about one mile apart.[17] Consequently, Shanghai Municipal Council constructed Singapore Road Park in 1931, Soochow Road Children's Garden in 1933, and Poyang Park in 1935 (Figure 31.2).[18] The British Municipal Council in Tianjin constructed Jubilee Park and Queen's Park in 1937 (Figure 31.3).[19] The designs of these neighborhood parks were modeled on those of other public parks: Singapore Road Park in Shanghai mirrored Wayside Park, also in Shanghai, while Queen's Park in Tianjin reflected the arrangement of the large municipal parks that provided lavatories and other facilities.[20] These neighborhood parks were as popular as the large municipal parks, meeting the demands of residents and attracting hundreds of visitors each week.

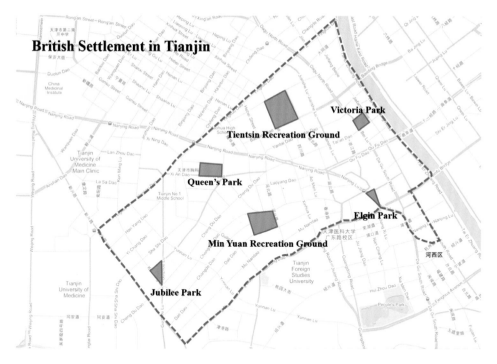

FIGURE 31.3: Layout of public parks in the British settlement of Tianjin in the 1930s. (Drawing by Yichi Zhang.)

Conclusion

The British settlements provided places where British settlers could import and implement European planning ideas in China. Following the disaster of the Hong Kong Plague outbreak in 1894, consideration of public health was positioned as an essential element of urban construction. The idea of public health facilities had drawn little attention when the British first founded their urban settlements, but the introduction of lavatories and drinking fountains was gradually promoted. Practices that could harm or improve public health began to change in the post-plague period. As a result, the physical construction and functions of the municipal parks in the settlements were shaped for the long term and became synonymous with public health rather than merely decorative social spaces, as in the early settlement days.

The plague and its consequences continued to influence urban planning and design even after the outbreak had abated by embedding the significance of public health into the social life of the settlements. The concept of a park system included the widespread construction of small public parks to ventilate the urban setting without the need to purchase large areas of vacant land. The parks of the settlements became a necessity of the city, reshaping urban planning strategies. The advancement of these parks popularized ideas about public health and public spaces and imported the public health concept through the parks themselves. As a direct result of the pestilence, the relationship between urban design and public health changed the lives of the residents of Shanghai and Tianjin.

Acknowledgement: This work was supported by the 2015–2016 Summer Fellowship of the Dumbarton Oaks Research Library and Collection, the Trustees for Harvard University, and the European Research Council (ERC) under the European Union's Horizon 2020 Research and Innovation Programme [No 802070].

NOTES

1. "Foreigners Discuss the Plague," *Shen Pao* (Shanghai), May 25, 1894, 115.

2. B. W. Brown, "Plague: A Note on the History of the Disease in Hongkong," *Public Health Reports (1896–1970)* 28, no. 12 (1913): 552.

3. George Chadwick, *The Park and the Town: Public Landscape in the 19th and 20th Centuries* (London: Architectural Press, 1966), 19.

4. Xidong Guo, Tong Zhang, Yan Zhang, eds., *Tianjin Historical Famous Gardens* (Tianjin: Tianjin Ancient Book Press, 2008), 102.

5. Ruth Rogaski, *Hygienic Modernity: Meanings of Health and Disease in Treaty-Port China* (Berkeley: University of California Press, 2004), 86.

6. "To the Editor of the Peking & Tientsin Times," *Peking and Tientsin Times*, April 5, 1902, 2.

7. Ibid.

8. Ibid.

9. "Prevent Disease by Removing Waste," *Shen Pao* (Shanghai), June 27, 1894, 1.

10. Shanghai Municipal Council, *Annual Report of the Shanghai Municipal Council 1914* (Shanghai: Shanghai Municipal Council, 1914), 70B.

11. Yichi Zhang, "The First British Concession Garden of Tianjin- Victoria Garden," *Modern Landscape Architecture*, no. 5 (2010): 45.

12. Peng Zhang, *Physical Foundations of City Form: A Study on the Relationship between Municipal Construction and Transformation of Urban Space in the International Settlement of Shanghai* (Shanghai: Tongji University Press, 2008), 175.

13. Arthur Stanley, "Health Officer's Report," in *Annual Report of the Shanghai Municipal Council, 1899*, ed. Shanghai Municipal Council (Shanghai: Shanghai Municipal Council, 1899), 101.

14. Shanghai Municipal Council, *Annual Report of the Shanghai Municipal Council 1914*, 70B.

15. Tianjie Zhang, Ze Li, and Yuan Sun, "Hybrid Modernity and Public Space: An Investigation on Public Park Development in Modern Tianjin," *New Architecture*, no. 5 (2012): 37.

16. Zhi Chen, *The Theory of City and Park* (Beijing: The Commercial Press, 1930), 12.

17. "Construct Additional Parks in the International Settlement," *Shen Pao* (Shanghai), October 25, 1931, 15.

18. Shanghai Municipal Council, *Annual Report of the Shanghai Municipal Council 1933* (Shanghai: Shanghai Municipal Council, 1933), 237.

19. Editorial Team of Tianjin Landscape and Greening, *Tianjin Landscape and Greening* (Tianjin: Tianjin Science and Technology Press, 1989), 8.

20. "The Settlement Will Construct Two Public Parks in the East and the West and Construct a Children's Playground," *Shen Pao* (Shanghai), August 10, 1931, 15.

32

Rebuilding the British Seamen's Hospital at Smyrna in the Wake of Smallpox and Cholera Epidemics, 1892

Işılay Tiarnagh Sheridan Gün and Erdem Erten

Changes in the modes and speed of transportation during the 19th century created an unprecedented movement of people in various parts of the world and dramatically affected urban populations. As meeting points of mobile communities including merchants, sailors, and travelers, port cities had always been vulnerable to epidemics, but in the 19th century the spread of infectious diseases acquired a global character with the introduction of maritime steam-liners and railway lines that crossed international boundaries.[1]

Now known as İzmir in the Republic of Turkey, Smyrna of Asia Minor (Anatolia) was one of those port cities that experienced the rise of epidemics toward the end of the 19th century, which eventually led its local government to establish principles for a sanitary urban environment. After the Anglo-Ottoman Commercial Treaty of 1838, the city became an open port for free trade and eventually transformed into the most important port of the Ottoman Empire, well connected to global networks of exchange.[2] During this transformation, Smyrna's multiethnic, multilingual, multireligious population was made up of Muslim, Greek, and Armenian Orthodox and Jewish communities as well as Venetian, French, Dutch, and British colonial merchants. These demographics increased the complexity of Smyrna's sociocultural and economic makeup.[3] Under the influence of all these groups, a new port was built and new railway lines were extended out to the hinterland, resulting in the fast expansion of the city.

Each of the ethno-religious groups living in Smyrna responded to infectious diseases differently. Accounts record that in times of epidemics, the Muslim population continued with their everyday lives within the city, while some of the non-Muslim members of colonial communities left the center for their residences in the growing suburbs of Buca and Bornova, which were connected to the city center via the new railway lines.[4] Those who did not have this opportunity remained in voluntary quarantine. The ethno-religious diversity was almost directly reflected in Smyrna's hospitals that were associated with these distinct communities. At times of epidemics, the victims were quickly buried in or near these hospital enclaves in shallow and hastily prepared graves that ended up contaminating these enclaves and making them the first targets of urban interventions.[5]

Located outside the city center when they were first built, these hospital enclaves were surrounded by urban expansion as the rise of trade brought in more people. Hospitals suddenly finding themselves within the developing urban center failed to comply with sanitary regulations, which were legislated towards the end of the 19th century. The first British Seamen's Hospital, built in 1816, was among these contaminated hospital enclaves in Smyrna. Relocated and reconstructed in 1894, the new hospital represented a turn toward prioritizing medical expertise and the development of sanitary urban space over lucrative real estate investment.

Case study: The hospital and sanitary urban space, 1894

Toward the end of the 19th century the complete shutdown of port cities became unthinkable during epidemics and the increase in infections became inevitable. The Ottoman Empire started to implement quarantine measures in 1831 for the first time, in response to a cholera outbreak twenty years before[6] the first International Sanitary Conference took place in Paris on July 23, 1851, which aimed to establish an international consensus on urban sanitation.[7] Ottoman imperial representatives attended this conference and the following ones regularly, and the third conference was held in İstanbul following the catastrophic 1861 and 1865 cholera outbreaks.[8] It was at this conference that the spread of cholera was connected to the movement of people as well as to the use of contaminated water.[9] The conferences pointed to the necessity of a new municipal organization to regulate the development of health facilities, sanitation, construction site selection, and the administration of quarantine measures as required by urban centers.

The municipality of Smyrna was established in 1868. The new governing body responded to epidemic measures and coordinated transportation systems, quarantine and accommodation facilities, and better health infrastructure demanded by the mobile, international merchant class of the city since outbreaks interrupted their economic activities.[10] The English comprised the majority of this merchant class as they managed half the trade from Smyrna's port, owned the railways that carried mining and agricultural products from the hinterland, and possessed up to one-third of the land in Western Anatolia.[11] Its economic, social, and spatial spheres being dominated by the British, Smyrna became part of Britain's "informal empire" where British seamen appeared as an important group of actors in the urban scene.[12]

280

Dedicated to the seamen, the British Seamen's Hospitals in Smyrna and in İstanbul were the most visible markers of British imperial interests in Ottoman cities.[13] The first British Seamen's Hospital in Smyrna was built by the Levant Company in 1816.[14] When the company dissolved in 1825, the hospital was transferred to the British government.[15] It remained in operation until 1891, when it was shut down due to failed expansion efforts. Smyrna had not experienced a serious cholera outbreak after 1865 at that time, and correspondence within the British government's Foreign Office noted that "there may be two or three infectious cases in five years."[16] While the construction of a new hospital was deemed unnecessary, the complete removal of the institution was also annulled: Mediterranean trade was too important and the seamen too vulnerable in times of epidemics to be without it. As result of the deliberations, drawings were prepared for the addition of an infectious disease ward above the existing mortuary in September 1891 (Figure 32.1).

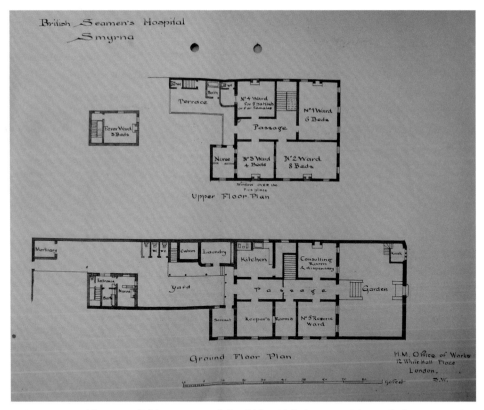

FIGURE 32.1: The monolithic massing of the Old British Seamen's Hospital, Smyrna, with a proposed infectious fever ward drawn in red, 1891. The plan shows the ground floor and the first floor of the existing hospital. In the back, a room for a nurse and a bath was added together with a staircase to reach the infectious fever ward built on top of the mortuary. (Courtesy of The National Archives (United Kingdom), Work 10/52/3.)

When the inspecting engineer of Her Majesty's Office of Works, R. H. Boyce, visited Smyrna in November 1891, he stated that the hospital was in the "most unhealthy quarter" and advised building a new one on a "healthy site" in the outskirts of the city (Figure 32.2) regardless of the drawn project for the existing hospital.[17] The 1892 outbreaks of smallpox and cholera in Smyrna proved the inspector right and made the British Foreign Office reconsider the rate of the spread of infection from adjacent hospitals in the existing quarter during these epidemics.[18] After a year spent fighting these two important outbreaks, the Ottoman government also appointed a special Sanitary Commissioner and a local Sanitary Board on November 19, 1892, granting them the power to ban all unsanitary arrangements on streets and in residences, as well as any ward additions to hospitals in December 1892.[19] Although the building of a new hospital was indispensable, the epidemics rendered any construction work in the city impossible until the end of 1893. In the meantime, a Syrian-born British architect living in Smyrna, Albert Frederick William Werry (1839–1906), was commissioned to undertake the work in March 1893. Werry sought to build the new hospital outside the center, noting that the sewers near the current hospital site were "nothing more than stagnant cesspools and have constantly to be cleaned out, [and] are a standing cause of infections to the whole neighborhood" (Figure 32.3).[20]

In correspondence dated October 6, 1893, Werry announced with joy that the 1892 cholera outbreak had ceased. He therefore recommended that Boyce, the inspecting engineer, could now sail to Smyrna via Marseilles but that he should avoid the overland route via Istanbul, as cholera restrictions still applied there.[21] The British government remained in control of overseas projects, even from a distance. Once the quarantine was lifted in November, the Ottoman Railway Company proposed to the British government that the new hospital to be built on a plot next to the British-owned railway station at Punta (Figure 32.4).[22] After the construction of the station in 1858, this site, which was relatively outside the city center, was expected to become a new development area for investors[23] instead of the densely built city center, and the company also anticipated other hospitals to buy adjacent plots.[24] However, the head surgeon of the hospital strongly opposed this swampy neighborhood, which was conducive to malaria.[25] Therefore, a site on the other side of the railway, which Werry described as isolated, healthy, and having a sufficient supply of good water for drinking and sanitary purposes, was chosen.[26]

This site was purchased in October 1894 and construction began.[27] Learning from the 1892 outbreaks, the monolithic mass of the old hospital was rejected in favor of a design that featured a hospital building, infirmary, and infectious ward surrounded by a vast garden (Figure 32.5). A map of Smyrna from 1919 shows that other hospitals were relocated on separate parts of the city as well, at considerable

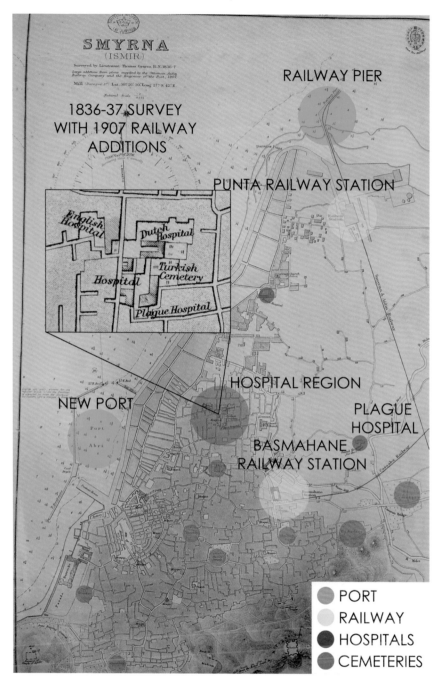

FIGURE 32.2: Map published in 1844 with the authors' overlay indicating the hospital cluster on the edge of urban Smyrna. "The City of Ismir or Smyrna ... Port Saip, Etc. [Admiralty Chart]," 1844. (Courtesy of The British Library, System number: 004925234, Shelfmark[s]: Cartographic Items Maps SEC.5., 1521.)

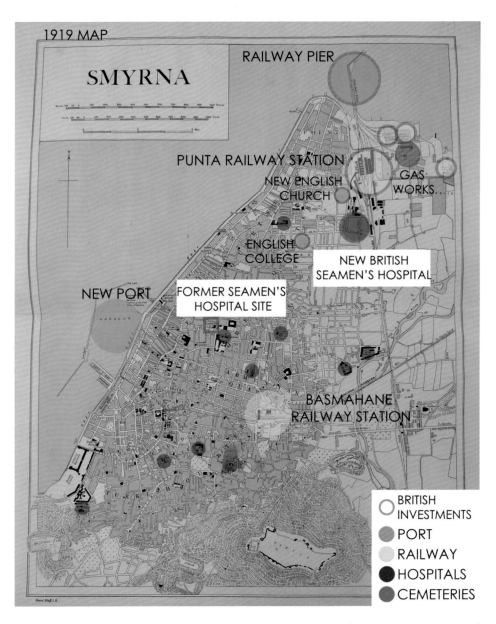

FIGURE 32.3: 1919 map, with the authors' overlay, showing the Old British Seamen's Hospital site in the middle of the newly populated part of the city, scattered hospitals, and enlarged railway facilities. The red outlined dots indicate the British investments to emphasize their dominance over the urban sphere. (Courtesy of The National Archives [United Kingdom], FO 925/41249.)

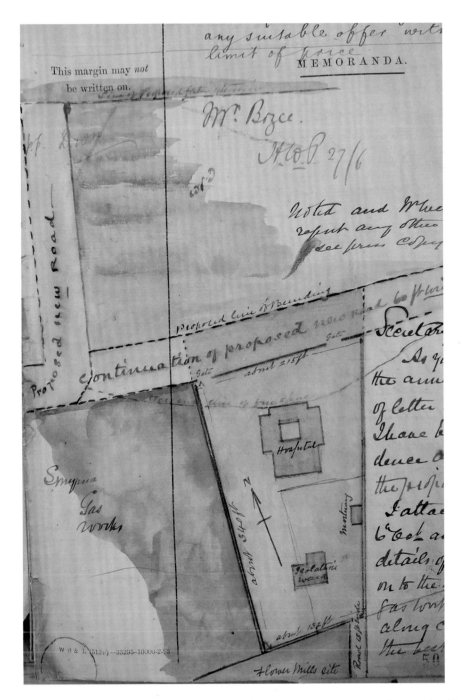

FIGURE 32.4: Proposed British Seamen's Hospital construction site on partial swampland by the British-owned Ottoman Railway Company next to its pier and a British gas works. (Courtesy of The National Archives [United Kingdom], Work 10/52/3.)

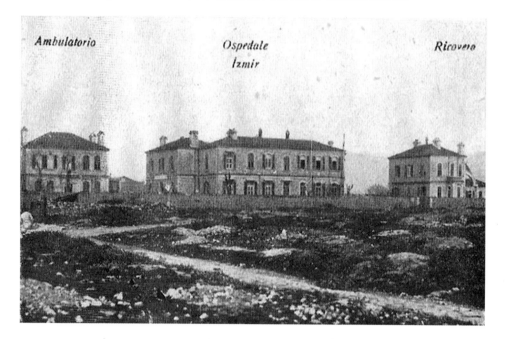

FIGURE 32.5: Separate structures in the garden setting of the new British Seamen's Hospital, Smyrna. The Italian names for the buildings written on the photograph date from the rental of the site by St. Antonio Italian Hospital between World War I and World War II. (Courtesy of Levantine Heritage Foundation and Okan Çetin, http://levantineheritage.com/seamans-hospital.html [accessed September 12, 2020].)

distances from one another, in order not to form an unhealthy cluster of medical facilities that could facilitate rather than curb the spread of disease.

Conclusion

Smyrna's integration into the globalized 19th-century market caught the city off guard. Although the city made full use of advanced transportation systems to quickly meet the demands of industrial production, it was incapable of dealing with the flow and sheltering of the large number of people the trade expansion entailed. The smallpox and cholera outbreaks in 1892 clearly demonstrated the lack of proper health and sanitation infrastructure, especially in times of serious diseases. The relocation of the British Seamen's Hospital following these two outbreaks represents the rise of awareness for a healthier urban environment and the turn toward prioritizing sanitary urban space over financial gain.

While the efforts to rebuild the hospital should be seen as an act of honoring and protecting the mercantile marine who made it possible to expand Britain's informal empire, it should also be understood as an important episode in the Ottoman Empire's modernization and the city's role in it.[28] The hospital's relocation away from the heavily populated city center and the dissolution of the hospital cluster according to the regulations set by the local sanitary board marked the dawn of a new era in public health. The rule of medical expertise over the planning of hospital quarters and the architecture of the new hospital put an end to practices such as the interment of the deceased on the hospital grounds and required the analysis of soil and water conditions, and the construction of separate wards for infectious diseases. One striking outcome of the strong determination and organization of the city's multiethnic communities to create a sanitary urban environment was Smyrna's success in overcoming the 1892 epidemics before İstanbul, the Ottoman capital, where the majority of qualified infectious disease doctors resided. Therefore, the hospital's history emphasizes the important role that the health administration of the city had with regard to urban development in the fight against deadly epidemics.

NOTES

1. Coşkun Bakar, "Avrupa'da Dolaşan Koleranın Gölgesinde İstanbul Uluslararası Sağlık Konferansı, 1866" [Istanbul International Health Conference, 1866: In the Shadow of the Cholera That Wanders Europe], *Turkish Journal of Public Health* 18, no. 1 (2020): 68–82.

2. Sibel Zandi-Sayek, "Introduction," in *Ottoman İzmir The Rise of a Cosmopolitan Port 1840-1880*, ed. Sibel Zandi-Sayek (Minneapolis: University of Minnesota Press, 2012), 5–46.

3. Ibid.

4. Pelin Böke, "İzmir Karantina Teşkilatının Kuruluşu ve Faaliyetleri (1840–1900)," *Çağdaş Türkiye Tarihi Araştırmaları Dergisi* 8, nos. 18–19 (2009): 137–59.

5. Ibid.

6. Ibid.

7. Norman Howard-Jones, "Introduction," in *The Scientific Background of the International Sanitary Conferences, 1851-1938*, ed. Norman Howard-Jones (Geneva: World Health Organization, 1975), 9–12.

8. Bakar, "Avrupa'da Dolaşan Kolera," 68–82.

9. During these conferences there was debate on the cause of cholera as either a waterborne or soilborne disease. Howard-Jones, "Introduction."

10. Böke, "İzmir Karantina."

11. Orhan Kurmuş, *Emperyalizmin Türkiye'ye Girişi* [The Introduction of Imperialism to Turkey] (İstanbul: Bilim Yayınları, 1974), 148.

12. Abdullah Martal, *Değişim Sürecinde İzmir'de Sanayileşme 19.Yüzyıl* [Nineteenth-Century Industrialization in İzmir during the Process of Change] (İzmir: Dokuz Eylül Yayınları, 1999).

13. Correspondence, June 13, 1894, The National Archives (United Kingdom), Work 10/52/3: *"You have drawn our attention to the fact that while Government provide a Hospital at Smyrna, they do not do so at other Mediterranean ports with the exception of Constantinople."*

14. The British Seamen's Hospital was founded in England in the 17th century. Conrad Hepworth Dixon, "Seamen and the Law: An Examination of the Impact of Legislation on the British Merchant Seamen's Lot, 1588-1918." (Ph.D. diss., University College London, 1981), 18–19.

15. Correspondence, April 2, 1924, The National Archives (UK), Work 10/52/3.

16. Correspondence, September 12, 1891, The National Archives (UK), Work 10/52/3.

17. Correspondence, November 9, 1892, The National Archives (UK), Work 10/52/3.

18. Correspondence, December 18, 1893, The National Archives (UK), Work 10/52/3.

19. Correspondence, December 1, 1892, The National Archives (UK), Work 10/52/3.

20. Correspondence, March 20, 1893, The National Archives (UK), Work 10/52/3.

21. Correspondence, October 6, 1893, The National Archives (UK), Work 10/52/3.

22. Correspondence, June 23, 1893, The National Archives (UK), Work 10/52/3.

23. Cana Bilsel, "19. Yüzyılın İkinci Yarısında İzmir'de Büyük Ölçekli Kentsel Projeler ve Kent Mekanının Başkalaşımı" [Large-Scale Urban Projects and the Transformation of Urban Space in Izmir in the Second Half of the 19th Century], *Ege Mimarlık* 36 (April 2000): 34–37.

24. Correspondence, December 18, 1893, The National Archives (UK), Work 10/52/3

25. Correspondence, January 2, 1894, The National Archives (UK), Work 10/52/3.

26. Correspondence, October 5, 1894, The National Archives (UK), Work 10/52/3.

27. Ibid.

28. Ibid.

33

Spatial Change and the Cholera Epidemic in Manila, the Philippines, 1902–4

Ian Morley

On December 10, 1898, the Treaty of Paris transferred colonial governance of the Philippines from Spain to the United States. A week and a half later, on December 21, President William McKinley addressed the nation of the Philippines in a speech entitled the "Benevolent Assimilation Proclamation," in which he emphasized the altruistic intentions of the colonial authority of the United States. Filipinos, however, with hardened memories of life under an oppressive Spanish colonial administration, had different ideas in mind. By February, the country took up arms in revolt against its new colonial overlords. The resulting conflict, the Philippine-American War, lasted from February 1899 until July 1902 and established conditions ripe for the propagation of cholera, an intestinal illness caused by the ingestion of the bacterium *Vibrio cholerae* from contaminated water or food.

The first cases of the 1902–4 Philippine cholera epidemic were detected on March 20, 1902, in the Farola district of the capital city of Manila on the island of Luzon. With overcrowded, unsanitary neighborhoods and lacking a city-wide sewage system, Manila offered a dangerous breeding ground for the disease. From early 1902 to mid-1904, more than 4,000 of the 220,000 people then living in Manila died from cholera, and more than 200,000 people succumbed to the disease countrywide (Figure 33.1).[1]

The 1902–4 epidemic—one of the modern era's most severe outbreaks of cholera—revealed the weaknesses at the intersection of colonial politics, public health, and urban planning in Manila.[2] To comprehend American policy toward public health and architecture in the city at that time, four issues must be acknowledged. First, the Americans linked the spread of infection both to the rundown condition of the built environment and to the behaviors of Filipinos. Second, the American colonial regime thereafter passed rules to regulate the form of building types.[3] Third, new public works projects were immediately established. Fourth, Daniel Burnham and Peirce Anderson proposed a monumental City Beautiful–inspired plan for Manila in 1905. These four matters demonstrated the Americans' desire to reconstruct Manila's built fabric, which had fallen into neglect and disrepair over the course of the Spanish colonial age (1565–1898). Toward these ends, the colonizers were willing and eager to use modern medical and urban planning logic to rationalize the need for a divergent environmental organization. However, to enact a new sanitary and spatial order, the colonial state needed to convince Filipinos that its policies would elevate their condition, and to do that, it needed to quash competing sources of information. Hence, the Spanish colonial approach to urban design and extant Filipino attitudes toward public health were roundly condemned by the Americans. This situation provoked displeasure from the colonized population. Erroneous criticisms appeared in local newspapers, such as claims that Burnham and Anderson's city planning project focused on superficial aesthetics rather than uplifting the health of Manila's population.[4]

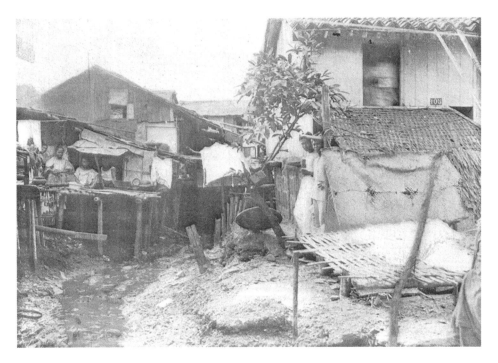

FIGURE 33.1: "Typical cholera house, over filthy drain," *Annual Reports of the War Department for the Fiscal Year Ended June 30, 1902*, vol. V. Report of the Philippine Commission, 1903, p. 320.

Case study: Managing contagion in the Manila City Plan of 1905

Environmental prophylaxes were introduced in Manila starting in 1902. The Americans utilized up-to-date epidemiological concepts in order to promote access to fresh air, clean water, and sanitation as the fundamentals of sound community health. Justifying their new hygienic practices and medical treatments, such as the administration of Benzozone to purge the *Vibrio cholerae* bacteria from infected people, the colonial system asserted cultural and scientific superiority over the Filipinos. The Americans torched districts where cholera was endemic, regulated architectonic control over buildings so that they conformed to contemporary sanitary notions, constructed the city's first crematorium, laid down pipes to supply clean water, and built public toilets, market buildings, hospitals, and reservoirs. They also introduced modern urban planning ideas to the suburbs of Malate and Ermita in 1905 and 1908. These neighborhoods embodied an environmentally conscious paradigm of wide footpath-lined streets and tree-covered lawns. This paradigm was augmented by Burnham and Anderson's City Beautiful plan and the colonial government's execution of the sanitary barrio concept, which was implemented to counteract the conspicuous squalor within Manila's least affluent quarters (Figure 33.2).

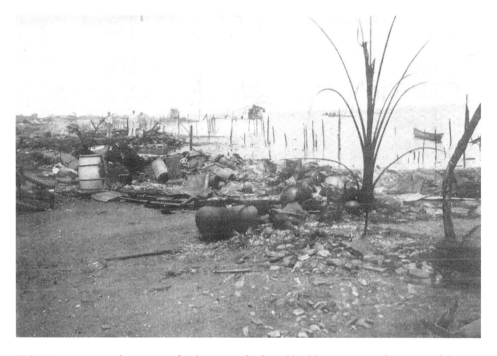

FIGURE 33.2: "Farola District after burning of infected buildings," *Annual Reports of the War Department for the Fiscal Year Ended June 30, 1902*, vol. V. Report of the Philippine Commission, 1903, p. 320.

In view of the many activities related to urban environmental improvement undertaken after 1902, it could be assumed that Burnham and Anderson's City Beautiful plan (adopted in 1905) simply broadened the existent American colonial health and urban management strategy (Figure 33.3). However, this supposition is incorrect. Under the leadership of Burnham and Anderson, the American colonial mission sought to reform Philippine civilization by means of education and example. Specifically, Burnham intended to establish an urban design template for future colonial construction based on landscape architecture and city planning already undertaken in the United States. His and Anderson's planning scheme envisioned a reformed colonial sense of place with "New Manila" being more picturesque and clean than it was before.[5]

The planners advocated a radial grid of roads to ameliorate the congested urban form. These roads were to be configured as circumferential parkways, crisscrossing districts and radiating from the new civic core with its Capitol Building and Mall, reminiscent of those in Washington, DC. Manila Bay's shoreline would be developed with a 250-foot-wide Ocean Boulevard, the port area enlarged, and resorts built on the uplands surrounding the city to furnish its denizens with the opportunity for a "change of air" without a "great cost of transportation."[6] In addition, new public buildings were to be erected and the local waterways revived. Burnham and Anderson suggested that dredging the *esteros* (estuarine inlets) and building up their banks with masonry would instigate commercial and visual benefits, stating that the *estero* was "not only an economical vehicle for the transaction of public business," but that it could also "become, as in Venice, an element of beauty."[7] Whereas during the Spanish colonial period Manila's numerous foul-smelling, polluted *esteros* functioned as sources for drinking water, fishing, laundry washing, and bathing—as well as waste disposal—from 1905 onward there were many public health benefits to cleaning up the watercourses. Rejuvenation measures, applied alongside new sanitary rules ensured that *esteros* were no longer associated with occurrences of contagious illness.

The new road layout further enhanced public health by avoiding north-south and east-west orientations, thereby allowing the façades of buildings "to have the advantage of direct sunlight at some time during the day, with consequent gain in ventilation and sanitation."[8] Green spaces were sited in all parts of the city, with small-sized tracts of open land designed as plazas, circles, and esplanades granting approaches for new buildings of importance. Fountains provided citizens with access to microclimates where they would find opportunities for refreshment from the tropical heat and humidity. Larger green areas and playing fields were used for leisure activities. Burnham and Anderson observed the value of Manila's natural water features and undulating suburban topography in recommending where such public spaces should be located.

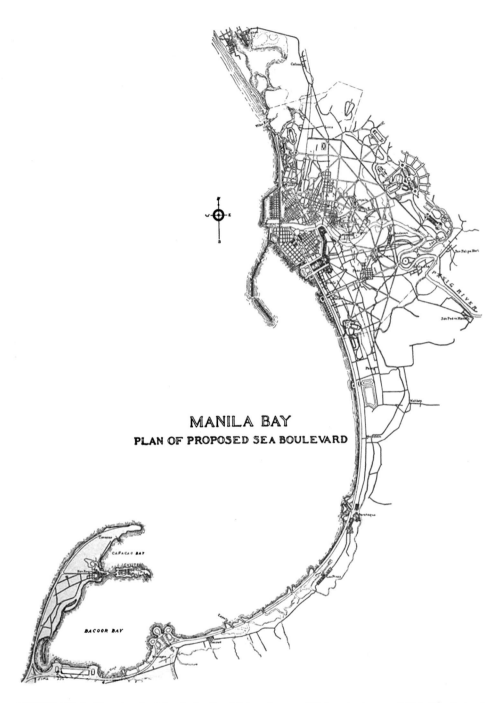

MANILA BAY
PLAN OF PROPOSED SEA BOULEVARD

FIGURE 33.3: City plan for Manila by Daniel Burnham and Peirce Anderson, 1905, *The Report of the Philippine Commission*, Part I, 1906.

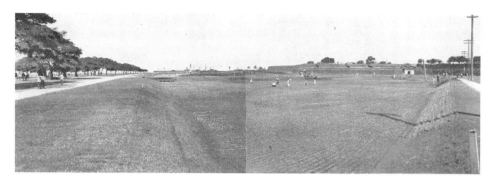

FIGURE 33.4: Photograph of the area of the former *Intramuros* moat after its transformation into a green lawn space. "Parking an old insanitary moat," *War Department Annual Reports*, 1909, vol. VIII. Report of the Philippine Commission, Part II, 1909, p. 128.

The 1905 city plan included a substantial green space downtown where the moat of the late sixteenth-century Spanish *Intramuros* (walled city) was formerly located (Figure 33.4). By filling in this trench, which was a known agent in the spread of disease, Burnham and Anderson gained the potential to create a vast lawn modeled on the greensward about the Ringstrasse in Vienna, Austria (see Figure 33.4).[9] Additionally, the two planners grasped the value of the *Intramuros* walls as a place for relaxation and to enjoy the sea breeze but realized that the entrances to the historic walled quarter required enlargement. While their proposal to widen the entrances may be read as a response to traffic circulation needs in the historic district, it was the matter of public health that most impacted their thought process. Around the year 1900 the *Intramuros* was widely considered unsanitary, and the average life expectancy in Manila at that time was less than 21 years; this was less than half of that in the United States at the same time.[10] Evidence of these conditions undoubtedly affected Burnham when he visited the Philippine capital in 1904–5; by widening the *Intramuros*' entrances, he could allow for a greater flow of air and the dissipation of noxious smells. By 1908 the idea of the hygienic district had been fortified via the invention of the sanitary barrio with its concrete gullies to drain surface runoff and symmetrically arranged houses placed in proximity to bath houses, latrines, water hydrants, and laundry facilities. The sanitary barrio, first developed on the San Lazaro Estate for a population in excess of ten thousand people, established a new benchmark in the American colonial quest to abate poor ventilation and overcrowding for the less well-off members of Manila society. By 1910, proposals to build such desirable neighborhoods had been presented in the districts of Paco, Pasay, Sampaloc, and Tondo; financial assistance was solicited through a municipal government ordinance.

Conclusion

Under the guidance of American colonial rule, environmental transition in early 1900s Manila exemplified a form of progress. The city became not only more beautiful but also more healthful. In some respects this transformation was unavoidable. Manila, when American colonization commenced, had a terrible reputation as "the filthiest place in the Orient."[11] Its waterways were severely polluted, many of its districts were congested and disease ridden, and almost 75 percent of all buildings were described as "shacks" in "poor condition."[12] Consequently, the 1902–4 cholera epidemic spurred the colonial administration to react decisively for the sake of improved public health. In activating architectural and spatial transformation, the Americans aligned Manila's new environmental character to contemporary epidemiological notions.[13] More significantly, in restructuring the city they inaugurated a new urban planning culture. Their new approach enabled a greater degree of control over infectious diseases than was hitherto possible. Subsequently, when cholera returned to Manila in 1908 and 1914, it affected considerably fewer people than during the outbreak of 1902–4; similarly, after 1905, Manila saw a massive decline in the mortality rate.[14]

Burnham and Anderson's plan intended to enhance livability.[15] As such, their scheme is an example of how cities today can recover from, and prepare for, future public health crises. Such awareness also helps to expose how technical, cultural, and political elements in the planning process interplay with local dynamics. Cognizance of this relationship can play a key role in assisting local governments to establish more inclusive, healthy, and resilient cities. Somewhat unsurprisingly, the Manila government during 2020–21 established new public spaces. The actions of the city government reflect the awareness that, now more than ever, citizens require green spaces to maintain good physical and mental health. So, as was apparent in 1905, urban planners in Manila are giving new priority to the need for green spaces.

NOTES

1. *Census of the Philippine Islands, Volume 3* (Washington, DC: United States Bureau of the Census, 1905), 10, 39, 47.
2. Victor G. Heiser, "American Sanitation in the Philippines and its Influence on the Orient," *Proceedings of the American Philosophical Society* 57, no. 1 (Spring 1918): 61.
3. These included Ordinances No. 16 (1902) and No. 53 (1904).
4. Ian Morley, *Cities and Nationhood: American Imperialism and Urban Design in the Philippines, 1898-1916* (Honolulu: University of Hawaii Press, 2018), 84.

5. David Brody, *Visualizing American Empire: Orientalism and Imperialism in the Philippines* (Chicago, IL: University of Chicago Press, 2010), 149.

6. Daniel Burnham and Peirce Anderson, "Report on Proposed Improvements at Manila," in *Report of the Philippine Commission, Part 1* (Washington, DC: Government Printing Office, 1906), 635.

7. Ibid., 634.

8. Ibid., 631.

9. Winand Klassen, *Architecture in the Philippines: Filipino Building in Cross-Cultural Context* (Cebu City: University of San Carlos Press, 2010), 257.

10. *Census of the Philippine Islands, Volume 3*, 73.

11. Bradford K. Daniels, "The Re-Making of Manila. Changing a Pest-Hole into a Healthful and Beautiful Capital of the Commerce of the East," *World's Work* 10, no. 5 (1905): 6629.

12. *A Pronouncing Gazetteer and Geographical Dictionary of the Philippine Islands* (Washington, DC: Government Printing Office, 1902), 184.

13. Ken De Bevoise, *Agents of Apocalypse: Epidemic Disease in the Colonial Philippines* (Princeton, NJ: Princeton University Press, 1995), 177.

14. Heiser (1918) remarked that Manila's death rate from 1904 to 1914 declined from 46.83 to 23.18 per 1,000 people.

15. Thomas Hines, "The Imperial Façade: Daniel H. Burnham and American Architectural Planning in the Philippines," *Pacific Historical Review* 41, no. 1 (1972): 53.

34

Plague, Housing, and Battles over Segregation in Colonial Dakar, Senegal, 1914

Gregory Valdespino

In May 1916, disgruntled residents of Dakar's Medina neighborhood wrote an angry petition to the colony's governor. They recounted frequent flooding, brutal winds, and a dire lack of municipal services.[1] These issues reflected the neighborhood's haphazard creation, emerging as it did amid a city-wide emergency: colonial planners designed the Medina during a 1914 outbreak of the bubonic plague. Officials saw the neighborhood as a key part of their efforts to use racialized zoning measures to contain the disease and transform the city. These segregationist policies fostered battles between French officials and Senegalese residents over how to design and inhabit this contested colonial capital.

The confrontations over segregationist urban reforms in plague-stricken Dakar reflected the city's centrality to France's empire. Capital of present-day Senegal, Dakar lies at the westernmost point of the African continent, the Cap-Vert peninsula. French colonists took control of the area from Indigenous Lebu communities in 1857. By the turn of the century, Dakar had become a major port and the capital of the French West African Federation. By 1914, almost thirty thousand city residents were composed of a small European population, Lebu inhabitants, and migrants from across French West Africa.[2] Many colonists sought to make Dakar an emblem of French imperialism by segregating the city into African neighborhoods filled with straw huts and a European quarter dotted with stone villas. However, this spatial and racial reorganization faced a major obstacle: the city's African residents themselves.

Dakar's African inhabitants deployed potent political weapons to challenge discriminatory urban reforms. Unlike most colonial subjects, African residents born in the coastal cities of Dakar, Gorée, Rufisque, and Saint-Louis, known as *originaires*, had many French citizenship rights. They regularly used elections and courts to hold onto lands coveted by French colonists. However, this did not fully stop French authorities from exerting political and economic domination. To challenge their growing marginalization, in 1914, Dakar's African voters mobilized a campaign that led to the election of France's first African parliamentarian, who promised to challenge colonial dispossession.[3] However, just after the election, the plague upended the city's political landscape.

Case study: Plague in Dakar, 1914

The bubonic plague that hit Dakar had been traveling the world for well over a decade. Caused by the bacterium *Yersina pestis*, the plague was typically spread by infected fleas carried on small animals, most famously rats. This third major bubonic plague pandemic in human history had its first recorded cases in southern China in the 1890s and quickly spread to ports around the world.[4] In Dakar, the disease killed roughly 1,500 people in its first few months alone.[5] As in many other colonial cities facing this pandemic, officials in Dakar pinned the plague's spread on unclean Indigenous dwellings.[6] This connection made urban design and planning key to official responses to the disease. French colonists advocated dividing the city between zones designated specifically for African or European style dwellings while presenting these racialized divisions as essential to stopping the disease.[7] However, efforts to enforce this discriminatory form of urban planning fostered widespread confrontations between Senegalese residents and French officials about who had the power to organize Dakar's built environment.

The use of racial zoning to combat the plague echoed policies found in cities across colonial Africa. From Cape Town to Nairobi, the plague produced what historian Maynard Swenson has called a "sanitation syndrome."[8] Many European authorities saw African dwellings as breeding grounds for disease and sought to protect Europeans colonists from contact with possible contagion. In Dakar, colonial authorities used this same logic to leverage public health concerns and to redesign the city in ways that had previously been impossible.

Colonial officials used plague-related measures to overcome previous challenges to urban segregation. The political rights of the city's *originaires*, as well as French republican limitations on explicitly race-based laws, challenged earlier efforts to racially divide the city. However, Dakar's city planners claimed that plague-related segregation was not based on race but rather domestic architectural style.[9] As documented in an early 20th-century postcard, homes lining the streets of Dakar were often made of diverse materials including cement, stone, and straw (Figure 34.1). However, soon after the disease's arrival, Dakar's government passed new laws requiring homes in the city to be built out of either stone or cement, which health experts deemed more hygienic than the inexpensive straw used by many of the

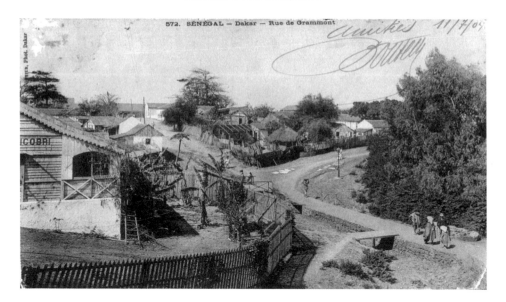

FIGURE 34.1: Postcard from the early 20th century identified as "Senegal – Dakar – Grammont Street." (Courtesy of the Archives Nationales du Sénégal.)

city's African residents. Officials openly acknowledged that these materials were too costly for most of Dakar's working-class African population and that these building requirements would inevitably displace most of the city's African residents and create de facto racial segregation.[10]

The government sought to move Dakar's African inhabitants and their supposedly insalubrious homes to the new Medina neighborhood on the city's northern edge, claiming that uprooted residents would be welcome to build homes with straw (Figure 34.2).[11] In this way, officials split Dakar between an African city of straw and a European city of stone. One French public works inspector declared that sorting out residences in this way would help people "feel at home" in the post-plague city, but the colonial government used home design dictates to produce racial segregation without ever invoking racial categories.[12]

Discriminatory policies in colonial Dakar were built on long-standing links between race, urban reform, and domestic design. One of Senegal's head medical officials, Dr. Leon d'Anfreville de la Salle, invoked this association in a speech given in 1908. "One recognizes people's degree of civilization," d'Anfreville declared, "by the beauty of their dwellings."[13] This same association of cultural progress and home design informed popular representations of Dakar. Many widely circulated postcards contrasted the supposedly simplistic huts used by Dakar's African residents with the ornate stone villas housing the city's affluent European inhabitants (Figures 34.3 and 34.4). In 1914, plague-related paranoia imbued these critiques with a sense of urgency.

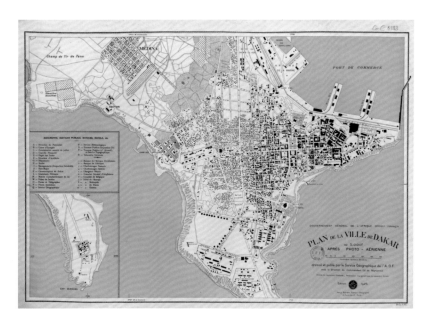

FIGURE 34.2: Map of Dakar indicating the location of the "Medina" in the city's northwestern edge, from Édouard de Martonne, *Plan de la ville de Dakar au 5.000e d'après photo-aérienne / dressé et publié par le Service géographique de l'A. O. F. sous la direction du Commandant Ed. de Martonne* (Paris, 1925). (Courtesy of the Bibliothèque Nationale de France.)

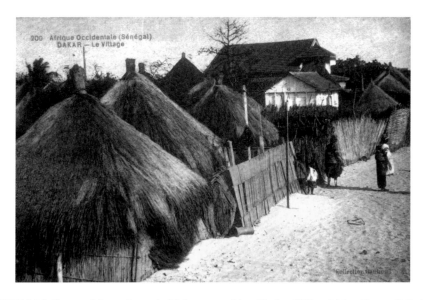

FIGURE 34.3: Postcard from the early 20th century identified as "West Africa (Senegal) Dakar – The Village." (Courtesy of the Archives Nationales du Sénégal.)

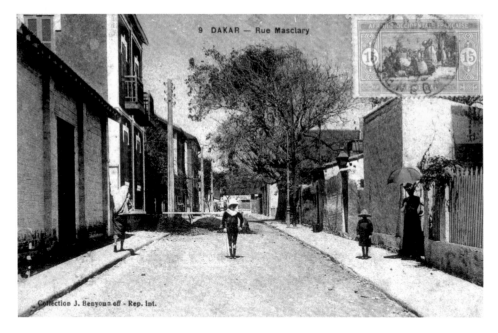

FIGURE 34.4: Postcard from the early 20th century identified as "Dakar – Masclary Street." (Courtesy of the Archives Nationales du Sénégal.)

Rumors circulated among French journalists and officials that Dakar's African residents were ignoring public health measures and burying dead relatives underneath their homes. "Do civilized people bury their dead in their huts," one journalist asked, "underneath a few centimeters of sand, at the foot of the bed of the living?"[14] Official archives do not record the frequency of home burials in Dakar during the plague, but regardless of their accuracy, descriptions of dead bodies beneath domestic floors turned African homes into perceived threats to the city's future. Saving Dakar from the plague meant displacing African residents and their dwellings.

Segregationist reforms caused massive disruptions to the lives of Dakar's African inhabitants. Colonial authorities burned any homes linked to plague diagnoses and hundreds of Senegalese houses went up in flames.[15] These incinerations were particularly upsetting to members of Dakar's Indigenous Lebu community, many of whom were enfranchised *originaires*. Many Lebu residents linked plague-related home destructions to decades of colonial land dispossession.[16] Urban reforms touted as public-health measures were often identified by Dakar's Lebu inhabitants as new tools in a long-standing French campaign to dominate the city.

This mix of suspicion and memory fueled widespread resistance to segregationist policies. Senegalese protestors and politicians frequently denounced home destructions. For five days in late May 1914, African workers brought the city to a standstill with the first general strike in French West Africa.[17] By July of that year, protest actions had achieved a settlement that slowed the rate of the ongoing house burnings and guaranteed a plot of land in the Medina for African residents who agreed to leave their homes. Homeowners also gained the right to indemnities for any destroyed property. Many officials hoped these measures would end the conflicts inspired by the colonial plague-control policies.[18] However, rather than withdrawing from anti-segregation protests, Senegalese residents used these promises to voice new critiques of government policies. As the plague and its destructive control measures traversed Dakar and Senegal more broadly, displaced residents used indemnity petitions to describe the consequences of plague-related home destructions. Patriarchs complained about losing the resources they needed to support dependents. Female household heads denounced the demolition of homes that provided the basis of their hard-fought autonomy.[19] Individuals used indemnity proceedings to document the losses caused by colonial health officials and urban planners. By debating the cost of a burned hut, bed, or crop bag, they demanded government support in rebuilding their lives.

Ultimately, widespread resistance and the assertion of the legal rights of the *originaires* prevented Dakar's total segregation. Thousands of Senegalese residents continued to live in what was intended to form the city's European quarter. Even those who did move to the Medina tried to shape their new urban environment to their own needs. Dozens of self-described "good citizens" filed a petition demanding that the government build the mosque and other public amenities that had been promised. These citizens emphasized that they had followed official health measures, even though compliance "forced us to leave the land where we were born, where our fathers lived and died, and where we hoped to stay ourselves."[20] They demanded that city planners respect these sacrifices and called on officials to build more public resources and to fulfill government promises to make the residents of the Medina "feel at home."

Conclusion

There was no quick end to the plague, nor to the debates about segregation that the plague had provoked. The plague became endemic to coastal Senegal and remained active for decades. French officials made home destructions their preferred measure of control, resulting in clashes over the discriminatory nature of public health and urban reform policies that influenced Senegalese politics for years. Colonial city officials in Dakar linked subsequent disease outbreaks to African homes as local newspapers and the minutes of municipal council meetings recorded colonists' revived calls to displace or destroy straw African dwellings.[21] In response, the city's African residents and their representatives invoked their right to live within the city and challenged racially discriminatory urban reforms and health policies.[22] Like the plague itself, battles over segregation remained part of Dakar's landscape long after 1914.

Pandemics can foment high-stakes confrontations about urban design, and health crises can incite battles between competing ideas about the government's role in managing urban landscapes. Urban built environments emerge out of both premade plans and unforeseen conflicts. The struggles that arose during the plague in Dakar in 1914 occurred in part because Senegalese residents and French officials held competing visions of how to construct and inhabit the city. French colonial planners used the language of public health to justify rearranging the city along racialized lines, separating Europeans in stone villas from Africans in straw huts. By contrast, Dakar's African residents argued that their legal status as *originaires* meant that they had a right to live where and how they saw fit. Dakar's plague and the colonial efforts to use disease to segregate the urban fabric transformed the city down to the very homes that lined the streets.

NOTES

1. Letter to Monsieur Gouverneur Général de l'Afrique Occidentale Française à Dakar, May 4, 1916, 3G2/160, Archives Nationales du Sénégal, Dakar.

2. Myron J. Echenberg, *Black Death, White Medicine: Bubonic Plague and the Politics of Public Health in Colonial Senegal, 1914-1945* (Portsmouth: Heinemann, 2002), 29.

3. Hilary Jones, *The Métis of Senegal: Urban Life and Politics in French West Africa* (Bloomington: Indiana University Press, 2013), 177–78.

4. Myron J. Echenberg, *Plague Ports: The Global Urban Impact of Bubonic Plague, 1894-1901* (New York: New York University Press, 2007), 6–9.

5. Echenberg, *Black Death, White Medicine*, 117.

6. Comité Local d'Hygiene Réunion du 7 Juillet, 1914, H73, Archives Nationales du Sénégal, Dakar, Senegal.

7. "A.S. de l'aménagement du nouveaux village de Dakar Le Lieutenant-Gouverneur p.i. du Sénégal à Monsieur le Gouverneur Général de l'Afrique Occidentale française," Saint-Louis July 18, 1915, 11D1-1284, Archives Nationales du Sénégal, Dakar, Senegal.

8. Maynard W. Swanson, "The Sanitation Syndrome: Bubonic Plague and Urban Native Policy in the Cape Colony, 1900–1909," *The Journal of African History* 18, no. 3 (1977): 387–410.

9. "Améliorations apporteees et à apporter à l'hygiène du Sénégal et surtout du port et de la ville de Dakar," Dakar, 19 Février 1915, 3G2-160, Archives Nationales du Sénégal, Dakar, Senegal.

10. "A.S. de l'aménagement du nouveaux village de Dakar Le Lieutenant-Gouverneur p.i. du Sénégal à Monsieur le Gouverneur Général de l'Afrique Occidentale française," Saint-Louis July 18, 1915, 11D1-1284, Archives Nationales du Sénégal, Dakar, Senegal.

11. Raymond F. Betts, "The Establishment of the Medina in Dakar, Senegal, 1914," *Africa: Journal of the International African Institute* 41, no. 2 (1971): 143–52.

12. "Envoi de deux projets de décret relatifs à Médina," September 16, 1916, 3G2-160, Archives Nationales du Sénégal, Dakar, Senegal.

13. Léon D'Anfreville de la Salle, *Conférences sur l'hygiène colonial, faites aux instituteurs et institutrices de Saint-Louis pour les élèves indigenes des colonies de l'Afriques occidentales (par M. le Dr. d'Anfreville. Préface de M. Camille Guy)* (Paris: A. Picard, 1908), 61.

14. "L'Elu et la Peste" *L.'A.O.F. Écho de la Cote Occidentale D'Afrique*, June 27, 1914, H-69, Archives Nationales du Sénégal, Dakar, Senegal.

15. Kalala J. Ngalamulume, *Colonial Pathologies, Environment, and Western Medicine in Saint-Louis-du-Senegal, 1867-1920* (New York: Peter Lang, 2012); Echenberg, *Black Death, White Medicine*, 99.

16. Elikia M'Bokolo, "Peste Et Société Urbaine à Dakar: L'épidémie De 1914" [The Plague and Urban Society in Dakar: The 1914 Epidemic], *Cahiers D'Études Africaines* 22, no. 85/86 (1982): 13–46.

17. Iba der Thiam, *Les Origines Du Mouvement Syndical Africain, 1790-1929* (Paris: L'Harmattan, 1993), 84–103.

18. Echenberg, *Black Death, White Medicine*, 75–84.

19. Examples of these indemnity claims from Dakar and other parts of Senegal can be found in files H-49, H-70, and H-78, Archives Nationales du Sénégal, Dakar, Senegal.

20. Letter to Monsieur Gouverneur Général de l'Afrique Occidentale Française à Dakar, May 4, 1916, 3G2-160, Archives Nationales du Sénégal, Dakar, Senegal.

21. For examples, see "Pour L'Assainissement de Dakar" *L'Ouest Africain Français: Organe Hebdomaire Socialiste*, December 26, 1927, SOM POM/f/645, Archives Nationales d'Outre-Mer, Aix-en-Provence, France; "Lutte Contre Les Taudis et Intervention de l'Office Des Habitations Economiques – Proces-Verbal de la conference tenue le 14 Décembre 1934 au Secretariat Général," December 14, 1934, Dakar, Senegal, 14Miom/2110 Archives Nationales d'Outre-Mer, Aix-en-Provence, France.

22. Aro Velmet, *Pasteur's Empire: Bacteriology and Politics in France, Its Colonies, and the World* (New York: Oxford University Press, 2020). See Chapter Six, "The Racial Politics of Microbes in Colonial Dakar," 170–88.

35

Urban Transformation and Public Health Policies in Post-Influenza Lagos, Nigeria, 1918

Timothy Oluseyi Odeyale

The city of Lagos, in the southwest corner of Nigeria, on the Gulf of Guinea, was the seat of government and the administrative headquarters of Nigeria during the colonial era. Lagos was annexed to the British Empire on August 6, 1861, following a series of invasions that began in 1851. Lagos was declared a colony on March 5, 1862. The Lagos colony was composed of Lagos Island, Iddo Island, Ebute Metta (The Three Harbours), Apapa, the neighborhood of Ikeja on the mainland, and the surrounding towns lying between the Lagoon and the Atlantic Ocean (Figure 35.1). Lagos later became the capital after the amalgamation of Northern and Southern Nigeria into the protectorate of Nigeria in 1914. Lagos's location and ports gave the city commercial importance and attracted people from the hinterland of Nigeria. The large concentration of settlers in Lagos led to the overcrowding of sites and dwellings, which contributed to poor sanitary conditions. Many houses and huts in the native areas were unfit for human habitation, which facilitated the spread of epidemic disease, especially during the influenza outbreak of 1918.

Influenza was first reported on the shores of Africa on August 15, 1918, having arrived in Freetown, Sierra Leone, then the capital of the British colony, with the armed merchant cruiser *HMS Mantua*. Two hundred of the ship's sailors, who had recently contracted influenza, reportedly came into close contact with a crew of hundreds of Sierra Leonean laborers as they loaded coal into the ship's bunkers. The ship set sail. Less than two weeks later, by August 24, 1918, the port's physicians started noticing many people with influenza-related symptoms. Shortly thereafter, two Freetowners died of pneumonia. Three days later, out of the 600 laborers who failed to appear for work, most were taking care of the sick or had succumbed to the disease themselves. In a similar story, the *SS Bida* arrived in the

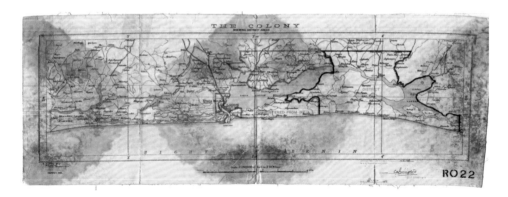

FIGURE 35.1: Map of Lagos Colony showing a densely populated area around the harbor of Lagos, *c.*1885–1920. (Courtesy of National Archives of Nigeria, Ibadan, Nigeria.)

Nigerian capital of Lagos from the Gold Coast (present-day Ghana) on September 14, docking with hundreds of infected passengers who quickly fanned out into Southern Nigeria and later spread the disease throughout the entire colony; just under five hundred thousand people died of influenza out of the entire colony of eighteen million (Figure 35.2).

The 1918–19 influenza pandemic, among the deadliest events in recorded human history, killed an estimated fifty million to one hundred million persons globally, five times more than the slaughter experienced during World War I.[1] The disease spread around the world, carried by troops deployed to fight in Europe, eventually making its way to Africa. A combination of the lack of adequate information and misinformation about the disease dispersed to the people by the colonial government also helped fuel the spread of the disease in the colony of Lagos. The colonial government focused more on World War I efforts than influenza, which greatly contributed to the lack of attention given to the disease.[2] This led to the local people looking inwardly to the use of herbs or potions, traditional medicine, and prayer houses for a solution.

Case study: Influenza in Lagos Colony, 1918

In parts of Lagos and the hinterland of Yoruba (an ethnic group of Western Africa) towns, the flu was known as *lukuluku* (killing by sudden stroke). Europeans were accused of bringing the infection. Deaths were so numerous in Lagos that desperate people dumped bodies on the streets or buried the dead in mass graves, both of which went against the culture of the Indigenous people of Lagos and Yorubaland. The disease affected people's sense of dignity and cultural sensibilities. It is difficult

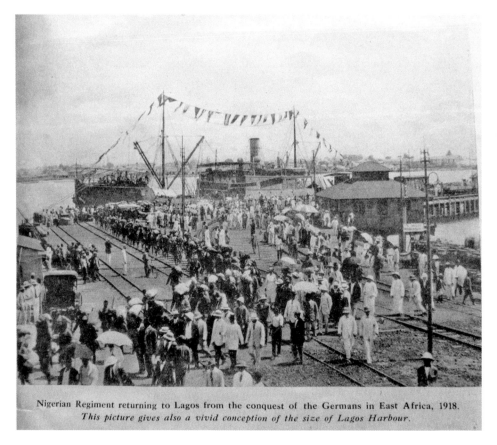

Nigerian Regiment returning to Lagos from the conquest of the Germans in East Africa, 1918.
This picture gives also a vivid conception of the size of Lagos Harbour.

FIGURE 35.2: Nigerian regiment returning to Lagos from victory over the Germans in East Africa in 1918, through the Lagos Harbor. (Courtesy of National Archives of Nigeria, Ibadan, Nigeria.)

to arrive at an accurate figure for the total dead, but the colonial administration attempted to derive an estimate based on the number of deaths reported in the Register of Death at each local colonial office. The 1918 colonial report notes that the death rate was highest among the impoverished and the illiterate. This was especially the case in the towns surrounding the greater Lagos colony, where medical aid was not available. The report asserts that an estimated 1.5 percent of the population of Lagos died of influenza between September 1918 and February 1919 (Figure 35.3).[3]

The living conditions and housing in towns and villages were often below a minimum standard, especially when compared to those seen in the areas where Europeans and colonials lived. Most of the population, especially in the old Lagos

Province	Total population	No of deaths	Percentage of deaths to population
Southern Province			
Lagos Township	82,000	1200	1.5
Lagos Colony excluding Lagos Township	148,000	2877	2.0
Abeokuta	328,000	3283	1.0
Benin	388,000	15,700	2.6
Calabar	1.182.500	35,175	2.9
Ogoja	923,360	62,832	6.8
Ondo	316,300	9490	3.0
Onitsha	1,970,000	39,510	2.0
Owerri	1,372,700	41,181	3.0
Oyo	1,550,000	29,750	1.9
Warri	614,400	14,663	2.3
Total	9,075,560	255,663	2.8
Northern Province			
Bauchi	949,461	17,102	1.8
Bornu	731.149	10,000	1.4
Ilorin	527,922	28.884	5.5
Kano	2,749,727	57,978	2.1
Kotangora	169,485	3580	2.1
Munshi	569,944	6695	1.2
Muri	222,258	6003	2.7
Nassarawa	266,248	10,442	3.9
Nupe	266,548	10,684	3.2
Sokoto	1,516,326	30,000	1.1
Yola	259,056	11,181	4.3
Zaria	327,242	6776	2.1
Total	8,615,376	199,325	2.3

Source: Public Record Office (PRO), C0583/77. 5 September 1919.
Reported by J. Beringer and M. Cameron Blair

FIGURE 35.3: Table of the colonial government record of death in the Lagos colony and other parts of colonial Nigeria in 1918–19. (Public Record Office, domiciled at National Archives of Nigeria, Ibadan, Nigeria.)

metropolis, lived in an unplanned, crowded, squalid, and unsanitary environment. Houses were not properly ventilated and many people lived next to open sewers.[4] The flu spread easily in these areas and among those that lived in such poor sanitary conditions. The squalid conditions of the houses and the environment could cause influenza victims to develop secondary infections that were likely to lead to death. As a result of the influenza outbreak, schools, shops, and all public places were closed in Lagos and other parts of Nigeria. The influenza epidemic in Africa was devastating. In many cases, entire households were infected, leaving only one or two persons to nurse or take care of others; in other cases, whole families succumbed to the disease without anyone to care for them. Hospitals and local dispensaries were quickly overwhelmed.

A series of epidemics in the colonies alerted the colonial authorities to the health problems of the people they governed. As a result, the colonial administration of Lagos instituted many sanitary reforms, such as the provision of pipe-borne water (mostly in the larger, regional capitals), town planning, swamp reclamation, and drainage. The colonial government in Lagos enacted the Public Health Ordinance and Rules to promote the cause of sanitation and enforced a program of Building Regulation to help with the proper layout of streets and drains. For example, under the Public Health Ordinance, new wells for water could not be dug in Lagos without permission from the Medical Officer of Health, who was appointed by the Colonial board of Lagos Town Council.[5]

Prior to 1918, West Africa faced shortages of doctors and nurses. The reform activities of the colonial government led to the development and expansion of medical and health services with large increases in the numbers of medical and subordinate staff. The epidemic of 1918 prompted the colonial government to institute networks of local dispensaries, mostly in rural towns and villages that were staffed with Indigenous doctors, nurses, auxiliary health workers, environmental sanitation officers, and sanitary health inspectors called *wole wole* (literally those who "poke [their] nose" to inspect the house and its environment). In the Lagos colony, the sanitary inspector wielded so much power over the populace and it was considered wise to have the fear of the *wole wole*.[6] The sanitary inspectors were trained by the colonial medical officers and were charged with delivering lectures, holding routine sanitary demonstrations for the local people, and charging those who broke the sanitation rules.[7] As a result of the influenza pandemic, elementary hygiene and sanitation were taught in the schools of the large towns under the watchful eyes of government officials.[8]

One of the dangers of a new influenza virus that leads to a pandemic is that the population has not previously been exposed and does not have any immunity. This results in a very high number of people becoming sick. During the 1918 influenza outbreak in Lagos, the railway system and modern transportation network helped to spread the disease, from the coast of Lagos to towns and provinces in to the hinterlands of Nigeria. The colonial administration introduced various segregation plans for townships across the Lagos colony, vestiges of which still exist till today. The colonial government began the introduction of town planning and the expansion of Lagos, from the city's islands to the mainland, including Ebute Metta in the greater Lagos area. In major Nigerian cities and towns, separate zones were introduced for Europeans. The British colonists and their immediate families were separated from the Indigenous population into Government Reserve Areas (GRAs). The GRAs in Nigeria following independence in 1960 have metamorphosed into modern housing zones for government officials and high-ranking people in the society. Yet, the broader question of ensuring adequate housing and infrastructure for Nigeria's population remains largely unresolved.

Conclusion

The 1918 influenza epidemic impinged on Nigerian society and its built environment. It was only following the impact of the epidemic that various missionary groups and private agencies established hospitals and dispensaries and several urban sanitary reforms, including the provision of pipe-borne water, drainage, swamp reclamation, and town planning measures. During the height of influenza in Lagos, the only safe place from contagion was considered to be inside a building, and residents were told to remain indoors. The only recourse for Nigerians was to avoid public spaces, such as town squares and large gatherings, and to quarantine.

The successful response to and conclusion of any pandemic requires medical intervention, including vaccination, as well as social design intervention, including the proper management of urban spaces and the built environment. However, it should be stressed that pandemics may end without these interventions but would take longer and almost inevitably lead to more death and disease. The 1918 influenza outbreak was largely left to run its course in Nigeria, which led to the deaths of many. The epidemic of 1918–19 alerted the colonial authorities to the need to pay attention to the sanitary and health needs of the Lagos colony and the people they governed. Some of the measures introduced in the Lagos colony were later adopted in other parts of West Africa, such as Accra in the Gold Coast colony (Ghana) and Freetown in the Sierra Leone colony. The changes in town planning rules and sanitary measures in Lagos led to greater progress and improvement in local health measures not only in the colonial city but also across different parts of Nigeria.

NOTES

1. The 1918–19 influenza pandemic has been attributed to a hyper-virulent influenza strain of the H1N1 subtype. Many influenza experts, policy-makers, and knowledgeable observers believe that a novel influenza A/H1N1 strain caused most of the deaths during the 1918–19 pandemic and that the source of this virus was avian. David Morens and Anthony Fauci, "The 1918 Influenza Pandemic: Insights for the 21st Century," *Journal of Infectious Diseases* 195, no. 7 (2007): 1018–28.

2. Florence E. Nkwam, "British Medical and Health Policies in West Africa C1920–1960," (Ph.D. thesis, University of London School of Oriental and African Studies, 1988).

3. See Colonial Reports-Annual. No- 1030. Nigeria. Report for 1918, presented to parliament by His Majesty Command April, 1920 (London: Published by His Majesty's Stationery Office). See also: A. D. Milne, "The Rise of a Colonial Medical Service," *The East African Medical Journal* 5, no. 1 (1928–29): 50–58; E. Burnet and W. R. Aykroyd, "Nutrition and Public Health," *Quarterly Bulletin of the Health Organization of the League of Nations* 4 (June 1935): 1–140; T. S. Gale, "British Medical and Health Policy in West Africa 1870-1930" (Ph.D. diss., University of London, 1976); G. W. Hartwig, "Health Policies and National Development in Kenya" (Ph.D. diss., University of Kentucky, 1975); D. G. Meredith, "The British Government and Colonial Economic Development with Particular Reference to West Africa" (Ph.D. diss., Exeter, 1976); C. R. Nordman, "Prelude to Decolonization in West Africa: The Development of British Colonial Policy, 1938-1947" (D. Phil., Oxford, 1976); Laura Spinney, *Pale Rider: The Spanish Flu of 1918 and how it Changed the World* (New York: Vintage, 2018), 36. Martin F. Shapiro, "Medicine in the Service of Colonialism: Medical Care in Portuguese Africa 1885–1974" (Ph.D. diss., University of California, Los Angeles, 1983); William N. M. Geary, Nigeria under British Rule (London: Methuen, 1927); Michael Crowder, West Africa under Colonial Rule (London: Hutchinson, 1970).

4. Liora Bigon, "Sanitation and Street Layout in Early Colonial Lagos: British and Indigenous Conceptions, 1851-1890," *Planning Perspectives* 20, no. 3 (2005): 247–69. See also Akin Mabogunje, "Lagos-Nigeria's Melting Pot." *Nigeria Magazine* 69 (1961): 128–55; Liora Bigon, "Bubonic Plague, Colonial Ideologies, and Urban Planning Policies: Dakar, Lagos, and Kumasi," *Planning Perspectives* 31, no. 2 (2016): 205–26.

5. Ayodeji Olukoju, "Population Pressure, Housing and Sanitation in Metropolitan Lagos: 1900–1939," in *Urban Transition in Africa: Aspects of Urbanization and Change in Lagos*, ed. Kunle Lawal (Lagos: Pumark Limited, 1994), 34–49.

6. Sandra Tomkins, "Colonial administration in British Africa during the influenza epidemic of 1918–19," *Canadian Journal of African Studies/La Revue Canadienne des Études Africaines* 28, no. 1 (1994): 60–83.

7. Ralph Schram, *A History of the Nigerian Health Services* (Ibadan: University Press, 1971).

8. Evelyn E. Sabben-Clare, David J. Bradley, and Kenneth Kirkwood, eds., *Health in Tropical Africa during the Colonial Period* (Oxford: Clarendon Press, 1980).

36

Urban Landscape Transformations and the Malaria Control Scheme in Mauritius, 1948–51

Nicole de Lalouvière

The malaria outbreak in Mauritius in 1865 set off a century-long battle with the disease on this small island, located approximately 800 kilometers (500 miles) to the east of Madagascar. Mauritius had no native inhabitants and thus provided a safe haven for commerce along trade routes running through the Indian Ocean. Various strains of malaria may have been imported to Mauritius prior to 1865 by slave ships originating from Madagascar or East Africa, indentured laborers from India, or British military personnel traveling through the colony.[1] Between 1866 and 1868, 13 percent of the population was killed by malaria (43,000 deaths out of a population of 330,000).[2] The cause of the disease was misunderstood until 1898, when British medical doctor Ronald Ross established the link between *Plasmodium* parasites, which cause malaria, and their carrier: the *Anopheles* mosquito.[3] Unlike bacteria and viruses, endoparasites like *Plasmodium* cannot survive outside a living host, making the elimination of the mosquito vector key to a successful eradication strategy for malaria.

The principal reason for the epidemic outbreak of 1865 remains unclear: it may have been due to population growth, new steamship transportation routes, deforestation, the growth of the sugarcane estates, genetic mutations and the emergence of new virulent forms of malaria, or all of the above.[4] There is little doubt that the intensification of landscape use (anthropization) in Mauritius was a crucial condition in the eruption of the disease. The establishment of a sugarcane monoculture entailed vast land use change, deforestation, the construction of canalization and road-building infrastructure, and the erection of new structures including factories and housing for day laborers. The transformation of the Mauritian landscape created the environmental conditions that allowed malaria to spread.[5] Alongside these landscape transformations, internal migrations took place as a result of the

efforts by inhabitants to escape malarial risk zones. This led to the urban reconfiguration of the island's settlements.

In spite of widespread larviciding campaigns and extensive civil works initiated in
1908, the disease still posed a threat by midcentury, particularly in the warm coastal
lowlands. Indeed, in the 40 years following the outbreak of 1865, 5,000–10,000
new malaria deaths were recorded annually in Mauritius. In response, the British
colonial powers and the local Mauritius government implemented the Malaria Control Scheme, an element of which was the Indoor Residual Spraying (IRS) campaign
of 1948–51. These efforts eradicated malaria as an endemic disease in Mauritius,
while also radically reshaping the landscape and urban fabric of the island as whole.

Case study: From sanitation works to indoor residual spraying in Mauritius

The malarial outbreak of 1865 led to the decimation of the population in the capital city of Port Louis and the reconfiguration of the island's urban spaces. Fleeing
disease, inhabitants left the coastal capital for the towns of the high plateau such
as Curepipe, Vacoas, and Quatre Bornes. This internal migration was supported by
a new rail connection that allowed commuting from residential to urban centers,
and as a result, the less economically stable Indo-Mauritian inhabitants, originally
brought to the island as indentured laborers, were able to acquire property in the
lowlands.[6] However, these areas remained high-risk zones for malaria, a disease
that was still poorly understood.

Physician Ronald Ross, a leading malaria expert, undertook an island-wide
epidemiological survey of Mauritius (Figure 36.1). Ross delivered his final report
in 1908, in which he recommended works of environmental "bonification." This
entailed ecological, infrastructural, and landscape interventions on both micro and
macro levels, with the aim of eliminating instances of standing water. Sanitation
works included bush-clearing, watercourse canalizations, and marsh drainage.[7]
Ross established the basis for decades of national larviciding campaigns, concerning himself not just with epidemiology but also with the financial and legal
pragmatics of the required civil works. By advocating for the drainage of the
Clairfond Marsh in the central highlands, Ross argued for the importance of saving
Curepipe, a nearby town to which many inhabitants of Port-Louis had previously
relocated (Figure 36.2). He stressed the urgency of addressing the malaria outbreak because it threatened one the island's wealthiest urban areas, established as
a safe haven in the cooler climatic zone of the highlands. Thanks to painstaking
larviciding campaigns set out by Ross, by the mid-twentieth century, Port Louis
and the central plateau were almost free of malaria.[8]

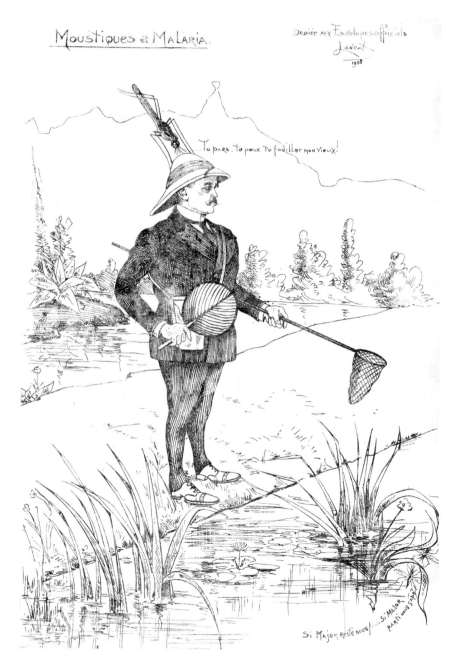

FIGURE 36.1: Cartoon published in local newspaper on Ronald Ross' departure from Mauritius, 1908. Figure from Leonard J. Bruce-Chwatt and Joan M. Bruce-Chwatt, "Malaria in Mauritius - as Dead as the Dodo," *Bulletin of the New York Academy of Medicine* 50, no. 10 (November 1974): 1078. (Courtesy of the London School of Hygiene & Tropical Medicine.)

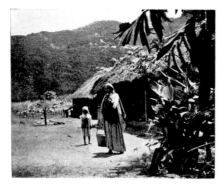

PHOTO. 9.—Indian's House. By Miss Lane.

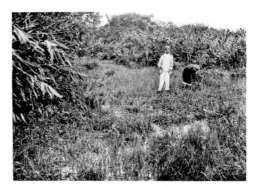

PHOTO. 11.—Moustiquiers at work in Marsh at Curepipe.

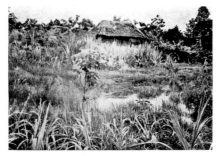

PHOTO. 10.—Indian's House near Clairfond Marsh.

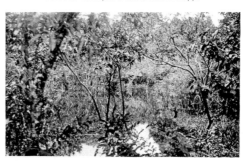

PHOTO. 12.—Marsh in Wood at Phœnix.

FIGURE 36.2: Breeding places of *Anopheles* mosquitoes at Clairfond Marsh, Curepipe, Phoenix. Photographs from Ronald Ross, *Report on the Prevention of Malaria in Mauritius* (London: J. & A. Churchill, 1908), 193–94. (https://wellcomecollection.org/works/rjj6m9qm. Courtesy of the London School of Hygiene & Tropical Medicine.)

However, in spite of extensive larviciding campaigns, malaria remained a threat in the coastal plains. This led the United Kingdom's Colonial Insecticides Committee to send a team to Mauritius and launch the Malaria Control Scheme (1948–51). The program further strengthened the island's urban and ethnic segregation through the implementation of the "MacGregor line" as a planning tool.[9] This line, approximately equivalent to the topographic line drawn at 1,000 feet above sea level, was derived from the island's physical geography: it mapped distinct climatic differences between the cooler and rainier central plateau, and the warmer and drier coastal plains (Figure 36.3). Based on empirical findings that had reliably established temperature as an important limiting factor in the spread of malaria, the "MacGregor line" demarcated at-risk/undesirable zones in the coastal lowlands, and safe/desirable zones in the central highlands.[10] This demarcation guided the distribution of financial and labor resources within the operations of the IRS campaign.

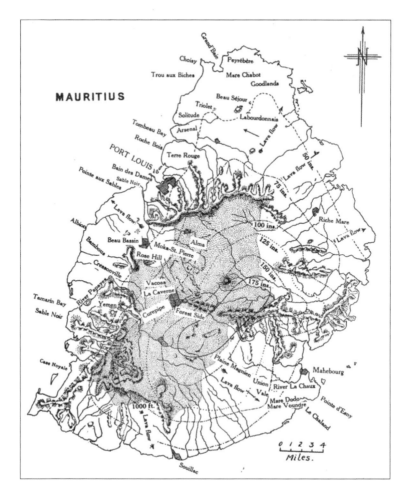

FIGURE 36.3: Map of Mauritius showing topography, rainfall, and main settlements, *c.*1947. Figure from W. F. Jepson, A. Moutia, and C. Courtois, "The Malaria Problem in Mauritius: The Bionomics of Mauritian Anophelines," *Bulletin of Entomological Research* 38, no. 1 (May 1947): 178. (Reproduced with permission from Cambridge University Press.)

The Malaria Control Scheme was led by British physician M. A. C Dowling, who directed a nationwide network of field officers, each with their team of "moustiquiers." These teams conducted indoor Dichlorodiphenyltrichloroethane (DDT) residual spraying for three consecutive years on a seasonal basis. The "MacGregor line" was translated into a zoning instrument. It differentiated areas to be sprayed with insecticides from the "unsprayed central zone" of the wealthier, residential area located on the cooler central plateau (Figure 36.4). Thus, climatic zoning used in the

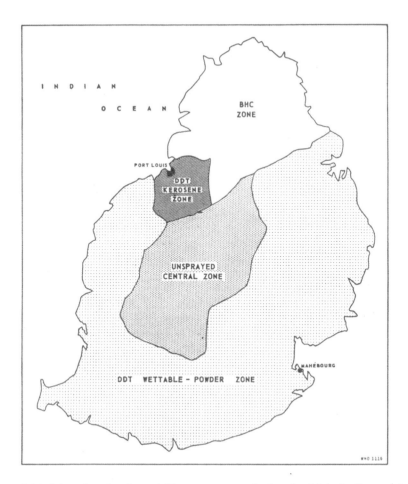

FIGURE 36.4: Map showing insecticide spray zones during the Malaria Control Scheme (1948–1951). Figure from M. A. C. Dowling, "An Experiment in the Eradication of Malaria in Mauritius," *Bulletin of the World Health Organization* 4, no. 3 (1951): 446. (Creative Commons BY 3.0 IGO.)

implementation of public health measures segregated the island along the lines of wealth, class, and ethnicity. Modest homes were subject to repeated insecticide spraying, while residences with painted walls (a sign of wealth) received special treatment. In these cases, in order to avoid staining the walls, the usual DDT wettable powder was replaced with the less destructive DDT solution in kerosene.[11] Particular operational challenges arose as the national public health measures were brought into the domestic realm. The following description by Dowling outlines the obstacles to spraying related to domestic furnishings, vernacular construction materials, and customary building practices:

317

It was the practice of spray gangs to cover all furniture and furnishings as thoroughly as possible to protect them from the spray. This procedure consumed a good deal of time as the average house contained a formidable array of bric-à-brac, but it was an important factor in maintaining the goodwill of the inhabitants. The custom of re-plastering the interior walls of houses immediately before the New Year, chiefly among the Indian community, presented a very serious obstacle, as this redecoration took place soon after spraying had been completed and at the beginning of the malaria epidemic season. A third difficulty was that spraying took place of necessity during the gathering of the sugar crop. Many families made their way at dawn to the cane-fields, leaving their houses locked, to return at dusk after the day's work.[12]

Although it was reported that only three households were prosecuted for refusal to allow entry during the spraying, the campaigns clearly entailed serious disruptions to work and domestic life, especially among day laborers.[13] The Malaria Control Scheme granted colonial authorities the right to enter the private domestic sphere and to repeatedly apply highly toxic substances to all building surfaces within the risk zones. The campaign was ultimately successful: by 1952, *Anopheles funestus* was considered eradicated through spraying, while *Anopheles gambiae* was being controlled by larviciding.[14] The local population saw a ten-year improvement in life expectancy, and malaria efforts switched to surveillance and treatment of imported cases. Local transmission came to a halt in 1969.[15]

Conclusion

The Malaria Control Scheme in Mauritius and the environmental control efforts that led up to it illustrate how advances in public health were deeply intertwined with landscape transformations and urban reconfigurations. Changes in the landscape and urban settlements were both cause and consequence of the spread of disease. Indeed, Mauritius's initial malaria outbreak of 1865 occurred in the context of widespread land use change linked to the establishment of the sugarcane monoculture. Part of the initial larviciding response utilized landscape interventions and civil works to eliminate mosquito breeding sites, systematically altering or destroying existing wetland ecosystems. Climatic zoning that differentiated warm coastal lowlands from the cool central plateau guided public health efforts, triggered internal human migrations, and firmly established the desirability of the highlands as a residential area. Together, this produced a large agglomeration of residential towns in the highlands, which remains a feature of the island's urban character to this day.

This demarcation based on climatic zoning would later be cemented through the implementation of the IRS campaign, which disproportionately affected inhabitants of the warmer coastal plains. Although it was successful in epidemiological terms, it further strengthened the divide between safe and danger zones in the urban environment. The malarial campaigns had a negative impact on marginalized members of society and intensified socio-economic and ethnic disparities. The malaria eradication scheme in Mauritius reveals how public health policies, especially those based on landscape interventions and territorial zoning, can exacerbate the inequitable effects of epidemiology and play an unanticipated role within urban planning. Further changes to the island's ecology, including the remediation of indigenous habitats, might likewise disrupt current environmental conditions and uncover new epidemiological threats. These impacts must be addressed through coordinated ecological, landscape, and urban planning approaches.

NOTES

1. For evidence of malaria on Mauritius before 1865, see Raj Boodhoo, *Health, Disease and Indian Immigrants in Nineteenth Century Mauritius* (Port Louis: Aapravasi Ghat Trust Fund, 2010), 173–91.

2. Leonard J. Bruce-Chwatt and Joan M. Bruce-Chwatt, "Malaria in Mauritius - as Dead as the Dodo," *Bulletin of the New York Academy of Medicine* 50, no. 10 (November 1974): 1075.

3. Ronald Ross, *Report on the Prevention of Malaria in Mauritius* (London: J. & A. Churchill, 1908), 24–29. For more on various *Plasmodium* parasites likely present in Mauritius, see: Edward A. Alpers, "Chikungunya and Epidemic Disease in the Indian Ocean World," in *Disease Dispersion and Impact in the Indian Ocean World*, ed. Gwyn Campbell and Eva-Maria Knoll, (Cham: Springer International, 2020), 222.

4. See ibid., 224.

5. See graph linking the establishment of a sugarcane monoculture to the malaria epidemic outbreak in: Jean Julvez, Jean Mouchet, and C. Ragavoodoo, "Epidémiologie Historique Du Paludisme Dans l'Archipel Des Mascareignes (Océan Indien)," *Annales Des Sociétés Belges de Médicine Tropicale, de Parasitologie et de Mycologie Humaine et Animale* 70, no. 4 (1990): 257. Ira Klein ties mortality due to malaria to British infrastructure development. Ira Klein, "Development and Death: Reinterpreting Malaria, Economics and Ecology in British India," *The Indian Economic & Social History Review* 38, no. 2 (June 1, 2001): 147–79.

6. Wolfgang Lutz and Anne Babette Wils, "People on Mauritius: 1638–1991," in *Population-Development - Environment: Understanding Their Interactions in Mauritius*, ed. Wolfgang Lutz et al. (Berlin: Springer-Verlag, 1994), 79.

7. Ross differentiates minor from major civil works. Ross, *Report on the Prevention of Malaria*, 113.

8. Ministry of Health and Quality of Life Mauritius and World Health Organization and the University of California, San Francisco, "Eliminating Malaria: Case Study 4. Preventing Reintroduction in Mauritius" (Geneva: The World Health Organization, 2012), 12.

9. The "MacGregor line" is named after entomologist Malcolm MacGregor. See his *Mosquito Surveys: A Handbook for Anti-Malarial and Anti-Mosquito Field Workers* (London: Baillière, Tindall & Cox, 1927). The appellation "MacGregor line" is employed in W. F. Jepson, A. Moutia, and C. Courtois, "The Malaria Problem in Mauritius: The Bionomics of Mauritian Anophelines," *Bulletin of Entomological Research* 38, no. 1 (May 1947): 185.

10. Ibid.

11. Ministry of Health and Quality of Life Mauritius and World Health Organization and the University of California, San Francisco, "Eliminating Malaria," 14.

12. M. A. C. Dowling, "The Malaria Eradication Scheme in Mauritius," *British Medical Bulletin* 8, no. 1 (January 1, 1951): 72.

13. Ministry of Health and Quality of Life Mauritius and World Health Organization and the University of California, San Francisco, "Eliminating Malaria," 13.

14. Lutz and Wils, "People on Mauritius," 72-3.

15. "When malaria was eradicated, life expectancy jumped by more than 10 years to 50 and 52 for men and women, respectively, in 1952–1953." Ibid., 90.

EPILOGUE

Right page: Social distancing circles at Domino Park, New York City. (Photograph by Jaclyn Skidmore, March 2021.)

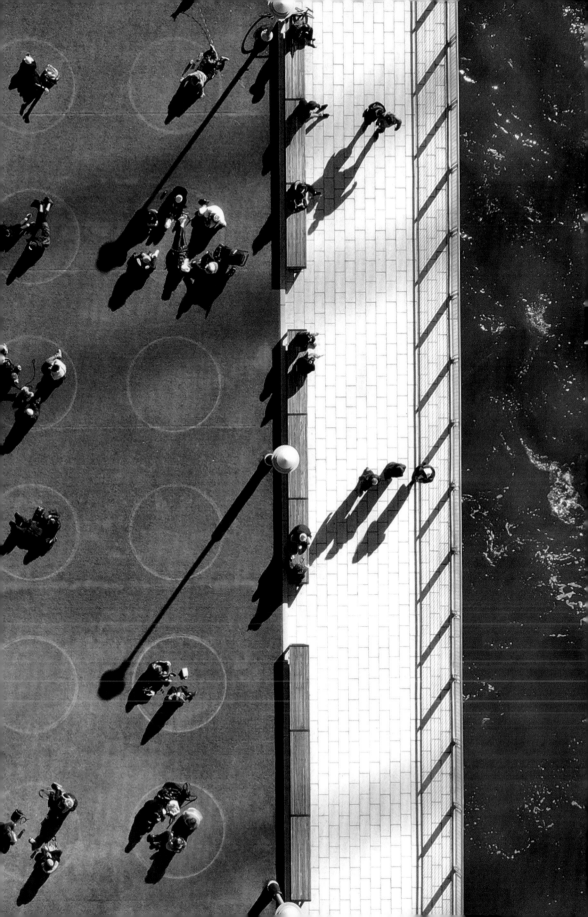

Epilogue:
Post-COVID Urbanism and Architecture

Richard J. Jackson

Learning *about* the past is important, but learning *from* the past is urgent.

The fine collection of essays in this volume on epidemics and urbanism teaches us that people, governments, and civilizations must learn from pandemics across the planet and across the centuries. As a physician who has served in a variety of public health leadership positions, I find these histories illuminating and at times astonishing. My own experience includes serving as the State Public Health Officer for California as well as the Director of the Centers for Disease Control and Prevention's National Center for Environmental Health in the United States. Disasters and epidemics tear away the cloak from comfortable social structures and daily routines. The public's demand for a "return to normal" and to "the way things were before" can rarely be met. And just as the adage "knowledge maketh a bloody entrance" suggests, a good deal of what these elegantly presented facts and studies have to teach us is distressing.

As I reviewed this volume, the churning confluence of the most noble and the most despicable aspects of human behavior became evident to me. Many people living through epidemics embody a spectrum of traits, even fluctuating between polar opposite behaviors from hour to hour. On the positive side, some epidemic histories illuminate persons with a deep regard for preventing human suffering by maintaining social order, by building hospitals and care facilities for the sick and dying, by assuring food and other support for the starving and destitute, and by bringing gentle care to those who are traumatized and bereft. At the other extreme, we see humanity's most negative traits: ignorance, greed, cruelty, and racism. Over the centuries, in some cultures there was a belief that those who lived in dank, impoverished, dangerous conditions were subjected to that way of life not because of social structures and misfortune but because God thought of them as unworthy. And if God judged them in this way, then those in power could or even should do the same. Sadly, such archaic beliefs persist today.

Epidemics are inevitable, in part because humans cannot survive in aseptic environments. Species have proliferated and collapsed across biological history; likewise the organisms that cause illness in humans smolder for years at low levels of virulence and contagion, and with environmental or social change can erupt into epidemics. While biology imposes its own, inescapable priorities, its cycles often come as a shock to human society, if not to those who study these natural phenomena. Humanity faced its last acutely infectious pandemic in 1918, in the form of H1N1 influenza, misnomered the "Spanish" flu in the United States as it was associated with soldiers returning from the European front of World War I. Indeed, the source of such threats is more comfortably conferred upon the "other." Yet, there are no guarantees of a century-long reprieve before the next pandemic visitation.

Pandemic control methods of the past included quarantine practices for visitors and the ill, or countering contagion by fleeing infected areas. Indifference, namely in the acceptance of large die-offs of susceptible humans and animals, was another approach to epidemics, which often tapered off as human victims and vectors, such as the flea infested rats during the Black Death plague, succumbed to the disease. The tuberculosis epidemic of 19th-century England was attenuated by high lethality among the young, resulting in the early deaths of the six Brontë siblings, including the extraordinary authors Emily, Charlotte, and Anne. Herd immunity, which results when 80 percent of the population has achieved immunity thereby slowing or halting transmission to those without immunity, has attenuated epidemics including polio and measles. Finally, the elimination of specific vectors such as black flies in the case of river blindness, and mosquitoes for arboviral diseases, can suppress outbreaks.

Biology endlessly provides the planet with new organisms, including pathogens, and nature is engaged in a series of ruthless experiments to determine which species will survive. For example, at the end of the Cretaceous period 66 million years ago, the tree of life was cut to the stump as many species, including dinosaurs, were lost, yet other species soon emerged. In the current (and potentially very brief) Anthropocene period, human survival will likely depend more on the care of the planet and of each other than one's individual bodily fitness for existence.

Among the lessons that I gleaned from this volume are that epidemics are costly, demand new physical infrastructure, and require strong governance and effective leadership with an impetus for well-being and a narrative of recovery.

Cost: When leaders fail to recognize that epidemics are costly in terms of societal and personal wealth, workforce capacity, prestige, and resiliency against other threats, the population suffers. Past experience teaches that scientists must prepare for epidemics through tracking and surveying disease, improving rapid diagnostic tools, and developing treatments. In addition, the treatments should be as effective at protecting caregivers as they are at improving the patient's condition. It is equally important to head off inevitable, future epidemics by creating physical infrastructure to help mitigate risks. Advanced societies invest in providing safe, and ideally, abundant water supplies. Humans and their food and drinking water must be separated from waste, a need that is often neglected leading up to and in the early stages of an epidemic. The entire population requires adequate supplies of safe food, but nursing mothers, young children, the disabled, and the elderly experience the most urgent need. Epidemics continue and can be prolonged when emergency supplies are contaminated, for example, by the introduction of the cholera organism to emergency water deliveries or by toxicants in outdated food supplies. As a result, the public becomes mistrustful, and the social order disintegrates. The economic harms from the loss of critical members of the population, for example, young parents, require financial subvention and support from public funds. Whenever possible, vulnerable populations, especially children, must be protected.

New Physical Infrastructure: There are important roles for the built environment in responding to such threats. Structures should protect inhabitants from the elements, minimize moisture and pest intrusion, and hold water and food sources safe from contamination. Malaria is the leading global cause of infectious disease deaths, and preventing that disease requires exclusion of mosquitoes from dwellings and sleeping areas, as well as the elimination of mosquito incubation sources like standing water. Purpose-built hospitals and hospices are essential, although very large epidemics inevitably require preexisting public structures like sports stadiums and armories to be repurposed for clinical care. In situations of large-scale death, mortuary facilities are also essential to maintain health and social order.

Governance and Leadership: Epidemics require strong governance. Disorder and lawlessness can have lethal consequences that are rarely controlled by mere words. In disasters, there is a human desire to seek scapegoats, a distraction that is doomed to fail. Decisions based on good science and best available data are essential. It is important for there to be a trusted leader, preferably one who has a vision of recovery. Researchers have found during recent major disasters that a public narrative of recovery is essential. Under effective governance, societies are able to make increasing use of preventive measures such as immunization, disease surveillance, and clinical treatment. Population growth and mobility is a factor. In the 50 years following the first moon landing in 1969, the global population more than doubled; 56 percent of the global population is urban at the time of writing. Over the same period, air transport passenger numbers increased nearly tenfold, reaching 4.4 billion in 2020.[1] The vast increase in population density and movement has enabled novel infections originating in remote settings to spread globally with astonishing lethality and speed.

The Future

Population density and increased travel and crowding due to urbanization tend to enhance disease spread. While urbanization brings benefits such as opportunities for education, employment, women's empowerment, and a reduction in the pressure to create the large families needed in subsistence agriculture, it also brings challenges. Proximity is one challenge as everyone who has tried to practice distancing as a method of disease prevention has learned. It is unclear whether the immense increase of intercontinental travel will continue to accelerate following the COVID-19 pandemic. As audiovisual technology grows increasingly effective at simulating in-person meetings and the need to reduce the human carbon footprint increases, it may be that business travel will never return to previous levels. Prior to the pandemic, tourist travel generated about 10 percent of travel revenues, but it remains to be seen whether humans will again seek to experience different cultures and geographies in such numbers. It is likely that people will continue to return to travel patterns to join family and visit familiar settings for celebrations and life transitions.

Climate change and attendant drought, famine, floods, intolerable heat, and the presence of new disease vectors, for example, malarial mosquitoes at higher altitudes and latitudes, will drive population movement. Large human migrations of impoverished and persecuted peoples will amplify fears of new diseases in previously unexposed regions and vulnerable populations. The jingoistic notion that "foreigners" bring disease has generated fearsome pogroms and backlash. Thoughtful leaders will work toward humane responses, but anxious populations have been and will continue to be exploited by would-be dictators and their followers as they act in ways to demonize minoritized racial groups and immigrants.

Increasing water levels due to climate change will require construction above anticipated flood levels, net-zero energy use must be nonnegotiable, and structures will need to be served by protected utility infrastructure. Among the lessons from the COVID-19 epidemic is the benefit of adequate daylight, outdoor space, and ventilation. Modern hospitals now strive to have "one pass" air-handling systems while limiting heating and cooling costs by using high-efficiency heat exchangers. Such systems must also be employed in homes, schools, work places, restaurants, and other public settings. Viricidal ultraviolet-C (UV-C) light can also be used to reduce the airborne viral load. With the advance of air-quality threats, for example, those generated by the massive wildfires in the western United States in 2020, many homes are now equipped with high-efficiency air filtration systems.

New realities including global climate change bring other epidemic threats. Scientists studying the global thawing of boreal permafrost worry about the release of not only deep-frozen greenhouse gases but also pathogens that have long been locked in the ground. I predict that the threat to humans from such organisms will likely be manageable, but the impacts on other species, including migrating herbivores, could be catastrophic.

Human-made threats will loom large. The benefits of antibiotics, the "wonder drugs" of the mid-20th century, are being squandered at an alarming rate. Increasing numbers of patients suffer from multidrug resistant infections. Immense amounts of antibiotics are used in agriculture, both to treat active disease in individual animals and as feed additives to promote fattening and growth. Epidemiological studies have uncovered serious infections in humans from antibiotic resistant organisms associated with overuse in agriculture. For example, a child who sustained mere skin scratches at home went on to develop fulminant infections requiring intensive care; the infecting organism was resistant to the five antibiotics used in hog feeding operations just a few miles away.

Laboratories worldwide contain dangerous pandemic-threat-level organisms. The smallpox virus, arguably the most lethal virus in human history, is still contained in highly secure facilities in the United States and Russia. Many laboratories have *Bacillus anthracis* (anthrax), *Yersinia pestis* (plague), *Clostridia botulinum* (botulism), and numerous other pathogens in storage. These organisms need to be used for study, not merely to prepare for outbreaks of the specific agent, but to examine their utility in other circumstances. Viruses understood to be common, such as the highly infectious common cold coronavirus, have the potential to be genetically combined with lethal zoonotic viruses, for example, those seen in bats. Laboratory security and safety may sound routine and ordinary, but the world continues to learn that these controls are a matter of life and death, not merely to the laboratorians but to entire cities and populations.

Human-made threats are a part of a continuum with natural threats. Humanity must embrace genomic manipulation cautiously. The genomics revolution has brought human benefits, for example, mRNA-based vaccines that can stimulate antibodies that respond to the proteins on the surface of the SARS CoV-2 virus. Predictably, the potential to create dangerous scenarios appear here as well, including the ability of a laboratory to synthesize a dangerous virus simply by using DNA sequence data. Smallpox killed 300 million people in the 20th century. The biotech firm Tonix synthesized the related horsepox virus by utilizing published data on its DNA sequence. The ability of malign actors to create new or older viral threats is a reality.

Future historians will research epidemics that come in many forms. The lessons learned in the last generation, and in the last 30 generations, cannot be ignored. Civic leaders must develop ongoing, all-hazard preparedness. Governmental agencies, private industry, and the academy must recruit and develop superb scientific, medical, and academic experts who possess strong ethical commitments to service and duty. And architects and historians must be among the scenario planners and disaster preparedness experts.

Two millennia ago, the architect and engineer Marcus Vitruvius Pollio (c.80–15 BCE) taught that buildings must embody *firmitas*, *utilitas*, and *venustas* (stability and resilience, usefulness and efficiency, and beauty) along with comfort for the human spirit. It is noteworthy that these are characteristics of good health and well-being. In the post-COVID-19 era, our homes, workplaces, transportation networks, cities, and nations must embody these essential characteristics. Humanity has been transformed by the past. So too, we must use what we have learned to transform the present and future.

NOTE

1. International Civil Aviation Organization, Civil Aviation Statistics of the World and ICAO staff estimates, https://data.worldbank.org/indicator/IS.AIR.PSGR.

Glossary

Built environment

The **built environment** refers to all human-made structures or spaces, including parks, buildings, streets, and other architectural and infrastructural elements of cities. This volume centers on the role the built environment plays, from a macro scale (cities) to a micro scale (interior design), in shaping human health both directly and indirectly.

Cholera

Caused by an intestinal infection by the bacterium *Vibrio cholerae* and transmitted via contaminated water or food, **cholera** is characterized by acute diarrhea and vomiting that can lead to rapid and significant dehydration.

Endemic

A disease that is **endemic** to a place is generally understood to be one that maintains a relatively constant presence among a population in a particular region. An example of a disease endemic to the United States is the seasonal flu (influenza), which arises in predictable patterns. Disease outbreaks cease being endemic when they expand beyond a typical occurrence rate, geographical region, or population in a short amount of time. A disease endemic to one place may be relatively unproblematic in that context but may become more severe or grow to an epidemic when introduced to another geographic context.

Epidemic

An **epidemic** is an outbreak of disease, typically over a short amount of time, that affects a greater number of people than usual for a given place. A disease epidemic may also refer to the sudden spread of an illness from one region in which the illness is endemic to another region in which it is not. The role of place is essential to these definitions; as such, natural and physical environments have long been seen as important contextual factors for understanding and describing illnesses, factors promoting the spread of illness outbreaks, or as sources of possible intervention to quell the spread or impact or illness.

Health and well-being

This volume embraces a broad perspective of **health and well-being**, including not only physical health but also mental, emotional, social, economic, and spiritual dimensions of health. Epidemics and pandemics have obvious implications for physical health; however, the varied chapters and case studies in this volume also demonstrate that these other aspects of health are similarly affected with infectious illness and indeed are also key to the healing process at individual and societal levels.

Hygiene

Hygiene generally refers to the practice of preventing illness and disease transmission through the promotion of cleanliness. One example is personal health hygiene, which includes practices such as handwashing that are meant to help reduce germs. Hygienic practices are seen as important to reduce and quell outbreaks of infectious illness; however, as this volume illustrates, when the design, provision, and/or location of infrastructures that aid hygienic practices, including access to clean water, are not equally distributed across urban environments, these hygienic practices are not equally accessible to all inhabitants, thereby rendering some more prone to infection than others.

Influenza

A contagious viral infection, **influenza** (commonly referred to as the flu) is a respiratory disease that affects the nose, throat, and lungs and is characterized by symptoms including fever, chills, and fatigue.

Leprosy

Caused by the bacteria *Mycobacterium leprae*, **leprosy** (or Hansen's disease) is an infection that affects the skin, nerves, and the mucous membranes of the eyes, throat, and nose.

Malaria

Malaria is a disease most commonly characterized by fever, chills, and other flu-like symptoms, as well as anemia and the swelling of the spleen. Malaria is caused by parasites, transmitted to humans via mosquitoes, that take hold in the blood or other tissues.

Meningitis

The term **meningitis** describes a disease in which the meninges, the membranes surrounding the brain and spinal cord, become inflamed. This disease can be viral or bacterial, meaning it can be caused by a virus or bacterial infection.

Pandemic

A disease epidemic becomes a **pandemic** when it spreads to a large geographic area—for example, across multiple countries or even continents—and, in so doing, affects a large number of people. The COVID-19 pandemic is an example of one such disease that has spread across the world and caused significant deaths world-wide. As this volume demonstrates, the notion of place, and of the connections between places—facilitated by and through air travel, maritime trade, and global tourism, to name just a few—are of particular importance in considering the outbreak and containment of pandemic illnesses.

Plague

Plague is an infectious disease that affects both humans and animals. There are three forms of plague. **Bubonic plague**, the most common, is characterized by the swelling and soreness of lymph nodes (buboes) and is caused by the bacterium *Yersenia pestis*, which can be transmitted between people (or between people and infected mammals such as rats or squirrels) via fleas that act as carriers of plague bacteria. When plague bacteria affect the host's lungs, the severe lung infection that results is called **pneumonic plague**. Importantly, this type of plague infection can be transmitted between people through the air. **Septicemic plague** occurs when the plague bacteria causes an infection of the blood called (septicemia).

Public health

As opposed to medical interventions, which typically target individuals, the concern for and the promotion and management of health at the population level are a primary foci of **public health** efforts, which are broad in focus, including (but not limited to) the monitoring of disease outbreaks and the prevention of illness and injury. One branch of public health is **epidemiology**, or the study of the patterns of health in populations, which is central to studies of disease outbreaks and helps us understand why and how populations become ill. Another branch, **social epidemiology**, foregrounds the ways in which social structures, conditions, and relationships pattern or shape health outcomes and disease risk (e.g., racism and social inequities). Efforts to promote or intervene in public health have long included interventions into the built and natural environments, especially the places in which people live, work, and play; yet, as this volume demonstrates, governmental policies, institutional resources, and social practices that govern and define these spaces also play a significant role in public health efforts.

Quarantine

The act of **quarantine** refers to the separation and limiting of interaction with or movement of people or goods due to feared, suspected, or confirmed illness or infection. For example, both material products and people traveling from a place suspected of or confirmed to be experiencing a disease outbreak to another place may be quarantined for a period of time to minimize the possibility of the goods or people affecting inhabitants of the destination location. The built environment factors significantly into the practice of quarantine, through the delineation or construction of spaces to hold or separate quarantined goods or people, as do instruments of governmentality to enforce quarantine practices.

Sanitation

Sanitation is the practice keeping places clean in order to promote public health. Common sanitation practices include garbage and waste disposal and the provision of clean water. Importantly, these sanitary infrastructures are essential for enabling people to practice good, health-promoting hygienic practices.

Smallpox

Part of the poxvirus family of diseases and caused by the variola virus, **smallpox** is an illness characterized by high fever and a severe skin rash or eruption known as pox.

Urban design

The practice of **urban design** involves the creation and arrangement of buildings, streets, parks, transportation systems, and other spaces within neighborhoods, towns, and cities. As with the built environment more broadly, urban design plays an important role in shaping and promoting health, both directly and indirectly.

Vaccine

A **vaccine** is a biological product, often a weakened version of a disease, that is introduced into a person's body to produce immunity from that disease, thereby offering them protection from the disease later on. Vaccines exist for a variety of illnesses and are a major and important mechanism for public health efforts to prevent and stem outbreaks of infectious illnesses. Importantly, this volume demonstrates the need for governmental, architectural, and infrastructural interventions that support the distribution of vaccines as well as broader structural, social, and political actions beyond vaccine distribution that also help prevent and respond to epidemic illnesses.

Vector

In its broadest sense, a disease **vector** is a pathway that facilitates disease transmission. Most commonly, vectors are identified in biological terms, referring to organisms (such as fleas, ticks, rodents, or mosquitoes) that transmit pathogens between humans (or between humans and animals). This book encourages us to consider the concept of a disease vector in a broad sense by recognizing the broader built and social environments (e.g., housing, infrastructure) that enable these vectors to transmit illnesses between people.

Bibliography

Afkhami, Amir. "Disease and Water Supply: The Case of Cholera in Nineteenth-Century Iran." In *Transformations of Middle Eastern Natural Environments*, edited by Jeff Albert, Magnus Bernhardsson, and Roger Kenna, 206–20. New Haven, CT: Yale University Press, 1998.

Afkhami, Amir. *A Modern Contagion: Imperialism and Public Health in Iran's Age of Cholera*. Baltimore, MD: John Hopkins University Press, 2019.

Agrawal, Hem Narayan. *The Administrative System of Nepal: From Tradition to Modernity*. New Delhi: Vikas, 1976.

Ahmed, Abubakari, and Romanus D. Dinye. "Impact of Land Use Activities on Subin and Aboabo Rivers in Kumasi Metropolis." *International Journal of Water Resources and Environmental Engineering* 4, no. 7 (2012): 241–51.

Ahmed, Sharif Uddin. "Dhaka under the British Crown (1858–1947) - Aspects of Urban History." In *400 Years of Capital Dhaka and Beyond: Politics, Society, Administration*, edited by Abdul Momin Chowdhury and Sharif Uddin Ahmed, 45–70. Dhaka: Asiatic Society of Bangladesh, 2011.

Ahmed, Sharif Uddin. "The History of the City of Dacca, c. 1840-1885." Ph.D. diss., School of Oriental and African Studies, University of London, 1978.

Ahmed, Sharif Uddin. *Mitford Hospital and Dhaka Medical School – History and Heritage, 1858-1947 (in Bengali)*. Dhaka: Academic Press, 2007.

Ahuja, Neel. *Bioinsecurities: Disease Intervention, Empire, and the Government of Species*. Durham, NC: Duke University Press, 2016.

Albuquerque, Teresa. *Bombay: A History*. New Delhi: Promilla, 1992.

Alibrandi, Rosamaria. "Ut Sepulta Surgat Veritas: Giovan Filippo Ingrassia e Fortunato Fedeli sulla Novella Strada della Medicina Legale" [Ut Sepulta Surgat Veritas: Giovan Filippo Ingrassia and Fortunato Fedeli on the New Path of Forensic Medicine]. *Historia et ius rivista di storia giuridica dell'età medievale e moderna*, no. 2 (November 2012): 5.

Alpers, Edward A. "Chikungunya and Epidemic Disease in the Indian Ocean World." In *Disease Dispersion and Impact in the Indian Ocean World*, edited by Gwyn Campbell and Eva-Maria Knoll, 211–36. Cham: Springer International, 2020.

Andō Yūichiro. "Shuto Tōkyō no kankyō eisei gyōsei: Shinyō shori shisuteme no henben to jōyaku kaisei" [The Administration of the Environment and Public Health in the Capital

City Tokyo: Changes in the Waste Disposal System and Treaty Revision]. *Hikaku toshishi kenkyū* 22, no. 1 (2003): 47–61.

Andō Yūichiro. "Tōkyō shiku kaisei izen no shinyō shori taisaku: Ushigome-ku gaitō benjo sojinin Nakamura Kametarō no dōkō wo chūshin ni" [Waste Disposal Measures before the Tokyo Urban Reforms: With a Focus on Nakamura Kametarō, a Toilet Cleaner in Ushigome Ward]. In *Kankyō to rekishi*, edited by Ishi Hiroyuki et al., 197–218. Tokyo: Shinseisha, 1999.

Arcilla, Jose A. "The Culion Leper Colony, 1900s–1970s." *Philippine Studies* 57, no. 2 (2009): 307–26.

Arhin, Kwame. "The Economic Implications of Transformations in Akan Funeral Rites." *Africa* 64, no. 3 (1994): 307–22.

Arnold, David. *Colonizing the Body: State Medicine and Epidemic Disease in Nineteenth-Century India*. Berkeley: University of California Press, 1993.

Ateş, Sabri. "Bones of Contention: Corpse Traffic and Ottoman-Iranian Rivalry in Nineteenth-Century Iraq." *Comparative Studies of South Asia, Africa and the Middle East* 30, no. 3 (2010): 512–32.

Bakar, Coşkun. "Avrupa'da Dolaşan Koleranın Gölgesinde İstanbul Uluslararası Sağlık Konferansı, 1866" ["Istanbul International Health Conference, 1866: In the Shadow of the Cholera That Wanders Europe"]. *Turkish Journal of Public Health* 18, no. 1 (2020): 68–82.

Barata, Rita de Cássia Barradas. "Epidemia de Doença Menigogócia, 1970/1977" ["Meningococcal Disease Epidemic, 1970–1977"]. *Revista de Saúde Pública* 22, no. 1 (1988): 19–23.

Barata, Rita de Cássia Barradas. *Meningite: Uma Doença Sob Censura?* [Meningitis: A Disease under Censorship?]. São Paulo: Cortez, 1988.

Barone, Ana Claudia Castilho. "A Periferia como Questão: São Paulo na Década de 1970" ["The Periphery as an Issue: São Paulo in the 1970s"]. *Revista da Pós* 20, no. 33 (2013): 64–85.

Barret-Kriegel, Blandine. "L'hôpital comme équipment" ["The Hospital as Equipment"]. In *Les Machines à guérir: aux origines de l'hôpital modern* [The Healing Machines: The Origins of the Modern Hospital], edited by Michel Foucault, 19–30. Bruxelles, Liège: Pierre Mardaga, 1979.

Barry, John M. *The Great Influenza: The Story of the Deadliest Pandemic in History*. New York: Penguin, 2005.

Barry, Jonathan. "The Politics of Religion in Restoration Bristol." In *The Politics of Religion in Restoration England*, edited by Tim Harris, Paul Seaward, and Mark Goldie, 163–89. Oxford: Oxford University Press, 1990.

Bashford, Alison. *Imperial Hygiene: A Critical History of Colonialism, Nationalism and Public Health*. Basingstoke: Palgrave Macmillan, 2014.

Belin, François-Alphonse. *La Latinité de Constantinople: champs du repos, rites funéraires d'après les Comptes-rendus du Cimetière latin* [Constantinople of the Latins: Cemeteries, and Funerary Rites according to the Records of the Latin Cemetery], edited by Rinaldo Marmara. Montpellier: Université Paul Valéry, Université Montpellier III, 2004.

Betts, Raymond F. "The Establishment of the Medina in Dakar, Senegal, 1914." *Africa: Journal of the International African Institute* 41, no. 2 (1971): 143–52.

Bigon, Liora. "Bubonic Plague, Colonial Ideologies, and Urban Planning Policies: Dakar, Lagos, and Kumasi." *Planning Perspectives* 31, no. 2 (2016): 205–26.

Bigon, Liora. "Sanitation and Street Layout in Early Colonial Lagos: British and Indigenous Conceptions, 1851-1890." *Planning Perspectives* 20, no 3 (2005): 247–69.

Bilsel, Cana. "19. Yüzyılın İkinci Yarısında İzmir'de Büyük Ölçekli Kentsel Projeler ve Kent Mekanının Başkalaşımı" [Large-Scale Urban Projects and the Transformation of Urban Space in Izmir in the Second Half of the 19th Century]. *Ege Mimarlık* 36 (April 2000): 34–37.

Bishop, Isabella. *Journeys in Persia and Kurdistan Including a Summer in the Upper Karun Region and a Visit to the Nestorian Rayahs.* London: John Murray, 1891.

Bliss, Katherine Elaine. *Compromised Positions: Prostitution, Public Health, and Gender Politics in Revolutionary Mexico City.* University Park: Pennsylvania State University Press, 2001.

Böke, Pelin. "İzmir Karantina Teşkilatının Kuruluşu ve Faaliyetleri (1840-1900)." *Çağdaş Türkiye Tarihi Araştırmaları Dergisi* 8, nos. 18–19 (2009): 137–59.

Bolaños, Isacar A. "The Ottomans during the Global Crises of Cholera and Plague: The View from Iraq and the Gulf." *International Journal of Middle East Studies* 51, no. 4 (2019): 603–620.

Bonastra, Joaquim. "Ciencia, Sociedad y Planificación Territorial en la Institución del Lazareto" [Science, Society and Territorial Planning in the Lazareto Institution]. Ph.D. diss., Universitat de Barcelona, 2006.

Bonastra, Joaquim. "Health Sites and Controlled Spaces. A Morphological Study of Quarantine Architecture." *Dynamis* 30 (2010): 17–40.

Boodhoo, Raj. *Health, Disease and Indian Immigrants in Nineteenth Century Mauritius.* Port Louis: Aapravasi Ghat Trust Fund, 2010.

Bowers, Kristy Wilson. *Plague and Public Health in Early Modern Seville.* Rochester: University of Rochester Press, 2013.

Brentjes, Sonja. "Introduction." In *Travellers from Europe in the Ottoman and Safavid Empires, 16th – 17th Centuries: Seeking, Transforming, Discarding Knowledge*, edited by Sonja Brentjes, ix–xxix. London: Routledge, 2016.

Bristow, Nancy. *American Pandemic: The Lost Worlds of the 1918 Influenza Epidemic.* Oxford: Oxford University Press, 2012.

Brody, David. *Visualizing American Empire: Orientalism and Imperialism in the Philippines.* Chicago, IL: University of Chicago Press, 2010.

Bruce-Chwatt, Leonard J., and Joan M. Bruce-Chwatt. "Malaria in Mauritius - as Dead as the Dodo." *Bulletin of the New York Academy of Medicine* 50, no. 10 (November 1974): 1069–80.

Bruyère, Louis. *Études Relatives à L'art des Constructions.* Paris: Chez Bance Aîné, 1823.

Bugalhão, Jacinta, and André Teixeira. "Os canos da Baixa de Lisboa no século XVI: leitura arqueológica" [The Sewers of Downtown Lisbon in the 16th Century: An Archaeological Approach]. *Cadernos do Arquivo Municipal* 2, no. 4 (2015): 89–122.

Bullock, Nicholas, and James Read. *The Movement for Housing Reform in Germany and France, 1840–1914.* Cambridge: Cambridge University Press, 1985.

Burgess, Perry. *Who Walk Alone.* New York: Henry Holt, 1940.

Burghardt. "Nachricht über die Behandlungsweise der Pestkranken in den Pestspitälern zu Konstantinopel" [Information on How the Plague-Infected are Treated in the Plague Hospitals of Constantinople]. *Medizinische Jahrbücher des kaiserlichen königlichen österreichischen Staates* 4, no. 1 (1817): 109–14.

Burt, Jonathan. *Rat.* London: Reaktion Books, 2006.

Bynum, William F. "The Evolution of Germs and the Evolution of Disease: Some British Debates, 1870–1900." *History and Philosophy of the Life Sciences* 24, no. 1 (2002): 53–68.

Calvi, Giulia. *Histories of a Plague Year: The Social and the Imaginary in Baroque Florence.* Berkeley: University of California Press, 1989.

Cancila, Rossella. "Salute Pubblica e Governo dell'Emergenza: la Peste del 1575 a Palermo" [Public Health and Government of the Emergency: The Plague of 1575 in Palermo]. *Mediterranea – ricerche storiche* 37 (August 2016): 231–72.

Carmichael, Ann G. "Plague Legislation in the Italian Renaissance." *Bulletin of the History of Medicine* 57, no. 4 (1983): 508–25.

Carmona García, Juan Ignacio. *El sistema de hospitalidad pública en la Sevilla del antiguo regimen* [The System of Public Hospitals in Seville during the Old Regime]. Sevilla: Excma. Diputación Provincial de Sevilla, 1979.

Carmona García, and Juan Ignacio. *Crónica urbana del malvivir. Insalubridad, desamparo y hambre en la Sevilla de los siglos XIV-XVII* [Chronicle of Urban Misery: Sickness, Destitution and Hunger in Seville from the Fourteenth to Seventeenth Centuries]. Sevilla: Universidad de Sevilla, 2018.

Chadwick, George. *The Park and the Town: Public Landscape in the 19th and 20th Centuries.* London: Architectural Press, 1966.

Chapman, Ronald F. "Leonard Wood and Leprosy in the Philippines: The Culion Leper Colony, 1921–1927. A Review." *Journal of the History of Medicine and Allied Sciences* 38, no. 4 (1983): 468–70.

Chaves, Cleide de Lima. "As Convenções Sanitárias Internacionais Entre o Império Brasileiro e as Repúblicas Platinas (1873 e 1887)" [International Health Conventions between the Brazilian Empire and the Platinum Republics (1873 and 1887)]. Ph.D. diss., Universidade Federal do Rio de Janeiro, 2009.

Chen, Zhi. *The Theory of City and Park.* Beijing: The Commercial Press, 1930.

Churchill, Winston. *My African Journey.* Toronto: William Briggs, 1909.

Cipolla, Carlo. *Public Health and the Medical Profession in the Renaissance.* London: Cambridge University Press, 1976.

Clark, Gracia. "Consulting Elderly Kumasi Market Women about Modernization." *Ghana Studies* 12, no. 1 (2009): 97–119.

Clark, Gracia. *Onions Are My Husband: Survival and Accumulation by West African Market Women.* Chicago, IL: University of Chicago Press, 1994.

Cohn, Samuel, Jr. *Cultures of Plague. Medical thinking at the end of the Renaissance.* Oxford: Oxford University Press, 2010.

Cohn, Samuel K. *The Black Death Transformed: Disease and Culture in the Early Renaissance.* London: Edward Arnold, 2002.

Collier, Richard. *The Plague of the Spanish Lady: The Influenza Pandemic of 1918–1919.* New York: Atheneum, 1974.

Collins, Yolande. "The Provision of Hospital Care in Country Victoria 1840s–1940s." Ph.D. diss., University of Melbourne, 1999.

Cook, Alexandra Parma, and Noble David Cook. *The Plague Files: Crisis Management in Sixteenth- Century Seville.* Baton Rouge: Louisiana State University Press, 2009.

Cook, Sherburne Friend, and Woodrow Borah. *The Indian Population of Central Mexico, 1531–1610.* Ibero-Americana 44. Berkeley: University of California Press, 1960.

Cranworth, Lord. *A Colony in the Making, or, Sport and Profit in British East Africa.* London: Macmillan, 1912.

Crawshaw, Jane Stevens. "The Renaissance Invention of Quarantine." In *Society in an Age of Plague,* edited by Linda Clark and Carole Rawcliffe, 161–73. Woodbridge: Boydell, 2013.

Critchley, A. Michael. "The Health of the Industrial Worker in Iraq." *British Journal of Industrial Medicine* 12, no. 1 (1955): 73–75.

Crosby, Alfred D. *America's Forgotten Pandemic: The Influenza of 1918.* Cambridge: Cambridge University Press, 2003.

Cuenya Mateos, Miguel Ángel. *Puebla de los Ángeles en tiempos de una peste colonial: una mirada en torno al matlazahuatl de 1737* [Puebla de los Ángeles during a Colonial Plague: A Look at the *Matlazahuatl* Plague of 1737]. Puebla, Mexico: El Colegio de Michoacán-Benemérita Universidad Autónoma de Puebla, 1999.

Cueto, Marcos, and Steven Paul Palmer. *Medicine and Public Health in Latin America: A History.* New York: Cambridge University Press, 2015.

Davidovici, Irina. "Recoding Reform: Ideology and Urban Form in London's Early Housing Estates, 1865–1900." In *Recoding the City: Thinking, Planning, and Building the City of the Nineteenth Century,* edited by Britta Hentschel and Harald R. Stühlinger, 82–94. Berlin: Jovis, 2019.

Davidovici, Irina. "The Depth of the Street." *AA Files,* no. 70 (2015): 103–23.

Daws, Karen. "Framing the Capricious: The Built Response to Infectious Diseases in Victoria between 1850 and 1950." Ph.D. diss., University of Melbourne, 2017.

De Bevoise, Ken. *Agents of Apocalypse: Epidemic Disease in the Colonial Philippines.* Princeton, NJ: Princeton University Press, 1995.

De Viana, Lorelei D. C. "Early Encounters between the Spanish Religious Missionaries and Leprosy in the Philippines." In *Hidden Lives, Concealed Narratives: A History of Leprosy in the Philippines*, edited by Maria Serena I. Diokno, 23–35. Manila, Philippines: National Historical Commission of the Philippines, 2016.

Dewachi, Omar. *Ungovernable Life: Mandatory Medicine and Statecraft in Iraq*. Stanford, CA: Stanford University Press, 2017.

Diokno, Maria Serena. "Fear of Contagion, Punishment, and Hope." In *Hidden Lives, Concealed Narratives: A History of Leprosy in the Philippines*, edited by Maria Serena I. Diokno, 1–20. Manila, Philippines: National Historical Commission of the Philippines, 2016.

Dixit, Hemang. *Nepal's Quest for Health*. Kathmandu: Educational Publishing House, 2014.

Dixon, C. W. *Smallpox*. London: J. & A. Churchill, 1962.

Dollo, Corrado. *Modelli Scientifici e Filosofici nella Sicilia Spagnola* [Scientific and Philosophical Models in Spanish Sicily]. Napoli: Guida, 1984.

Dossal, Miriam. *Imperial Designs and Indian Realities: The Planning of Bombay City, 1845–1875*. Bombay: Oxford University Press, 1991.

Duffy, John. "The Social Impact of Disease in the Late 19th Century." In *Sickness and Health in America*, 3rd ed., edited by Judith Walzer Leavitt and Ronald N. Numbers, 418–25. Madison: University of Wisconsin Press, 1997.

Du, Lihong. "Qingmo Dongbei Shuyi Fangkong yu Jiaotong Zheduan" [The Prevention and Control of Plague and Shut-Down of Transportation in Northeast China in the Late Qing Dynasty]. *Lishi Yanjiu* [Historical Research] 4 (2016): 74–82.

Durey, Michael. *The First Spasmodic Cholera Epidemic in York, 1832*. York: St Anthony's Press, 1974.

Earle, Rebecca. *The Body of the Conquistador: Food, Race, and the Colonial Experience in Spanish America, 1492–1700*. Cambridge: Cambridge University Press, 2012.

Echenberg, Myron J. *Black Death, White Medicine: Bubonic Plague and the Politics of Public Health in Colonial Senegal, 1914–1945*. Portsmouth: Heinemann, 2002.

Echenberg, Myron J. *Plague Ports: The Global Urban Impact of Bubonic Plague, 1894-1901*. New York: New York University Press, 2007.

Editorial Team of Tianjin Landscape and Greening. *Tianjin Landscape and Greening*. Tianjin: Tianjin Science and Technology Press, 1989.

Elkins, Caroline. *Imperial Reckoning: The Untold Story of Britain's Gulag in Kenya*. New York: Henry Holt, 2005.

Elliot, Charles. *The East Africa Protectorate*. London: Edward Arnold, 1905.

Engels, Friedrich. "The Great Towns." In *The Condition of the Working-Class in England in 1844: With Preface Written in 1892*, translated by Florence Kelley Wischnewetzky, 23–74. Cambridge: Cambridge University Press, 2010.

Escamilla González, Iván, Julieta García, and Ana María Huerta. *Remedio contra el olvido: Un acercamiento a la arquitectura del ex Hospital de San Pedro* [A Remedy against Oblivion: A

Close Look at the Architecture of San Pedro Hospital]. Edited by Beatriz Mackenzie. Puebla: State Government of Puebla, 1999.

Evans, R. J. W. *The Making of the Habsburg Monarchy, 1550–1700: An Interpretation.* Oxford: Clarendon Press, 1979.

Evans, Robin. "Rookeries and Model Dwellings." In *Translations from Drawing to Building and Other Essays*, vol. 2, 93–118. London: Architectural Association, 1997.

Eyler, John M. "Scarlet Fever and Confinement: The Edwardian Debate over Isolation Hospitals." *Bulletin of the History of Medicine* 61, no. 1 (1987): 1–24.

Farhan, Sara. "The Making of Iraqi Doctors: Reproduction in Medical Education." Ph.D. diss., York University, 2019.

Feng, Alice Y. T., and Chelsea G. Himsworth. "The Secret Life of the City Rat: A Review of the Ecology of Urban Norway and Black Rats (*Rattus norvegicus* and Rattus rattus)." *Urban Ecosystems* 17 (2014): 149–62.

Few, Martha. "Circulating Smallpox Knowledge: Guatemalan Doctors, Maya Indians and Designing Spain's Smallpox Vaccination Expedition, 1780–1803." *British Journal for the History of Science* 43, no. 159 (2010): 519–37.

Floor, Willem. *Public Health in Qajar Iran.* Washington, DC: Mage, 2004.

Flóra, Ágnes. *The Matter of Honour: The Leading Urban Elite in Sixteenth-Century Transylvania.* Turnhout: Brepols, 2019.

Fodor, Pál. *The Unbearable Weight of Empire: The Ottomans in Central Europe – a Failed Attempt at Universal Monarchy (1390–1566).* Budapest: Research Centre for the Humanities, Hungarian Academy of Sciences, 2016.

Fonseca, Maria Rachel Fróes da. "A Saúde Pública no Rio de Janeiro Imperial" [Public Health in Imperial Rio de Janeiro]. In *História da Saúde no Rio de Janeiro: Instituições e Patrimônio Arquitetônico (1808–1958)* [History of Health in Rio de Janeiro: Institutions and Architectural Heritage (1808–1958)], edited by Ângela Porto, Gisele Sanglard, Maria Rachel Fróes da Fonseca, and Renato da Gama-Rosa Costa, 31–58. Rio de Janeiro: FIOCRUZ, 2008.

Fontes, Paulo. *Migration and the Making of Industrial São Paulo.* Durham, NC: Duke University Press, 2008.

Foster, William, ed. *Early Travels in India 1583–1619.* London: Oxford University Press, 1921.

Frangakis-Syrett, Elena. "Commerce in the Eastern Mediterranean from the Eighteenth to the Early Twentieth Centuries: The City- Port of İzmir and Its Hinterland." *International Journal of Maritime History* 10, no. 2 (December 1998): 125–54.

Gaide, Laurent Joseph, and Henri Désiré Marie Bodet. *La Peste en Indochine.* Hanoi: Imprimerie d'Extrême-Orient, 1930.

Gaitors, Beau. "Commerce, Conflict, and Contamination: Yellow Fever in Early-Independence Veracruz in the US Imaginary, 1821–1848." *História, Ciências, Saúde-Manguinhos* 25, no. 3 (September 2018): 779–95.

Gealogo, Francis A., and Antonio C. Galang Jr. "From Collection to Release: Segregated Lives in the Culion Colony, 1906–1935." In *Hidden Lives, Concealed Narratives: A History of Leprosy in the Philippines*, edited by Maria Serena I. Diokno, 163–89. Manila, Philippines: National Historical Commission of the Philippines.

Gecser, Ottó. "Understanding Pestilence in the Times of King Matthias: The Plague Tract in the Manuscript of János Gellértfi of Aranyasi." In *Matthias Rex 1458–1490: Hungary at the Dawn of the Renaissance*, edited by István Draskóczy et al. Budapest: Eötvös Loránd University Faculty of Humanities, Centre des hautes études de la Renaissance, 2013, http://renaissance.elte.hu/wp-content/uploads/2013/10/Otto-Gecser-Understanding-Pestilence-in-the-Times-of-King-Matthias-The-Plague-Tract-in-the-Manuscript-of-Janos-Gellertfi-of-Aranyas.pdf (online only; accessed September 14, 2020).

Geltner, Guy. *Roads to Health: Infrastructure and Urban Wellbeing in Later Medieval Italy.* Philadelphia: Pennsylvania University Press, 2019.

Gharipour, Mohammad, ed. *Health and Architecture: Designing Spaces for Healing and Caring in the Pre-Modern Era.* London: Bloomsbury Press, 2021.

Goldberg, Sylvie Anne. *Crossing the Jabbok: Illness and Death in Ashkenazi Judaism in Sixteenth-through Nineteenth-Century Prague.* Berkeley: University of California Press, 1996.

Green, Adrian, and Barbara Crosbie. *Economy and Culture in North-East England 1500–1800.* Suffolk: Boydell and Brewer, 2019.

Green, Henry. "The Wooden Walls of England." *Morning Chronicle and London Advertiser*, June 25, 1773.

Greenblatt, Rachel L. *To Tell Their Children: Jewish Communal Memory in Early Modern Prague.* Stanford, CA: Stanford University Press, 2014.

Guo, Xidong, Tong Zhang, and Yan Zhang, eds. *Tianjin Historical Famous Gardens.* Tianjin: Tianjin Ancient Book Press, 2008.

Gutiérrez, Gerardo. "Identity Erasure and Demographic Impacts of the Spanish Caste System on the Indigenous Populations of Mexico." In *Beyond Germs: Native Depopulation in North America*, edited by Catherine M. Cameron, Paul Kelton, and Alan C. Swedlund, 119–45. Tucson: University of Arizona Press, 2015.

Haj, Samira. *The Making of Iraq, 1900–1963: Capital, Power, and Ideology.* Social and Economic History of the Middle East SUNY series. Albany: State University of New York Press, 1997.

Hass, Jennifer Carrie. "Press Coverage of Three Epidemic Diseases: Influenza, Polio and Measles." MA thesis, University of Minnesota, 2004.

Heiser, Victor G. "American Sanitation in the Philippines and its Influence on the Orient." *Proceedings of the American Philosophical Society* 57, no. 1 (Spring 1918): 60–8.

Hepworth Dixon, Conrad. "Seamen and the Law: An Examination of the Impact of Legislation on the British Merchant Seamen's Lot, 1588–1918." Ph.D. diss., University College London, 1981.

Hernández-Sáenz, Luz María. *Carving a Niche: The Medical Profession in Mexico, 1800–1870.* Montreal: McGill-Queen's University Press, 2018.

Hervé, Francis. *A Residence in Greece and Turkey with Notes on the Journey through Bulgaria, Servia, Hungary and the Balkan*, vol. 2. London: Whittaker, 1837.

Heudebert, Luycien. *L'Indo-Chine Francaise*. Paris: G. Dujarric, 1909.

Hiep, Buu. *La Médicine française dans la vie annamite* [The French Doctor in the Vietnamese World]. Hanoi: Imprimiére Le-van-Phuc, 1936.

Hillary, Sir Edmund. *Schoolhouse in the Clouds*. London: Hodder and Stoughton, 1964.

Hines, Thomas S. "The Imperial Façade: Daniel H. Burnham and American Architectural Planning in the Philippines." *Pacific Historical Review* 41, no. 1 (February 1972): 33–53.

Hoffman, Monica Ann. "Malaria, Mosquitoes, and Maps: Practices and Articulations of Malaria Control in British India and WWII." UC San Diego, 2016.

Honingsbaum, Mark. *The Pandemic Century: One Hundred Years of Panic, Hysteria, and Hubris*. New York: W. W. Norton, 2019.

Howard-Jones, Norman. "Introduction." In *The Scientific Background of the International Sanitary Conferences, 1851–1938*, edited by Norman Howard-Jones, 9–12. Geneva: World Health Organization, 1975.

Hu, Cheng "Quarantine Sovereignty during the Pneumonic Plague in North China (November 1910–April 1911)." *Frontiers of History in China* 5, no. 2 (2010): 294–339.

Huerta, Ana María. "La cirugía y sus instrumentos en el Real Hospital de San Pedro de Puebla, 1796–1826" [Surgery and Its Instruments at the Royal Hospital of San Pedro in Puebla, 1796–1826]. In *El Hospital de San Pedro: pilar de la medicina en Puebla*, edited by José Ramón Eguibar, Ma. del Carmen Cortés, and Ma. del Pilar Pacheco, 53–68. Puebla: BUAP-Academia Nacional de Medicina, 2012.

Hughes, Jessica, and Claudio Buongiovanni. *Remembering Parthenope: The Reception of Classical Naples from Antiquity to the Present*. Oxford: Oxford University Press, 2015.

Ingrassia, Giovan Filippo. *Informatione del pestifero et contagioso morbo* [The Information of the Pestiferous and Contagious Disease]. Edited by Luigi Ingalisio. Milano: Franco Angeli, 2005.

Iqbal, Iftekhar. *The Bengal Delta: Ecology, State and Social Change, 1840–1943*. London: Palgrave Macmillan, 2010.

Ishizuka Hiromichi. "Tōkyō no toshi suramu to kōshū eisei mondai" [Urban Slums in Tokyo and Public Health Problems]. In *Kokuren Daigaku Ningen to shakai no hatatsu puroguramu kenkyū hokoku*. Tokyo: United Nations University, 1981.

Itō Yōichi. *Edo jōsuidō no rekishi* [The History of Edo's Water System]. Tokyo: Yoshikawa Kōbunkan, 2010.

Jackson, Richard J. "Foreword." In *Extreme Weather, Health, and Communities*, edited by Sheila Lakshmi Steinberg and William A. Sprigg, v–ix. Switzerland: Springer International, 2016.

Jaffary, Nora E. *Reproduction and Its Discontents in Mexico: Childbirth and Contraception from 1750 to 1905*. Chapel Hill: University of North Carolina Press, 2017.

Jahangir, Nuruddin Muhammad. *The Jahangirnama: Memoirs of Jahangir, Emperor of India*. Translated, edited, and annotated by Wheeler M. Thackston. Washington D.C: Smithsonian Institute; New York and Oxford: Oxford University Press, 1999.

Jahangir, Nuruddin Muhammad. *The Tuzuk-i Jahangiri*. Translated by Alexander Rogers, edited by Henry Beveridge. Delhi: D.K. Fine Art Press, 1989.

Jepson, W. F., A. Moutia, and C. Courtois. "The Malaria Problem in Mauritius: The Bionomics Of Mauritian Anophelines." *Bulletin of Entomological Research* 38, no. 1 (May 1947): 177–208.

Jones, Hilary. *The Métis of Senegal: Urban Life and Politics in French West Africa*. Bloomington: Indiana University Press, 2013.

Julvez, Jean, Jean Mouchet, and C. Ragavoodoo. "Epidémiologie Historique Du Paludisme Dans l'Archipel Des Mascareignes (Océan Indien)." *Annales Des Sociétés Belges de Médicine Tropicale, de Parasitologie et de Mycologie Humaine et Animale* 70, no. 4 (1990): 249–61.

K'Akumu, O. A., and W. H. A. Olima. "The Dynamics and Implications of Residential Segregation in Nairobi." *Habitat International* 31, no. 1 (2007): 87–99.

Karskens, Grace. *The Colony: A History of Early Sydney*. Crow's Nest, Australia: Allen and Unwin, 2010.

Khan, Enayatullah. "Visitations of Plague in Mughal India." *Proceedings of the Indian History Congress* 74 (2013): 305–12.

Klassen, Winand. *Architecture in the Philippines: Filipino Building in Cross-Cultural Context*. Cebu City: University of San Carlos Press, 2010.

Klein, Ira. "Development and Death: Reinterpreting Malaria, Economics and Ecology in British India." *The Indian Economic & Social History Review* 38, no. 2 (June 2001): 147–79.

Klein, Ira. "Imperialism, Ecology and Disease: Cholera in India, 1850–1950." *The Indian Economic & Social History Review* 31, no. 4 (1994): 491–518.

Klein, Ira. "Urban Development and Death: Bombay City, 1870–1914." *Modern Asian Studies* 20, no. 4 (1986): 725–54.

Kosambi, Meera. *Bombay in Transition*. Stockholm: Almqvist and Wiskell International, 1986.

Kurmuş, Orhan. *Emperyalizmin Türkiye'ye Girişi* [The Introduction of Imperialism to Turkey]. İstanbul: Bilim Yayınları, 1974.

Kusaka, Wataru. "Discipline and Desire: Hansen's Disease Patients Reclaim Life in Culion, 1900–1930s." *Social Science Diliman* 13, no.2 (2017), 1–30.

Latimer, John. *The Annals of Bristol in the Seventeenth Century*. Bristol: William George's Sons, 1900.

Lee, Jonathan, ed. *The Journals of Edward Stirling in Persia and Afghanistan, 1828–29, from Manuscripts in the Archives of the Royal Geographical Society*. Naples: Istituto Universitario Orientale, 1991.

Lewis, Miles. *Melbourne: The City's History and Development*. Melbourne: City of Melbourne, 1995.

Leys, Norman. *Kenya*. London: The Hogarth Press, 1924.

Link, Bruce, and Jo Phelan. "Social Conditions as Fundamental Causes of Disease." *Journal of Health and Social Behavior*, Extra Issue (1985): 80–94.

Long, Cheng. "Fangyi yu Boyi: Qingmo Shuyi Beihou de Daguo Waijiao" [Epidemic Prevention and Gaming: The Great Power Diplomacy behind the Late Qing Plague]. *Dushu* 7 (2020): 6–7.

Long, Esmond R. "Forty Years of Leprosy Research History of the Leonard Wood Memorial (American Leprosy Foundation) 1928 to 1967." *International Journal of Leprosy* 35, no. 2 (1967): 239–89.

Lord, Evelyn. *The Great Plague: A People's History*. New Haven, CT: Yale University Press, 2014.

Louthan, Howard. *Converting Bohemia: Force and Persuasion in the Catholic Reformation*. Cambridge: Cambridge University Press, 2009.

Lugard, Frederick John Dealtry. *The Rise of Our East African Empire: Early Efforts in Nyasaland and Uganda*. London: W. Blackwood and Sons, 1893.

Lupescu, Radu. "The Medieval Fortifications of Sibiu." In *"Vmbringt mit starken turnen, murn:" Ortsbefestigungen im Mittelalter* ["Encircled by Strong Towers and Walls:" Fortifications of Cities and Towns in the Middle Ages], edited by Olaf Wagener, 351–62. Frankfurt am Main: Peter Lang, 2010.

Lutz, Wolfgang, and Anne Babette Wils. "People on Mauritius: 1638–1991." In *Population — Development — Environment: Understanding Their Interactions in Mauritius*, edited by Wolfgang Lutz, J. Baguant, C. Prinz, F. L. Toth, and Anne Babette Wils, 75–97. Berlin: Springer-Verlag, 1994.

M'Bokolo, Elikia. "Peste Et Société Urbaine à Dakar: L'épidémie De 1914" [The Plague and Urban Society in Dakar: The 1914 Epidemic]. *Cahiers D'Études Africaines* 22, no. 85/86 (1982): 13–46.

Mabogunje, Akin. "Lagos-Nigeria's Melting Pot." *Nigeria Magazine* 69 (1961): 128–55.

Macgregor, Malcolm. E. *Mosquito Surveys: A Handbook for Anti-Malarial and Anti-Mosquito Field Workers*. London: Baillière, Tindall & Cox, 1927.

Maclean, Charles. *Results of an Investigation Regarding Epidemic and Pestilential Diseases Including Researches in the Levant Concerning the Plague*, vol. 1. London: Thomas and George Underwood, 1817.

Magyary-Kossa, Gyula. *Magyar orvosi emlékek: Értekezések a magyar orvostörténet köréből. III. kötet: Adattár 1000–1700-ig* [Hungarian Medical Records: Treatises on Hungarian Medical History, vol. 3: Repertory 1000–1700]. Budapest: Magyar Orvosi Könyvkiadó Társulat, 1931.

Majorossy, Judit, and Katalin Szende. "Hospitals in Medieval and Early Modern Hungary." In *Europäisches Spitalwesen: Institutionelle Fürsorge in Mittelalter und Früher Neuzeit* [The System of Hospitals in Europe: Institutional Care in the Middle Ages and the Early Modern Period], edited by Martin Scheutz et al., 409–54. Vienna: Oldenbourg, 2008.

Malta, Renato, Alfredo Salerno, and Aldo Gerbino. "L'Informatione del pestifero et contagioso Morbo: Processi diagnostici" [The Information of the Pestiferous and Contagious Disease: Diagnostic Processes]. In *Atti Convegno Primaverile Società Italiana di Storia della Medicina*, 48–52. Dogliani: Dogliani Castello, 2010.

Marín Bosch, Miguel. *Puebla neocolonial, 1777–1831: Casta, ocupación y matrimonio en la segunda ciudad de Nueva España* [Neocolonial Puebla: Caste, Occupation, and Marriage in New Spain's Second City]. Puebla, Mexico: El Colegio de Jalisco-Instituto de Ciencias Sociales y Humanidades, BUAP, 1999.

Martal, Abdullah. "XIX. Yüzyılın İkinci Yarısında İzmir'İn Sosyo-Ekonomik Yapısında Gerçekleşen Değişmeler." *Çağdaş Türkiye Araştırmaları Dergisi* 1, no. 3 (1993): 117–31.

Martal, Abdullah. *Değişim Sürecinde İzmir'de Sanayileşme 19. Yüzyıl* [Nineteenth-Century Industrialization in İzmir during the Process of Change]. İzmir: Dokuz Eylül Yayınları, 1999.

Martínez Shaw, Carlos, ed. *Sevilla, siglo XVI: el corazón de las riquezas del mundo* [Seville in the Sixteenth Century: The Heart of the World's Riches]. Madrid: Alianza Editorial, 1993.

McCaskie, Tom C. " 'Water Wars' in Kumasi, Ghana." In *African Cities: Competing Claims in Urban* Spaces, edited by Francesca Locatelli and Paul Nugent, 135–55. Leiden: Brill, 2009.

McCrea, Heather. *Diseased Relations: Epidemics, Public Health, and State-Building in Yucatán, Mexico, 1847–1924*. Albuquerque: University of New Mexico Press, 2011.

Miller, John. *Cities Divided: Politics and Religion in English Provincial Towns, 1660–1722*. Oxford: Oxford University Press, 2007.

Ministry of Health and Quality of Life Mauritius, and World Health Organization and the University of California, San Francisco. "Eliminating Malaria: Case Study 4. Preventing Reintroduction in Mauritius." Geneva: The World Health Organization, 2012.

Mitman, Gregg. *Breathing Space: How Allergies Shape Our Lives and Landscapes*. New Haven, CT: Yale University Press, 2008.

Moe, Nelson. *The View from Vesuvius: Italian Culture and the Southern Question*. London: University of California Press, 2006.

Moote, A. Lloyd, and C. Dorothy. *The Great Plague: The Story of London's Most Deadly Year*. Baltimore, MD: Johns Hopkins University Press, 2004.

Moraes, José Cássio de Moraes, and Rita de Cássia Barradas Barata. "A Doença Meningocócica em São Paulo, Brasil, no século XX: Características Epidemiológicas" [Meningococcal Disease in São Paulo, Brazil in the 20th Century: Epidemiological Features]. *Cadernos de Saúde Pública* 21, no. 5 (September–October 2005): 1458–71.

Morens, David M., and Anthony S. Fauci. "The 1918 Influenza Pandemic: Insights for the 21st Century." *Journal of Infectious Disease* 195, no. 7 (2007): 1018–28.

Morley, Ian. *Cities and Nationhood: American Imperialism and Urban Design in the Philippines, 1898-1916*. Honolulu: University of Hawaii Press, 2018.

Müller, Ulrike. *Thimi: Social and Economic Studies on a Newar Settlement in the Kathmandu Valley*. Giessen: Geographical Institute, Justus Liebig University, 1981.

Munkhoff, Richelle. "Poor Women and Parish Public Health in Sixteenth-Century London." *Renaissance Studies* 28, no. 4 (2014): 579–96.

Muriel, Josefina. *Hospitales de la Nueva España: Tomo I. Fundaciones del siglo XVI*. Mexico City: UNAM-Instituto de Investigaciones Históricas-Cruz Roja Mexicana, 1990.

Murphy, Michael. "In Search of the Water Pump: Architecture and Cholera." *Harvard Design Magazine: Architecture, Landscape Architecture, Urban Design and Planning*, no. 40 (Spring–Summer 2015): 148–53.

Naikaku Kirokukyoku, ed. *Hōki bunrui dai taizen* [A Complete Compilation of Laws and Regulations, Classified], *vol. 32: Eisei*. Tokyo: Hara Shobō, 1981.

Needham, J. P. *Facts and Observations Relative to the Disease Commonly Called Cholera as It Has Recently Prevailed in the City of York*. London: Longman, Rees, Orme, Brown, Green, 1833.

Newman, Kira L. S. "Shutt Up: Bubonic Plague and Quarantine in Early Modern England." *Journal of Social History* 45, no. 3 (2012): 809–34.

Newton, Diana, and A. J. Pollard, eds. *Newcastle and Gateshead before 1700*. Chichester: Phillimore, 2009.

Ngalamulume, Kalala J. *Colonial Pathologies, Environment, and Western Medicine in Saint-Louis-du-Senegal, 1867–1920*. New York: Peter Lang, 2012.

Nkwam, Florence E. "British Medical and Health Policies in West Africa c.1920–1960." Ph.D. thesis, University of London School of Oriental and African Studies, 1988.

Nowrojee, Pheroze. *A Kenyan Journey*. Nairobi: Manqa Books, 2019.

Offner, Robert. "Johannes Saltzmann, der Stadtarzt von Hermannstadt, ließ 1510 in Wien seine Pest-Ordnung drucken" [Johannes Saltzmann, the town physician of Sibiu had his plague tract printed in Vienna in 1510]. *Kaleidoscope* 2, no. 2 (2011): 127–32.

Olukoju, Ayodeji. "Population Pressure, Housing and Sanitation in Metropolitan Lagos: c1900–1939." In *Urban Transition in Africa: Aspects of Urbanization and Change in Lagos*, edited by Kunle Lawal, 34–49. Lagos: Pumark Limited, 1994.

Opdyke, Sandra. *The Flu Epidemic of 1918: America's Experience in the Global Health Crisis*. New York: Routledge, 2014.

Ortholan. "La peste en Indo-Chine. (Historique)." *Annales d'Hygiène et de Médecine Coloniale* 11 (1908): 633–38.

Osborne, Thomas. "Security and Vitality: Drains, Liberalism and Power in the Nineteenth Century." In *Foucault and Political Reason. Liberalism, Neo-liberalism and Rationalities of Government*, edited by A. Barry, T. Osborne, and N. Rose, 99–123. London: UCL Press, 1996.

Osei, Frank Badu, and Alfred Stein. "Temporal Trend and Spatial Clustering of Cholera Epidemic in Kumasi-Ghana." *Scientific Reports* 8, no. 1 (2018): 1–11.

Pach, Zsigmond Pál. "Hungary and the Levantine Trade in the Fourteenth-Seventeenth Centuries." *Acta Orientalia Academiae Scientiarum Hungaricae* 60, no. 1 (2007): 9–31.

Pakucs-Willcocks, Mária. *Sibiu-Hermannstadt: Oriental Trade in Sixteenth-Century Transylvania*. Cologne: Böhlau, 2007.

Pandey, M. R., I. L. Acharya, and A. Moyeed. "Clinical Survey of Small Pox." *Journal of Nepal Medical Association* 2, no. 1 (1964): 8–11.

Pansieri, Guido. "La nascita della polizia medica" [The Birth of the Medical Police]. In *Storia d'Italia: Annali 3: Scienza e tecnica nella cultura e nella società dal Rinascimento a oggi*, edited by Gianni Micheli. Torino: Einaudi, 1980.

Parco De Castro, Maria Eloisa G. "Rediscovering a Paradigm: The Fransciscan Order's Response to Leprosy and the Afflicted in the Philippines, 1578–1898." In *Hidden Lives, Concealed Narratives: A History of Leprosy in the Philippines*, edited by Maria Serena I. Diokno, 37–62. Manila, Philippines: National Historical Commission of the Philippines, 2016.

Patterson, David K. "The Influenza Epidemic of 1918–1919 in the Gold Coast," *The Journal of African History* 24, no. 4 (1983): 485–502.

Peckham, Robert, ed. *Empires of Panic: Epidemics and Colonial Anxieties*. Hong Kong: Hong Kong University Press, 2015.

Pelsaert, Francisco. *Jahangir's India: The Remonstrantie of Francisco Pelsaert*. Translated by W. H. Moreland and P. Geyl. Cambridge: W. Heffer & Sons, 1925.

Petrucciolo, Attilio. "Fathpur Sikri, Akbar's Capital and Construction Models for Mughal Towns." In *Akbar: The Great Emperor of India*, edited by Gian Carlo Calza, 41–51. Milan: Fondazione Roma and Skira Editore, 2012.

Phillips, Doris G. "Rural-to-Urban Migration in Iraq." *Economic Development and Cultural Change* 7, no. 4 (1959): 405–21.

Phillips, Howard, and David Killingray, eds. *The Spanish Influenza Pandemic of 1918–1919: New Perspectives*. London: Routledge, 2013.

Pike, Ruth. *Aristocrats and Traders: Sevillian Society in the Sixteenth Century*. Ithaca, NY: Cornell University Press, 1972.

Pinkney, David. H. *Napoleon III and the Rebuilding of Paris*. Princeton, NJ: New Jersey, 1958.

Prince, Ruth J., and Rebecca Marsland, eds. *Making and Unmaking Public Health in Africa: Ethnographic and Historical Perspectives*. Athens: Ohio University Press, 2014.

Prokeš, Jaroslav, and Anton Blaschka. "Der Antisemitismus der Behörden und das Prager Ghetto in nachweißenbergischer Zeit" [The Anti-Semitism of the Authorities and the Prague Ghetto in the Post-White Mountain Era]. *Jahrbuch der Gesellschaft für Geschichte der Juden in der Čechoslovakischen Republik* 1 (1929): 41–262.

Rachmuth, Michael. "Der Plan einer Verlegung des Prager Ghettos nach Lieben 1680" [The Plan to Move the Prague Ghetto to Lieben in 1680]. *Jahrbuch der Gesellschaft für Geschichte der Juden in der Čechoslovakischen Republik* 6 (1934): 145–56.

Ramírez, Paul F. *Enlightened Immunity: Mexico's Experiments with Disease Prevention in the Age of Reason*. Stanford, CA: Stanford University Press, 2019.

Reid, Donald. *Paris Sewers and Sewermen: Realities and Representations*. Cambridge, MA: Harvard University Press, 1991.

Risse, Guenter. "Hospitals." In *Europe 1450 to 1789: Encyclopedia of the Early Modern World*, vol. 3, 204–6. New York: Charles Scribner's Sons, 2004.

Rockafellar, Nancy. "'In Gauze We Trust': Public Health and Spanish Influenza on the Home Front, Seattle, 1918–1919." *Pacific Northwest Quarterly* 77, no. 3 (July 1986): 104–5.

Rodríguez Álvarez, María de los Ángeles. "La aparición de los muertos" [The Apparition of the Dead]. In *El Hospital de San Pedro: pilar de la medicina en Puebla* [The Hospital of San Pedro: A Pillar of Medicine in Puebla], edited by José Ramón Eguibar, Ma. del Carmen Cortés, and Ma. del Pilar Pacheco, 91–111. Puebla: BUAP-Academia Nacional de Medicina, 2012.

Roesel, Kristina, and Delia Grace, eds. *Food Safety and Informal Markets: Animal Products in Sub-Saharan Africa*. New York: Routledge, 2015.

Rogaski, Ruth. *Hygienic Modernity: Meanings of Health and Disease in Treaty-Port China*. Berkeley: University of California Press, 2004.

Ross, Ronald. *Report on the Prevention of Malaria in Mauritius*. London: J&A. Churchill, 1908.

Rothenberg, Gunther E. "The Austrian Sanitary Cordon and the Control of the Bubonic Plague: 1710–1871." *Journal of the History of Medicine and Allied Sciences* 28, no. 1 (1973): 15–23.

Rouffiandis, M. le V. "La peste bubonic au Tonkin" [Bubonic Plague in Tonkin]. *Annales d'Hygiène et de Médincine Coloniale* [Annals of Colonial Hygiene and Medicine] 8 (1905): 609–30.

Royle, Edward. *Modern Britain: A Social History 1750–1997*. London: Arnold, 1997.

Runming, Jiao. "Gengxu Shuyi Yingdui yu Zhongguo Jindai Fangyi Tixi Chujian" [Responding to the Plague in Northeast China and the Beginning of a Modern Epidemic Prevention system in China]. *Lishi Yanjiu* [Historical Research] 2 (2020): 15–18.

Sabben-Clare, E. E., David J. Bradley, and Kenneth Kirkwood, eds. *Health in Tropical Africa during the Colonial Period*. Oxford: Clarendon Press, 1980.

Salgado de Barros, António Augusto. "Os canos na drenagem da rede de saneamento da cidade de Lisboa antes do terremoto de 1755" [The Sewerage of Lisbon before the Earthquake of 1755]. *Cadernos do Arquivo Municipal* 2, no. 1 (2014): 85–105.

Salgado de Barros, António Augusto. *O Saneamento da cidade pós-medieval—o caso de Lisboa* [The Sanitation of the Post-Medieval City—the Case of Lisbon]. Lisbon: Ordem dos Engenheiros, 2014.

Santos, Myrian Sepúlveda dos. "Lazareto da Ilha Grande: Isolamento, Aprisionamento e Vigilância nas Áreas de Saúde e Política (1884–1942)." [The Ilha Grande Lazaretto: Isolation, Imprisonment and Surveillance in the Health and Political Fields (1884–1942)] *História, Ciências, Saúde – Manguinhos* 14, no. 4 (2007): 1173–96.

Schram, Ralph. *A History of the Nigerian Health Services*. Ibadan: University Press, 1971.

Schwarcz, Lilia Moritz. *O Espetáculo das Raças – cientistas, instituições e questão racial no Brasil 1870–1930* [The Spectacle of the Races – Scientists, Institutions and Racial Issues in Brazil 1870–1930]. São Paulo: Cia das Letras, 1993.

Scott, Susan, and Christopher J. Duncan. *Biology of Plagues: Evidence from Historical Populations*. Cambridge: Cambridge University Press, 2009.

Seyf, Ahmad. "Iran and Cholera in the Nineteenth Century." *Middle Eastern Studies* 38, no. 1 (January 2002): 169–78.

Shuhe, Guan. "Wu Lian De 1910–1911 Nian za Dongbei Fangyi zhong Renzhi 'Quanquanzongyiguan' Kao" [An Investigation of Wu Lien-teh as the Plenipotentiary General Medical Officer for Epidemic Protection in Northeast China from 1910 to 1911]. *Shixue Jikan* [Collected Papers of History Studies] 6 (2018): 85–97.

Sinclair, Iain. *Charles Booth's London Poverty Maps: A Landmark Reassessment of Booth's Social Survey*. London: Thames & Hudson, 2019.

Slack, Paul. *The Impact of Plague in Tudor and Stuart England*. Oxford: Oxford University Press, 1990.

Slack, Paul. *The Impact of Plague in Tudor and Stuart England*. London: Routledge, 1985.

Snow, John. *On the Mode of Communication of Cholera*, 2nd ed. London: John Churchill, 1855.

Snowden, Frank M. *Epidemics and Society: From the Black Death to the Present*, revised ed. New Haven, CT: Yale University Press, 2020.

Snowden, Frank. M. *Naples in the Time of Cholera, 1884–1911*. Cambridge: Cambridge University Press, 2002.

Spinney, Laura. *Pale Rider: The Spanish Flu of 1918 and How It Changed the World*. New York: Vintage, 2018.

Stepan, Nancy. *The Hour of Eugenics: Race, Gender, and Nation in Latin America*. Ithaca, NY: Cornell University Press, 1991.

Stronge, Susan. "Jahangir's Itinerant Masters." In *Indian Painting: Themes, Histories, Interpretations: Essays in Honour of B.N. Goswamy*, edited by M. Sharma and P. Kaimal, 125–35. Ahmedabad: Mapin, 2013.

Suetonius. *The Life of Nero*. In *Suetonius, Lives of the Caesars, Vol. 1*, trans. J. C. Rolfe. Cambridge, MA: Harvard University Press, 1914.

Summers, William C. *The Great Manchurian Plague of 1910–1911: The Geopolitics of an Epidemic Disease*. New Haven, CT: Yale University Press, 2012.

Swanson, Maynard W. "The Sanitation Syndrome: Bubonic Plague and Urban Native Policy in the Cape Colony, 1900-1909." *The Journal of African History* 18, no. 3 (1977): 387–410.

Szende, Katalin. "Kraków and Buda in the Road Network of Medieval Europe." In *On Common Path: Budapest and Kraków in the Middle Ages*, edited by Judit Benda et al., 31–37. Budapest: Budapesti Történeti Múzeum, 2016.

Talton, Benjamin. " 'Kill Rats and Stop Plague': Race, Space, and Public Health in Postconquest Kumasi." *Ghana Studies* 22, no. 1 (2019): 95–113.

Tarn, John Nelson. *Five per Cent Philanthropy; an Account of Housing in Urban Areas between 1840 and 1914*. London: Cambridge University Press, 1973.

Thiam, Iba der. *Les Origines Du Mouvement Syndical Africain, 1790–1929*. Paris: L'Harmattan, 1993.

Tōkyō-fu, ed. *Tōkyō-fu shi: Gyōsei hen* [The History of Tokyo Prefecture: Administration]. 6 vols. Tokyo: Tōkyō-fu, 1935–37.

Tōkyo-to, ed. *Tōkyō-shi shikō: Shigai hen* [A Draft History of Tokyo: Urban Development]. 27 vols. Tokyo: Tōkyō-to, 1952–74.

Tomes, Nancy. "'Destroyer and Teacher': Managing the Masses during the 1918–1919 Influenza Pandemic." *Public Health Reports* 125, no. 3 (2010): 48–62.

Tomes, Nancy. *The Gospel of Germs: Men, Women and the Microbe, in American Life.* Cambridge, MA: Harvard University Press, 1999.

Tomkins, Sandra M. "Colonial Administration in British Africa during the Influenza Epidemic of 1918–19." *Canadian Journal of African Studies/La Revue Canadienne des Études Africaines* 28, no. 1 (1994): 60–83.

Trivedi, K. K. "The Emergence of Agra as a Capital and a City: A Note on Its Spatial and Historical Background during the Sixteenth and Seventeenth Centuries." *Journal of the Economic and Social History of the Orient* 37, no. 2 (1994): 147–70.

Turniansky, Chava. "Yiddish Song as Historical Source Material: Plague in the Judenstadt of Prague in 1713." In *Jewish History: Essays in Honour of Chimen Abramsky*, edited by Chimen Abramsky, Ada Rapoport-Albert, and Steven J. Zipperstein, 189–98. London: P. Halban, 1988.

Ullman, James Ramsey. *Americans on Everest.* Philadelphia, PA: J.B. Lippincott, 1964.

Van Andel, Tinde, Britt Myren, and Sabine Van Onselen, "Ghana's Herbal Market," *Journal of Ethnopharmacology* 140, no. 2 (2012): 368–78.

Varlık, Nükhet. "'Oriental Plague' or Epidemiological Orientalism? Revisiting the Plague Episteme of the Early Modern Mediterranean." In *Plague and Contagion in the Islamic Mediterranean*, edited by Nükhet Varlık, 57–86. Kalamazoo, MI: Arc Humanities Press, 2017.

Varlık, Nükhet. "İstanbul'da Veba Salgınları" [Plague Epidemics in Istanbul]. Translated by Ahmet Aydoğan. In *Antik Çağ'dan XXI. Yüzyıla Büyük İstanbul Tarihi Cilt IV (Toplum)*, edited by Coşkun Yılmaz, 146–51. Istanbul: İstanbul Büyükşehir Belediyesi Kültür Yayınları, 2015.

Varlık, Nükhet. *Plague and Empire in the Early Modern Mediterranean World: The Ottoman Experience 1347–1600.* New York: Cambridge University Press, 2015.

Velázquez y Sánchez, José. *Anales Epidémicos: Reseña Histórica de Las Enfermedades Contagiosas En Sevilla Desde La Reconquista Cristiana Hasta Nuestros Días (1866).* [Chronicle of Epidemics: Historical Review of Contagious Diseases in Seville from the Christian Conquest to Our Times]. Sevilla: Servicio de Publicaciones del Excmo. Ayuntamiento de Sevilla; Real e Ilustre Colegio Oficial de Médicos de la Provincia de Sevilla, 1996.

Velmet, Aro. *Pasteur's Empire: Bacteriology and Politics in France, Its Colonies, and the World.* New York: Oxford University Press, 2020.

Vesco, Maurizio. "Un piano di espansione per Palermo nel secondo Cinquecento: Guglielmo Fornaya e la fondazione del borgo di Santa Lucia" [An Expansion Plan for Palermo in the Second Half of the 16th Century: Guglielmo Fornaya and the Foundation of the Village of Santa Lucia]. In *Storie di Città e Architetture – Scritti in Onore di Enrico Guidoni*, edited by Giuglielmo Villa, 151–64. Roma: Edizioni Kappa, 2014.

Vilímková, Milada. *The Prague Ghetto*. Prague: Aventinum, 1993.

von Moltke, Helmuth. *Briefe über Zustände und Begebenheiten in der Türkei aus den Jahren 1835 bis 1839* [Letters about the Conditions and Occurrences in Turkey from the Years 1835 to 1839]. Berlin: Ernst Siegfried Mittler, 1841.

von Osten, Anton Prokesch. *Denkwürdigkeiten und Erinnerungen aus dem Orient* [Memorabilia and Memories from the Orient], vol. 1. Stuttgart: Hallberger'sche Verlagshandlung, 1836.

Wallis, Patrick. "Plagues, Morality and the Place of Medicine in Early Modern England." *English Historical Review* 121, no. 490 (2006): 1–24.

Weston, Gretchen. "Municipal Reform and Agitation: Terre Haute 1900–1910." MA thesis, Indiana State University Department of History, 1967.

Wheeler, Margaret Marion. "The Culion Leper Colony." *The American Journal of Nursing* 13, no. 9 (June 1913): 663–66.

Whelpton, John. *A History of Nepal*. Cambridge: Cambridge University Press, 2005.

Willen, Diane. "Women in the Public Sphere in Early Modern England: The Case of the Urban Working Poor." *The Sixteenth Century Journal* 19, no. 4 (1988): 559–75.

Williams, George Bransby. *Report on the Sanitation of Nairobi*. London: Waterlow, 1907.

Willrich, Michael. *Pox: An American History*. New York: Penguin Press, 2011.

Wrightson, Keith. *Ralph Tailor's Summer: A Scrivener, His City and the Plague*. New Haven, CT: Yale University Press, 2011.

Wu, Lien-teh, Chen, Yonghan, Bo, Lishi and Wu, Changyao. *Introduction to the Plague*. Shanghai: Harbor Quarantine Office, Department of Health, 1937.

Yamamoto, Shun'ichi. *Nihon korera shi* [A History of Cholera in Japan]. Tokyo: Tōkyō Daigaku Shuppankai, 1982.

Zakarian, A.V. "Organization and Conduction of Mass Smallpox Vaccination in Iraq with the Aid of the Soviet Union." *Voprosy Virusologii* 6 (1961): 733–35.

Zandi-Sayek, Sibel. "Introduction." In *Ottoman İzmir The Rise of a Cosmopolitan Port 1840-1880*, edited by Sibel Zandi-Sayek, 5–46. Minneapolis: University of Minnesota Press, 2012.

Zhang, Peng. *Physical Foundations of City Form: A Study on the Relationship between Municipal Construction and Transformation of Urban Space in the International Settlement of Shanghai*. Shanghai: Tongji University Press, 2008.

Zhang, Tianjie, Li, Ze, and Sun, Yuan. "Hybrid Modernity and Public Space: An Investigation on Public Park Development in Modern Tianjin." *New Architecture*, no. 5 (2012): 33–40.

Zhang, Yichi. "The First British Concession Garden of Tianjin- Victoria Garden." *Modern Landscape Architecture*, no. 5 (2010): 44–47.

Authors' Biographies

Danielle Abdon is a researcher specializing in early modern architecture on the Italian and Iberian Peninsulas. She earned her Ph.D. in Art History from Temple University. Her dissertation focused on 15th- and 16th-century hospitals in Italy, Iberia, and the Americas, specifically how contemporary ideas of poor relief and public and environmental health promoted architectural and infrastructural innovations in hospital buildings. As the recipient of the Carter Manny Award's Writing Citation of Special Recognition (2019), she has received grants from the Bibliotheca Hertziana—Max Planck Institute for Art History, the Countway Library of Medicine at Harvard University, the Getty Foundation, the Huntington Library, the John Carter Brown Library, and the Society of Architectural Historians.

Ann-Marie Akehurst is Programmes Officer and Trustee of the Society of Architectural Historians of Great Britain. She received her Ph.D. from the University of York in the United Kingdom. She formerly taught art and architectural history at the University of York and is now an independent researcher with interests in architecture related to place. She speaks internationally and has published on sacred space, urban identity, and the architecture of health, broadly defined, in early modern Britain and Europe.

Mary Anne Alabanza Akers is Dean and Professor at the School of Architecture and Planning at Morgan State University in Baltimore, USA. She earned degrees in Sociology and Urban Planning from the University of the Philippines, a graduate degree in Professional Writing (Creative) from Towson University, and a Ph.D. in Urban Planning from Michigan State University. She has published on topics related to health and design, biophilic and active classrooms, and

353

community-based development. She is the author of the book *Urban Environments and Health in the Philippines: A Retrospective on Women Street Vendors and their Spaces* (Routledge, 2021).

Kristy Wilson Bowers is Assistant Professor of History at the University of Missouri, USA. She received her Ph.D. from Indiana University. Her research focuses on the history of medicine in early modern Europe. She is the author of *Plague and Public Health in Early Modern Seville* (University of Rochester Press, 2013) as well as articles in the *Bulletin of the History of Medicine* and *The Sixteenth Century Journal*. Her current research examines surgeons and their texts in the late 16th century.

Juan Luis Burke is Assistant Professor of architectural history at the University of Maryland, College Park, USA. His book, *Architecture and Urbanism in Viceregal Mexico: Puebla de los Ángeles, Sixteenth to Eighteenth Centuries* (Routledge, 2021), traces the city of Puebla's historical development through an architecture and urban history lens. Juan Luis's research focuses on architecture and urbanism in the early modern period, particularly in Mexico and Latin America, as well as issues of sociological, artistic, and political impact in the region and their resonances with contemporary discussions on gender, social justice, decolonial theory, and race.

Susan L. Burns is Professor of Japanese History and East Asian Languages and Civilizations at the University of Chicago, USA. She works on the history of gender, medicine, and public health in early modern and modern Japan. Her recent publications include *Kingdom of the Sick: A History of Leprosy and Japan* (University of Hawaii Press, 2019) and "Reinvented Places: Tradition, Family Care, and Psychiatric Institutions in Japan," in the journal *Social History of Medicine*. She is currently completing a book titled *Cartographies of Care: Medicine and Public Health in Tokyo, 1868–1912*.

Yishen Chen is a doctoral candidate in the Department of History at Peking University, China. He is currently working on his dissertation entitled "A Foreign Land in the Homeland: Returned Overseas Chinese and Fuzhou Overseas Chinese Plastic Factory in the People's Republic of China (1958–2008)." Using a combination of traditional textual sources and ethnographic fieldwork, he works on the intersection of migration studies, ethnic identity, history of the People's Republic of China, and the history of Southeast Asia.

Yongming Chen is a research associate at the School of Architecture at The Chinese University of Hong Kong. His Ph.D. dissertation, "From the Cold War Front Line to the Global City: Everyday Politics in Urbanization of Boat People's Settlement, Xiamen," received the 2020 Anthony Sutcliffe Dissertation Award from the International Planning History Society. He is an executive member of the International Forum on Urbanism based in Delft University of Technology, The Netherlands.

Mehreen Chida-Razvi is the deputy curator and in-house editor for the Khalili Collection of Islamic Art in London, UK. As an art historian specializing in the art and architecture of Mughal South Asia, she serves as the associate editor for the *International Journal of Islamic Architecture*. She obtained her Ph.D. from SOAS, University of London, and has published extensively on Mughal art, architecture, and urbanism, most recently: "Lahore's *Badshahi Masjid*: Spatial Interactions of the Sacred and the Secular" (2020); "From Function to Form: *Chini-khana* in Safavid and Mughal Architecture" (2019); and "Patronage as Power, Power in Appropriation: Constructing Jahangir's Mausoleum" (2019).

Rachel Clamp is a doctoral student at Durham, UK. Her work is focused on plague nursing, policy, and the poor law in early modern England. She received her BA in History from Jesus College, Cambridge, in 2017 and her MA in History with distinction from Durham University in 2018. Rachel was awarded the Mitchie MA Prize in History for her dissertation on women and the plague in Newcastle (2018). Her research is funded by the Economic and Social Research Council via a NINE Doctoral Training Partnership Award.

Irina Davidovici is Senior Lecturer and researcher at Eidgenössische Technische Hochschule (ETH), Zurich, Switzerland, where she leads the Doctoral Programme in the History and Theory of Architecture. She was the Harvard Graduate School of Design Richard Rogers Fellow in 2018. In 2020, she obtained her Habilitation with the thesis "Collective Grounds: Housing Estates in the European City, 1865-1934." Her doctoral thesis on contemporary Swiss architecture from the University of Cambridge received the Royal Institute of British Architects President's Research Award for Outstanding Doctoral Thesis in 2009. She is the author of *Forms of Practice: German-Swiss Architecture 1980–2000* (gta Verlag, Zurich, 2012, second expanded edition published 2018) and numerous articles.

Karen Daws is a registered nurse working at a small hospital in Australia's remote far-North. She obtained her Ph.D. in 2017 from the Faculty of Architecture, Building & Planning at the University of Melbourne. Her thesis examined buildings constructed in response to infectious diseases in Victoria, Australia, between

355

1850 and 1950. Her interests include architectural history, especially hospital buildings, and factors that reveal and are revealed by examining health care practices.

Caitlin DeClercq is Assistant Director of Graduate Student Programs and Services at the Center for Teaching and Learning at Columbia University in the City of New York, USA. She also serves as a research fellow at the Interdisciplinary Center for Healthy Workplaces at the University of California, Berkeley. Her work on the history and practice of healthy campus design has been included in edited volumes and journals such as *Experiencing Architecture in the Nineteenth Century: Buildings and Society in the Modern Age* (Bloomsbury, 2018) and *Planning for Higher Education*. She is the author of a forthcoming volume, *Building Sound Bodies for Sound Minds: Architecture, Pedagogy, and Students' Sedentary Lives* (Routledge, 2022). She is the cofounder of the Epidemic Urbanism Initiative.

Niuxa Dias Drago is Professor of architecture at the Federal University of Rio de Janeiro, Brazil. She is also a researcher at the Laboratory for Architectural Narratives at the Architecture Graduate Program, the Federal University of Rio de Janeiro. She completed her Ph.D. in Performing Arts at the Rio de Janeiro State University. Her studies focus on urban and architectural history in Rio de Janeiro and on theater architecture and scenography.

Erdem Erten is Professor of architecture at the Izmir Institute of Technology, Turkey. His research interests include the theorization of culture and its impact on modern architecture and urban design, architectural journalism, and the problem of the avant-garde in architecture and romanticism. He is the coeditor of *Alternative Visions of Post-war Reconstruction: Creating the Modern Townscape* (Routledge, 2015). His work has been published as book chapters and in journals such as *The Journal of Architecture* and *The Design Journal* and *Planning Perspectives*.

Sandro Galea is Dean and Professor of Public Health at Boston University, USA. He holds a medical degree from the University of Toronto, graduate degrees from Harvard University and Columbia University, and an honorary doctorate from the University of Glasgow. He has published extensively in the peer-reviewed literature and is a regular contributor to a range of public media regarding social causes of health, mental health, and the consequences of trauma. He has been listed as one of the most widely cited scholars in the social sciences. He is chair of the board of the Association of Schools and Programs of Public Health and past president of the Society for Epidemiologic Research and of the Interdisciplinary Association for Population Health Science. He is an elected member of the National Academy of Medicine. He has received several lifetime achievement awards.

Ottó Gecser is Associate Professor at the Eötvös Loránd University in Budapest and was Humboldt Fellow at the Georg-August-Universität in Göttingen, Germany, in 2019–2020. He holds an MA and a Ph.D. in Medieval Studies from the Central European University, as well as an MA in Sociology from Eötvös Loránd University, Budapest. His research has focused on preaching and the cult of saints between the 13th and the 15th centuries, as well as on religious and medical interpretations of the plague in the late Middle Ages. His recent publications include *The Feast and the Pulpit: Preachers, Sermons and the Cult of St. Elizabeth of Hungary, 1235–ca. 1500* (Centro Italiano di Studi sull'Alto Medioevo, 2012).

Mohammad Gharipour is Professor and Director of Architecture Graduate Program at the School of Architecture and Planning at Morgan State University in Baltimore, USA. He has received grants and awards from various organizations including the Society of Architectural Historians, National Endowment in Humanities, Fulbright-Hays, Foundation for Landscape Studies, Council of Educators of Landscape Architecture, National Institute of Health, American Institute of Architects, and Fulbright. In addition to publishing numerous papers and reviews, he has authored and edited twelve books including *Health and Architecture: The History of Spaces of Healing and Care in the Pre-Modern Era* (Bloomsbury Press, 2021). Dr. Gharipour is the director and founding editor of the *International Journal of Islamic Architecture* and the cofounder of the Epidemic Urbanism Initiative.

Sofia Greaves is a doctoral candidate at the University of Cambridge, UK. Her research is part of the "Impact of the Ancient City Project," fully funded by the European Research Council, under the European Union's Horizon 2020 research and innovation program. Her Ph.D. dissertation examines how Italian planners relied upon Greco-Roman thinking about health and infrastructure to regenerate cities between 1860 and 1914, particularly through urban layout and clean water systems. She has forthcoming articles in two edited volumes, *Rome and the Colonial City* (Oxbow, 2021), and *Remembering and Forgetting the Ancient City* (Oxbow, 2021).

Huma Gupta is the Neubauer Junior Research Fellow at the Crown Center for Middle Eastern Studies at Brandeis University, USA. She is currently writing two books: *The Architecture of Dispossession* and *Dwelling and the Wealth of Nations*. She obtained her Ph.D. in History, Theory, and Criticism of Architecture at the Massachusetts Institute of Technology. She has been a fellow of New York University–Abu Dhabi, the Social Science Research Council, and the Aga Khan Program for Islamic Architecture. Her work has been published in the *International Journal of Islamic Architecture*, *Thresholds*, and the *Journal of Contemporary Iraq and the Arab World*.

Fuchsia Hart is a D.Phil. Candidate in Oriental Studies at the Khalili Research Centre for the Art and Material Culture of the Middle East at the University of Oxford, UK. Her research focuses on the major shrines of Iran and Iraq during the reign of Fath 'Ali Shah (1797–1834). She obtained her M.Phil. in Islamic Art and Archaeology and her BA in Persian from the University of Oxford. She is the 2020–21 Hadid Scholar at the Middle East Centre, St. Antony's College, Oxford. She is also the editor of the *Journal of the Iran Society*.

Susan Heydon is Senior Lecturer in Social Pharmacy at the School of Pharmacy, University of Otago, New Zealand. She gained her master's degree and Ph.D. in History from the University of Otago. Much of her research focuses on Nepal, where she and her family were volunteers for two years. She is author of *Modern Medicine and International Aid: Khunde Hospital, Nepal, 1966–1998* (Orient BlackSwan Private Limited, 2009), as well as a number of book chapters and journal articles. She is a coeditor of *Health and History*. Her current project is "Himalayan Roots of a Global Programme: Smallpox in Nepal."

Mohammad Hossain is a doctoral student in History at Ibn Haldun University, Istanbul, Turkey. He completed his MA in Civilization Studies from the Alliance of Civilizations Institute at Ibn Haldun University. His MA thesis is entitled "Ecology, Epidemics and the Colonial State: Environmental change and Health in Eastern Bengal Delta, 1858–1947." His research interests include environmental history and epidemics in South Asia.

Louisa Iarocci is an associate professor in the Department of Architecture at the University of Washington in Seattle, USA. She obtained her master's degree at Washington University in St. Louis and her Ph.D. at Boston University. She is a licensed architect who has worked in architectural firms in Toronto, ON, New York, NY, and Cambridge, MA. She is the author of *The Urban Department Store in America* (Ashgate, 2014; Routledge, 2018) and editor of *Visual Merchandising: The Image of Selling* (Ashgate, 2013; Routledge, 2016). Her research focuses on the forms and operations of the material artifacts of the city, with a focus on commerce, storage and health.

Richard J. Jackson is Professor Emeritus at the Fielding School of Public Health at University of California, Los Angeles, USA. A pediatrician, he has served in many leadership positions with the California Health Department, including as the State Health Officer. He served as Director of the CDC's National Center for Environmental Health and is an elected member of the National Academy of Medicine of the US National Academy of Sciences. He lectures on issues related to children's health, climate heating, built environment, architecture, environmental policy, and more.

Fezanur Karaağaçlıoğlu is a doctoral student in History at Boğaziçi University in Istanbul, Turkey. She obtained her BA in History and Byzantine Archeology and Art History from the Ruprecht Karl University of Heidelberg, Germany, in 2016, followed by her MA in History from Boğaziçi University in 2019. Her research is focused on the history of the Catholics within the Ottoman Empire, social, cultural, and urban histories of medicine, the history of perceptions of classical languages, and the textual and artistic employments of authority figures.

Nicole de Lalouvière is a doctoral fellow at the Institute of Landscape and Urban Studies, Eidgenössische Technische Hochschule (ETH) Zürich, Switzerland. She holds a liberal arts degree from Colgate University, New York, USA, and a Master of Architecture from the University of British Columbia in Vancouver, Canada. She has practiced as a landscape architect at Vogt Landscape Architects in Zürich. Her doctoral research project is a landscape and material history of the communal irrigation systems of Canton Valais, Switzerland.

Ian Morley is Associate Professor of History at the Chinese University of Hong Kong. His research focuses upon the design of the built fabric in the Philippines during the American colonial era. His publications include *Cities and Nationhood: American Imperialism and Urban Design, 1898-1916* (University of Hawai'i Press, 2018) and *American Colonisation and the City Beautiful: Filipinos and Planning in the Philippines, 1916–35* (Routledge, 2019), the latter being awarded the 2020 International Planning History Society Koos Bosma Prize in Planning History Innovation. He currently serves as a member of the editorial board for the journal *Planning Perspectives*.

Catherine Odari is a lecturer of African History, African Diaspora and the World, and World History at Spelman College in Atlanta, USA. She obtained her BA in Political Science and History from the University of Nairobi, Kenya, her master's in History from Miami University in Oxford, Ohio, and her Ph.D. in African History at the Georgia State University in Atlanta, USA, where she wrote her dissertation entitled "The Unknown Nationalists: Indian Migration, Integration, and Involvement in the Creation of the Kenyan Republic, 1895–1970." Her research interests are colonialism, transnational liberation movements in Eastern Africa, migration and diaspora, and race and gender. She is the Humanities Scholar for the Black Money Exhibit Project.

Timothy Oluseyi Odeyale is Professor and the Head of Department at the Department of Architecture, University of Ibadan, Nigeria. He holds a Ph.D. in Architecture from the University of Lincoln, UK. He is a chartered member of the Nigerian Institute of Architects and member of England's Higher Education Academy. His research interests include the history and theory of architecture, sustainability, urban design, urban systems, and theories of place. His work explores and critiques the concept of health and culture in the transformation of African cities, from the traditional to the modern milieu.

George Marfo Osei is a doctoral student in history at Stony Brook University, USA. He holds an M.Phil. degree in History from the University of Ghana. He received a Diploma in Education from the University of Education, Winneba, in 2019. In 2015, he was awarded a bachelor's degree in History from Kwame Nkrumah University of Science and Technology. He is an Africanist with broader research interests in human rights, the history of witch camps, women, gender, and sexuality.

Fernando Delgado Páez is Professor in the Faculty of Architecture of the Federal University of Rio de Janeiro, Brazil. He completed his master's degree in Architecture at the Postgraduate Program in Architecture at Federal University of Rio de Janeiro, where he is currently a Ph.D. candidate. His publications and research are focused on the history and theory of architectural design.

Ana Paula Polizzo is Professor of Architecture at the Federal University of Rio de Janeiro, Brazil. She is also a researcher at the Laboratory for Architectural Narratives at the Architecture Graduate Program. She completed her Ph.D. in Social History of Culture at the Pontifical Catholic University in Rio de Janeiro. Her studies focus on Brazilian and Latin-American architecture and landscape design.

Daniela Sandler is Associate Professor of Architectural and Urban History at the University of Minnesota, USA. She has a Ph.D. in Visual and Cultural Studies from the University of Rochester and a professional degree in Architecture and Urbanism from the University of São Paulo. She has published on grassroots urbanism, public space in São Paulo, squatting and gentrification in Berlin, contemporary affordable housing in Brazil, and the historiography of Brazilian modernism. Her book, *Counterpreservation: Architectural Decay in Berlin since 1989* (Cornell University Press, 2016), investigates how Berlin residents appropriated architectural decay to engage a difficult past, resist gentrification, and create alternative housing and cultural spaces.

Shobana Shankar is Associate Professor of History at Stony Brook University, USA. She is a sociocultural historian of modern West Africa. She is the author of *Who Shall Enter Paradise? Christian Origins in Muslim Northern Nigeria, c.1890–1975* (Ohio University Press, 2014) and coeditor of two essay collections on religion and global interactions. Her numerous articles include a piece in *The Conversation* about Nigeria's polio immunization experience and another in *The Washington Post* on eugenicist practices at the Mississippi State Penitentiary. Her book, *An Uneasy Embrace: Africa, India and the Spectre of Race* (Hurst, 2021), examines how Africans and Indians have navigated their racial tensions in spheres like religion, science, and education in order to find solidarity and autonomy from Euro-American power.

Işılay Tiarnagh Sheridan Gün is a student and research assistant in the Department of Architecture at the Izmir Institute of Technology, Turkey. As a conservation specialist, her work focuses on industrial history and heritage, architectural history, the urban development of Western Anatolia by British investors, and architectural practice under British influence during the second half of the 19th and the early 20th centuries. Her archival work on the Seamen's Hospital in Smyrna was conducted at the School of Architecture, Planning and Landscape at Newcastle University within the 2019–20 academic year as a visiting Ph.D. researcher.

Allen Shotwell is Professor of History and Director of the Center for Humanities and Medicine at Ivy Tech Community College, Terre Haute, USA. He earned his Ph.D. in the History and Philosophy of Science from Indiana University, USA. He has published a number of works on the history of medicine and specializes in the history of medicine in the early modern period. His interest in medicine and society in progressive-era Terre Haute arises from his work from the Vigo County Historical Society Museum.

Katalin Szende is Professor of Medieval Studies at the Central European University, Hungary and Austria. She holds degrees in history, archaeology, and Latin philology. She is a board member of the International Commission for the History of Towns, founding member and president of the Medieval Central Europe Research Network, member of the Lendület (Momentum) Medieval Hungarian Economic History Research Group, and recipient of a research fellowship at the

Max-Weber-Kolleg, University of Erfurt, Kollegforschungsgruppe "Religion and Urbanity Reciprocal Formations" (2020–21). She published *Trust, Authority and the Written Word in the Royal Towns of Medieval Hungary* (Brepols, 2018) and coedited the volumes *Medieval Buda in Context* (Brill, 2016) and *Medieval East Central Europe in a Comparative Perspective* (Routledge, 2016).

Joshua Teplitsky is Associate Professor of History at Stony Brook University, USA. His research is about Jewish life in Central Europe in the early modern period. His book, *Prince of the Press: How One Collector Built History's Most Enduring and Remarkable Jewish Library* (Yale University Press, 2019), was named a finalist for the National Jewish Book Award and the winner of the Salo Baron Prize (2019) and Jordan Schnitzer Book Award (2020). He coleads a digital humanities project called *Footprints: Jewish Books Through Time and Place*, which tracks the movement of Jewish books since the inception of print. He is currently at work on a book reconstructing a plague epidemic in 18th-century Prague and its impact on Jewish social and cultural life in the city.

Carlo Trombino is a doctoral candidate in heritage studies at the University of Palermo, Italy. He holds an MA in World History from the University of Bologna. He is currently working on a research project on the 16th- and 17th-century Mediterranean slave trade, with a focus on the Mercedarian Order and other redeeming institutions in Sicily and Catalunya. He has coauthored, along with Claudia Martino, the historical documentary *Furio Jesi - Man from Utopia*, on the life of Italian essayist and mythologist Furio Jesi (2018).

Gregory Valdespino is a doctoral candidate in history at the University of Chicago, USA. His dissertation project is entitled "At Home in Empire: Dwelling, Domesticity, and Welfare in France and Senegal, 1914–1974." His research examines the interconnectedness of African and European histories with a particular focus on material culture, imperialism, domesticity, and welfare. His work, including the following chapter, is supported by the Committee on African Studies at the University of Chicago and the George Lurcy Charitable and Educational Trust.

Michael G. Vann is Professor of History at California State University, Sacramento, USA. He earned his Ph.D. at the University of California, Santa Cruz. Vann has received three Fulbright awards for research in France, Vietnam, and Cambodia, as well as fellowships from the Council of American Overseas Research Centers, the Center for Khmer Studies, and the Korea Society. Vann is the author of three books: *The Great Hanoi Rat Hunt: Empire, Disease, and Modernity in French Colonial Vietnam* (Oxford University Press, 2018), *"The Colonial Good*

Life:" A Commentary on Andre Joyeux's Vision of French Indochina (White Lotus Press, 2008), and *Twentieth Century Voices: Selected Readings in World History* (Cognella, 2012). He served as President of the French Colonial Historical Society.

Emily Webster is a doctoral candidate in History at the University of Chicago, USA. She is currently finishing her dissertation project, entitled "Microbial Empires: Changing Ecologies and Multispecies Epidemics in the Urban British Empire, 1837–1910." She has a master's degree in Public Health Science. She works at the intersection of health studies, environmental history, urban history, and imperialism. She serves as a review editor for *Environmental History Now*. Her work is supported by the Social Science Research Council and the National Science Foundation.

Andrew Wells is an independent scholar based in Leipzig, Germany. He studied at the Universities of Bristol and British Columbia and obtained his doctorate from the University of Oxford. He has written a dozen articles and book chapters on various topics in modern cultural and intellectual history, particularly the history of race, urban history, and the history of animals. He is coeditor of *Interspecies Interactions: Animals and Humans between the Middle Ages and Modernity* (Routledge, 2018). He has two monographs forthcoming on race and reproduction in the 18th-century British Empire, and on urban cultures of freedom in the British Atlantic world.

Julie Willis is a Redmond Barry Distinguished Professor of Architecture and Dean of the Faculty of Architecture, Building & Planning at the University of Melbourne, Australia. Her research concentrates on the history of Australian architecture and encompasses issues of gender equity in the profession and contemporary health care design. Her books include the *Encyclopedia of Australian Architecture* (Cambridge University Press, 2011), *Designing Schools: Space, Place and Pedagogy* (Routledge, 2017), and *Architecture and the Modern Hospital: Nosokomeion to Hygeia* (Routledge, 2019).

Farren Yero is Postdoctoral Associate in Gender, Sexuality, and Feminist Studies at Duke University, USA. She obtained her master's degree in Latin American Studies from Tulane University and her Ph.D. from Duke University, where she studied the history of medicine in Latin America and the Caribbean. Her current book project, a study of smallpox vaccination in the Atlantic world, follows the introduction of the world's first vaccine to explore questions about the racial and gender politics of preventative and public health and parental and patient rights amid anti-colonial and anti-slavery revolutions. Her research has been supported by the American Council of Learned Societies, Fulbright-Hays, Andrew W. Mellon Foundation, the John Carter Brown Library, and the Newberry Library.

Yichi Zhang is Postdoctoral Fellow at the Department of Culture Studies and Oriental Languages, The University of Oslo, Norway. Trained as a landscape architect, conservator, and garden historian, he has served as a postdoctoral fellow at the Paul Mellon Centre for Studies in British Art at Yale University (2016) and a research fellow in Garden and Landscape Studies at Dumbarton Oaks Research Library and Collection, Trustees for Harvard University (2015). He was awarded the 13th Annual Mavis Batey Essay Prize by the Garden Trust, UK (2017) and the Annual Award for Postdoctoral Scholars from the Geographical Society of New South Wales, Australia (2017).

Index

Note: *Italic* numbers denote reference to figures